CLEAN LIVING
MOVEMENTS

CLEAN LIVING MOVEMENTS

American Cycles of Health Reform

Ruth Clifford Engs

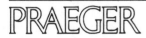

Westport, Connecticut
London

Library of Congress Cataloging-in-Publication Data

Engs, Ruth C.
    Clean living movements : American cycles of health reform / Ruth Clifford Engs.
        p. cm.
    Includes bibliographical references and index.
    ISBN 0–275–95994–5 (alk. paper)—ISBN 0–275–97541–X (pbk. : alk. paper)
    1. Health promotion—United States—History.   2. Health reformers—United
States—History.   3. Health behavior—United States—History.   I. Title.
RA427.8 E54 2000
613′.0973—dc21   99–043111

British Library Cataloguing in Publication Data is available.

Library of Congress Catalog Card Number: 99–043111
ISBN: 0–275–97541–X (pbk.)

First published in 2000

Praeger Publishers, 88 Post Road West, Westport, CT 06881
An imprint of Greenwood Publishing Group, Inc.
www.praeger.com

Printed in the United States of America

The paper used in this book complies with the
Permanent Paper Standard issued by the National
Information Standards Organization (Z39.48–1984).

10 9 8 7 6 5 4 3 2 1

This book is for

Mary Louise de Castro Macmillian (1879–1972)
My grandmother,
who taught me to wonder about many aspects of the universe

Irene Cushing (1898–1987)
My high school Latin teacher,
who showed me the interconnections between all realms of learning

Elinor K. Clifford (b. 1910)
My mother,
who allowed me to be an independent woman
even though it was against the norm

Contents

Preface

In the early 1970s, there began to be a clamor among health professionals for Americans to change their personal habits and lifestyles. Accompanying this "fitness craze" was an increase in articles, books, and media programming that urged the nation to exercise, give up smoking, and eat a more healthy diet. Concerns about nonmarital sex, alcohol and drugs, out-of-wedlock births, and the new HIV/AIDS epidemic in the early 1980s gave further cause for alarm about perceived risky behaviors and their consequences to the health of the nation. Some individuals and organizations began to advocate public-health programs and public policies to encourage Americans to adopt healthier behaviors. New legislation to effect behavior changes included severe penalties for drunken driving, mandatory use of motor-vehicle seatbelts, and warning labels on tobacco, alcoholic beverages, and other products. A "war on drugs," prohibition of smoking in public places, and legislation to curtail use of any alcohol and tobacco among youth and reduce its use among adults ensued.

Comments by my colleagues, government officials, and some public-health advocates suggested that we as a nation were finally realizing the serious nature of these problems. Based upon new scientific discoveries, it was realized that the time had finally come to eradicate these ills completely from society. However, more cautious scholars, including Jack Blocker, Dwight Heath, David Musto, Harry Levine,

David Pittman, and Robin Room, began to point out that agitation against alcohol and drugs, for instance, had arisen earlier and that these temperance movements might even be cyclical.

By the late 1980s, I realized that reform crusades against many health problems not only had occurred before, but also had been widely discussed by several authors. Works by Ronald Walters, Stephen Nissenbaum, James Whorton, and Harvey Green noted that reform crusades for the elimination of a variety of perceived health problems had emerged in the mid-nineteenth century and also at the turn of the twentieth century. Changes resulting from many of these reform efforts were now an acceptable part of our society. However, some of these measures were later rejected inasmuch as they led to other social problems.

The realization that we were repeating the actions of the past that in many cases had not been successful led to this book. I intend to discuss the rise and fall of health reforms, or "Clean Living" Movements; to propose that these movements come in cycles of approximately every seventy to ninety years; and to examine the issues and the commonalities among the three major health-reform movements that have emerged over the past 200 years. Another aim of this book is to examine changes made in past movements and their long-term effects. As will be noted, many of the same arguments for particular health issues have been used in all three movements. Some late-twentieth-century materials concerning fitness, diet, alcohol, tobacco, and sexual abstinence are nearly paraphrases of material written 100 and 150 years ago. Readers are urged to read the quotations at the beginning of each section and chapter to get a sense of this similarity.

Besides the authors already mentioned, other publications have helped shape the essence of this work. Two years ago, John Burnham introduced me to his 1993 book, *Bad Habits,* as we waited in an airport. His book discusses our national obsession of telling others how to behave and gives insight about our puritanical reforming impulse against a variety of pleasurable personal behaviors that in the late twentieth century have become matters for social decision and public policy. He details the power of the media and industry in shaping public attitudes and opinions concerning drinking, smoking, sexual activities, and so on. In the summer of 1998, when my first draft was almost complete, I discovered a provocative work, *The Fourth Turning,* by William Strauss and Neil Howe, which supports the cyclical hypothesis and implies that the present reform era is likely at its peak. Others in the past, such as Arthur Schlesinger Jr. (1950, 4), have also noted "cycles of reform and repost," in terms of social movements. I also found Michael Goldstein's (1992) work, *The Health Movement,* that covers some aspects of the current fitness and health surge. He also notes that a resurgence in spirituality, alternative medicine, and feminism is associated with the current movement.

This book has drawn upon information from many disciplines, including history, sociology, public health, health education, anthropology, and medical history, among others. It is based upon a variety of scholarly works in addition to information from popular magazines, books, tracts, and other publications of the time period examined. Today, some of the language, and even ideas, of earlier reformers and writers may be construed as offensive and not "politically correct." However, it is important for the reader to get a feeling of how certain groups were perceived. Therefore, terms commonly found in middle-class popular and scholarly publications of the era will be used in this work. It was generally the middle-class fear of a particular health problem associated with a particular ethnic group infecting "respectable people" and children that pushed reformers into action for education and legislation to eliminate a perceived problem.

Throughout this book, two Victorian terms, *moral suasion* and *coercion*, are used to describe the activities of reformers and the two activist phases of specific health movements. In general, moral suasion constitutes education and social pressure to change attitudes or behaviors (e.g., making smoking socially unacceptable). These efforts are fostered by individual activists, religious groups, schools, government bodies, activist organizations, and the media. Coercion includes procedures to force people to reduce or eliminate the activity or behavior (e.g., making it illegal to smoke on airplanes). Coercion entails social sanctions that are reflected in legislation, public policies, and laws to make substances or activities illegal. It also includes stiffer penalties for lawbreakers, increased taxes, the curtailment of advertisement, and so on.

The book is divided into three sections, one for each health reform movement. The author–date system is used, and each source is to be found in alphabetical order by author and date. Notes at the end of each chapter provide further clarification or reference. Within the notes, the author–date system is used, although with newspapers, popular magazines, and many government publications dates only are given.

Acknowledgments

Most of the material for this book was found within the immense Indiana University library system. This included the Special Collections section of the Medical School Library in Indianapolis, in addition to the Main Library, Lilly Library, and Kinsey Institute Library located in Bloomington, Indiana. Some organizations were also helpful in providing material, including the American Cancer Society, Lung Association, Planned Parenthood, and the YMCA.

As is customary in any scholarly work, I am indebted to a host of individuals who have helped in one way or another. Many individuals in all the libraries mentioned were most gracious with their time and help. I would especially like to thank Ann Bristow, David Frasier, Jeffrey C. Graf, Jian Liu, and Frank Quinn in the reference section of the Indiana University Main Library, who answered many questions and went out of their way to find me a variety of resources. A number of individuals in the circulation department were particularly helpful including Randy Lent, Marty Chambers, Jan Clinch, and John Pate. I would also like to thank Rita Rogers and other staff members in the interlibrary loan department.

I am indebted to several colleagues and authors who either kindly commented on specific sections or chapters or offered constructive ideas or references which clarified a fuzzy area or thought. Any errors, however, are mine. These include Rita Barsun, William D.

Engs, Bruce Horonic, Patrick J. Kiger, Stephanie Sanders, William Tresslar, Jan Shipps, Jacob Sullum, and William L. Yarber. John C. Burnham, a health and science historian, and Mary Lou Remley, a physical-education historian, read the entire manuscript. I am especially indebted to John Burnham for his many valuable suggestions, even though he did not always agree with my point of view.

A special thanks is offered to my dedicated and efficient student helpers, who spent many hours copying sources and other mundane tasks essential to this work. These wonderful assistants over a three-year period included Shadia Garrison, Gail Grundermann, Sarah Hoffman, Malea Jochim, Jamie M. Kaplan, Tiffany Kinney, and Brandy Reid. Jennifer E. Susoreny in particular was most efficient. I am indebted to Indiana University history doctoral students Daphne L. Cunningham and Damon Freeman, not only for their data collection, but also for the whispered conversations on the "quiet floor" of the library, which helped clarify some details.

I would also like to thank my academic unit, the Department of Applied Health Science, for some funding in support of this project and for allowing me a reduced load for one semester so I could focus on finishing the manuscript. Special thanks is also due to Elaine Hehner for keyboarding the final draft, to Robert W. Baird for his detailed critique, and to Jay and Laura Wilkerson for indexing and checking references.

Finally, I would like to thank my husband, Jeffrey Franz, for just being there.

Awakenings of the Jacksonian (1830–1860), the progressive (1890–1920), and the current millennial (1970–2005?) reform eras. Most of the individual health crusades within each of these movements have been fostered by reformers with a zeal for a specific health issue. Some reformers in each era have supported several crusades. However, on the whole, the varying health crusades within a reform era have tended to be single-issue campaigns. Crusades for a particular health issue have also emerged at different times over the course of the reform era. As will be seen in subsequent chapters, temperance was the first concern to emerge in the first two movements, while antismoking was the initial thrust of the late twentieth-century movement.[4] A hereditarian movement to explain social problems and disease has tended to reach its peak of power after the main thrust of the movement. Perhaps reformers have reasoned that when both moral suasion (education and social pressure) and coercion (public policies) have not changed behaviors or eliminated health problems, the root causes must be hereditary.

This book strives to discuss the three cycles of health reform, their ebb and flow, and the transitory nature—from thirty to forty years—of the reforming phase in each cycle. For example, what was a burning issue during the peak of the reform phase often became forgotten or was considered a quaint eccentricity years later. In the 1950s, the use of tobacco and alcohol increased among the middle class so that smoking and the two-martini lunch were considered socially acceptable and even sophisticated. The antismoking laws of the first decade of the century became only a distant memory of a few older individuals and Prohibition had become a national joke. In the late 1950s and early 1960s, few would have predicted that smoking would not be allowed in most public places and that there would be limitations on alcohol consumption thirty years hence. In addition, most Americans, other than a few students of history, had forgotten that at the end of the Jacksonian era most of the states north of the Mason–Dixon line had state prohibition and tobacco use was frowned upon.[5]

Some observers might argue that health reform has experienced a steady uphill march since colonial times. Only in the past generation have we finally realized the dangers, based upon new scientific knowledge, of unhealthful activities such as smoking, heavy drinking, lack of exercise, and so on. However, this continuous-reform hypothesis culminating in ever-increasing health campaigns is not supported, as will be seen in the following chapters. A major focus of this book is to discuss the observation that health-reform crusades tend to ebb and flow. Advances have tended to progress in steps. After a reform campaign, a plateau of interest or compliance occurred, followed by increasing apathy on the issue until some perceived problems began to reemerge again. This has in particular occured for more controversial reform issues such as drinking and smoking.

Sociologists Ralph H. Turner and Lewis M. Killian (1957, 333) have suggested that all social movements "have two broad directions in which the program and ideology may point. They may point toward changing *individuals* directly or toward changing *social institutions*" (italics added). Within each of the three Clean Living Movements, as will be seen, some movements have been aimed at individual reform, some at societal reform, and some at both. For example, there has been advocacy against alcohol consumption in all three movements, which resulted in legislation to prohibit alcohol for certain groups. On the other hand, advocacy to reduce fat in the diet, become a vegetarian, or avoid premarital sex has not been imposed by public policy.

The Popularization of Health Issues

Health reform crusades have served to "popularize" a health concern. At any given period of time, a few individuals have usually been concerned about any given health issue and a few articles concerning the topic could be found in scholarly journals. However, it was not until the educated public perceived a problem that the movement began. Burnham (1984, 190–191) has suggested that the most important institutions for popularizing health have been the schools and the press. The media first raised the issue with the "public," which, traditionally, has been the middle class. When the middle class became concerned, the reform phase of the cycle emerged. Education of schoolchildren and the masses to change behaviors then followed.[6]

During the surge phase of a health-reform movement, activists have had an exhilarating sense that society has finally awakened to the issue more so than at any time in history, and/or that profound changes will finally occur. For example, Luther H. Gulick, an early twentieth-century physician and physical educator, in an article "The High Tide of Physical Conscience" in the June 1908 *World's Work*, noted that the nation was amidst a "physical well-being" movement. He commented that "interest runs higher in this direction than ever before in the history of our civilization." Similar comments could be found in the late twentieth-century movement.

Belief Systems and Ideologies

Health historian James C. Whorton (1981b, 60) has suggested that "health-reform movements must be understood as hygienic ideologies, idea systems which identify correct personal hygiene as the necessary foundation for most, even for all, human progress, and which invite acceptance by incorporating both certain universal feelings about man and nature, and the popular values and anxieties peculiar to distinct eras." These belief systems have specified both the grievances to which the movement was responding as well as its objectives. The ideas and beliefs that underlied a movement developed into an ideology, or a set of norms, to which many believers adhered.

Turner and Killian (1957, 331–333) have argued that a movement's ideology has facilitated collective action in a number of ways. It provided internal guidance for the movement's members in selecting and carrying out their tactics. It offered a sense of identification and membership, as well as a single viewpoint—a "clear message" to the millennial movement's antialcohol, antitobacco, and antidrug campaigns—with boundaries to the outside world. The ideology sought to strengthen the movement's legitimacy by invoking logic, emotion, and identification with core values of a society. It also developed negative images of those who did not share or who opposed their views. The health crusades within each of the three Clean Living Movements developed their own ideologies which will be discussed in subsequent chapters.

PHASES OF HEALTH-REFORM MOVEMENTS

Health-reform cycles have exhibited different phases—stages or "turnings"—within the overall cadence of the movement. Each phase has lasted about a generation. These stages have been found for campaigns addressing alcohol, tobacco, other mood-altering substances, diet, exercise, certain foods, and adolescent virginity. For any particular reform issue, however, stages may have occurred simultaneously or even been skipped. The phases within a health crusade's cycle have been *moral suasion, coercion, backlash,* and *complacency.* The clearest example of these phases, and the most documented, has been the temperance, or antialcohol cycle. At the beginning of the movement, a general change in attitude toward alcohol was observed. A drinking-related problem was then identified: "ardent spirits" in the first, "saloons" in the second, and "drunk driving" in the third Clean Living Movement.[7] This change in attitude began the moral suasion phase of the cycle, which used social pressure through emotional appeals and educational programs to what reformers considered the right position. In all three alcohol movements, this right position was the encouragement of more temperate, moderate, or responsible drinking behaviors. When these suasive efforts were perceived as being ineffective in changing behavior, abstinence was then championed and drinking in certain circumstances began to be presented as deviant.[8]

When abstinence messages for alcohol, tobacco, drugs, and other perceived risky health behaviors were ignored by certain segments of the population, the coercion phase of the cycle emerged. Even though the perceived problem—high per capita consumption, saloons, or drunk driving—began to decrease, the popular perception was that the situation had become worse. Reformers then mobilized political power in an attempt to enforced compliance through increased taxation, prohibition legislation, limited sales and distribution, and other laws to control consumption. Such measures, to force people to respond in a prescribed way "for their own good," have emerged in all three movements and were the common characteristic of each movement's peak. In terms of alcohol, during the first Clean Living Movement, thirteen states enacted prohibition laws. During the second, national prohibition was legislated. In the late twentieth-century movement, prohibition for those under twenty-one years of age, along with stiff penalties for drunken driving, were instituted.

The next phase of the cycle was a backlash against increasingly unpopular public policies. Laws became ignored by many, a lively black market emerged, and some legislation was repealed as being unenforceable. In terms of alcohol, the industry, through the media and advertisement, began to again portray drinking as an acceptable activity. Per capita alcohol consumption increased and became socially acceptable to the middle class. Many began to believe that alcohol itself posed little risk to life and health. During the end of this stage and the beginning of the next phase of the cycle, complacency, temperance advocates were derided as quaint, ignorant, or puritanical "do-gooders"; alcohol-related problems were ignored; and laws concerning alcohol use were increasingly disregarded. However, problems related to drinking again began to increase, thus completing the cycle.

For any given health-reform issue, the adoption of a new behavior or policy had the potential of creating both a positive or a negative result. Mandates for better sanitation, pure drinking water, and personal hygiene near the beginning of the second movement, for example, did much to reduce communicable diseases and were accepted by the population. On the other hand, overzealous or controversial efforts which were not acceptable to a large minority of the population, such as alcohol prohibition, were ignored or flaunted, resulting in other problems. Over the three Clean Living Movements, successful reforms were those that became completely integrated into society. They became common practice and acceptable by most, regardless of socioeconomic class, education, or ethnic background (i.e., handwashing after using the toilet, frequent bathing, etc.).

COMMONALITIES AMONG THE THREE
CLEAN LIVING MOVEMENTS

Many similarities have been apparent among the three Clean Living Movements. Some of the most common will be outlined in this section. Others, including profound political, technological, economic, and demographic changes, or the power and influence of the mass media and commercial interests in changing attitudes and perceptions concerning alcohol, tobacco, or sex-related activities are beyond the scope of this book.[9] As will be seen in subsequent chapters, health-reform movements, for the most part, have emerged in the wake of, or tangential to, a revival of religious interest. This religious climate and cultural awakening has yielded an evangelical fervor among some individuals or groups who then strove to eliminate a perceived problem. Whorton (1981b, 60) has suggested that health reformers have commonly regarded themselves as "physiological missionaries to spread the gospel of health to the gluttonous and indolent unhealthy of the world. This essential dogma binds American health reformers from all ages," but has given a unique expression within the cultural preoccupations of each reformer's contemporary society. Since 1800, the three Clean Living Movements have reflected the tenor of the time in which they developed. The hygienic ideology in Jacksonian America was molded by millennialism, romanticism, nationalism, feminism, and educational reforms. The progressive era provided optimism to change the world through modern science and to restore an America which had been weakened by urbanization, immigration, government corruption, and ruthless capitalism. The current millennial era emerged from the social stress of rapid population growth, profound technological changes, alterations in family structure, and anxieties stemming from the Cold War.

The Traits and a Typical Biography of a Health Reformer

Reformers in each of the three movements took it upon themselves to change other people's behaviors. They often garnered nicknames as zealots, busybodies, do-gooders, puritans, the food police, kooks, fanatics, health nuts, and cranks. In many instances, reformers sought to impose their beliefs and values on others through repression. John H. Knowles (1977, 76), a physician, remarked that "those who do work in the field of prevention and health education have too often stressed social control (some have called them 'health fascists') rather than social change and have become curiously indifferent to the needs and aspiration of families, communities, and particularly minority groups."

John C. Burnham (1972, 22), when discussing the tuberculosis movement, stated that "the use of education as a reform device has been
well understood and may be traditionally American. But the use of
social coercion to bring about widespread social change, individual
by ill individual, in the name of science was typical and indicative of
the ambitiousness of the reformers."

Reformers often made it clear that they felt they were right and those
who disagreed with them were wrong—for that matter, even "bad" or
evil. They attempted to control others' lives without regard to individual differences, values, or beliefs. This was particularly true for
health campaigns with moral overtones, such as those addressing the
use of mood-altering substances, sexuality issues, and even diet. Some
reformers have been extremely judgmental, even sadistic. For example,
Anthony Comstock, the anti-pornography crusader of the second Clean
Living Movement, delighted in the early deaths and suicides of some
of his arrestees. Eric Hoffer (1951, xi), in his *The True Believer*, suggested
that "most reformers irrespective of the doctrine they preach and the
program they project, breed fanaticism, fervent hope, hatred and intolerance. . . . All demand blind faith and singlehearted alliances."
They tended to see a simple solution for a complex problem. On the
whole, reformers have been strident individuals. They have pushed
through their agendas at the cost of careers, reputations, and liveli-
hoods, even if their repressive measures were unacceptable to a large
segment of the population or their reforms caused a backlash leading
to other social problems. Within each movement, certain individuals
have brought a perceived health problem to the public eye. These individuals have often founded or become leaders in organizations advocating a particular reform issue. Reformers have typically been
"native-born" Americans. In the first two movements, most were from
"old-stock" Protestant Anglo-Saxon backgrounds. In the late twentieth-
century movement, reformers tended to be middle-class and native
born. In this Clean Living Movement, however, "reformers" increasingly became "advocacy organizations" and not single voices with
minimum support such as Sylvester Graham, the diet and temperance crusader of the first movement.

For many but not all health reformers, there was a fairly typical
biography (Whorton 1982, 8–10). At some point in the person's life,
often in childhood or youth, he or she was sickly or near death. This
poor health was due to a weak constitution, a disease such as tuberculosis, or bad lifestyle habits. The illness and debilitation caused the
individual to search for a cure. A health revelation was found through
reading or self-experimentation. Fresh air, change in diet, physical activity, and/or the elimination of meat, alcohol, tobacco, or some other
substance was found as the cure. The well-being which followed this

conversion convinced the reformer that his or her program was the key to all individual and societal problems, and the reformer was driven to propagandize this truth through various media and political strategies.

Puritanism, the Religion of Health, and the Rise of New Religions

Since the country's Puritan beginnings, the case could be made that Americans have been obsessed by sin and vice. If it felt good, it must be bad. If it was bad it must be repressed.[10] Obsession with certain aspects of health turned into a "religion" or a religious campaign for moral perfection. Illness was considered unnatural and a consequence of the individual's violation of physiological laws. Good hygiene and health became a moral obligation. This religion of health implied that if a person lived a healthy lifestyle, he or she would live longer than normally expected (Whorton 1981b, 60). An illustration of this view was found in the titles of two articles, published a hundreu years apart in popular magazines, "Exercise and Longevity" (1897), and "How to Live to 100" (1997), from the second and third movements, respectively. Some individuals even spoke of health activities as a religion. For example, in the upsurge of the late twentieth-century movement, Richard Keelor (1978), in a popular magazine, quoted a jogging enthusiast who exclaimed, "Jogging is not a hobby, it's a religion." The report suggests that those participating in this activity "become evangelists who are eager to recruit others."

Each Clean Living Movement produced new religious sects in which health and dietary laws became an integral part of their belief systems. This included the Mormons and Seventh-Day Adventists in the first, and Christian Scientists in the second movement, all of whom eschewed alcohol, tobacco, and caffeinated beverages as part of their religious practices. Vegetarianism was also a religious principle among the Adventists. In the third movement, many newly formed sects embraced vegetarianism, the elimination of tobacco and sometimes alcohol and other drugs as part of their religious faith.[11]

Demonization, Scapegoating, and Militarization

An aspect of the religion of health was demonization. Demonization was the process in which a substance or activity associated with poor health or social problems was deemed evil (i.e., "demon rum," "the devil's weed," "fallen women," etc.). In this process, health and a healthy lifestyle were considered good, disease and an unhealthy lifestyle were considered bad or immoral. In all three movements, demonization occurred with alcohol, tobacco, other mood-altering substances, some aspects of sexuality, certain foods, and new diseases, such as cholera and HIV/AIDS. In addition, persons who engaged in these activities or succumbed to these diseases and the industries which manufactured these products were demonized and considered immoral. For example, advertisement campaigns using cartoons—"Joe Camel" and "Budweiser frogs"—were considered bad by many reformers during the late 1980s and 1990s on the grounds that they promoted smoking and drinking among youth.[12]

Not only was the activity demonized, it also became a scapegoat for other social problems. It was often blamed for the deterioration of the family, loss of traditional values, poor health, and increased crime. Blaming a substance for severe problems has been found, in particular, for alcohol and tobacco. Scapegoating occurred for alcohol in each of the three Clean Living Movements and for tobacco in the second and third movements. During the first movement, for example, the *Temperance Almanac* of 1838 remarked, "If the tavern or grocery man sells, by virtue of that license, and our fellow-citizen purchases and drinks and dies, or kills his neighbor, who is the murderer and what portion of the fault belongs to each?" During the second movement, the saloon was blamed for the deterioration of the family and the "smoking habit" for poor school performance. Both were blamed for increased crime. During the third movement, tobacco manufacturers were blamed for the early death of thousands of smokers. Scapegoating led to the destruction of saloons and to Prohibition in the second, and taverns being held liable for patrons' driving-while-intoxicated accidents in the third Clean Living Movement. It led to litigation against cigarette manufacturers by both individuals and states during the third movement.[13]

A secular aspect of demonization was militarization. Concern about an issue evolved into a military campaign, war, or "jihad." Combatants or soldiers of the health movement engaged in a battle, crusade, or campaign against the perceived problem. Examples of rhetoric used in health movements which have reflected militarization of a perceived health problem was the "modern health crusade" against tuberculosis in the second and the "war on drugs" and battle against the tobacco industry in the third movement. The health problem, as well as institutions and individuals who opposed the reformer's point of view, also became an enemy, opponent, adversary, or foe. Other militaristic phraseology, such as "tactical," "conflict," "strategic," "attack," and "extermination" have been common. All these terms will be seen throughout this work for various health issues. A symbolic illustration of turning health campaigns into a war against perceived health problems was the formation of the Public Health Service, which from its beginning had a military structure headed by a surgeon general (see Chapter 6).[14]

Battles against some health concerns in the second and third movements became more than symbolic military campaigns. They were actual wars as a result of military components of the U.S. government being enlisted to help eliminate the problem. In the third movement, drug interdiction by the U.S. Coast Guard and using military units against drug smugglers were examples of this. The December 17, 1989 *Washington Post*, for example, stated, "A Marine unit accompanying U. S. Border Patrol agents in Arizona exchanged gunfire with horse-riding drug smugglers near the Mexican border." In the second movement, the "revenuers," who were components of the Federal Bureau of Investigation and the Alcohol, Tobacco, and Firearms Bureau, were alleged to have engaged in gunfire with bootleggers.[15]

Politically Correct Health Opinions, Suppression of Data, and Hyperbole

Each Clean Living Movement has produced a "politically correct" health message for a given issue. Individuals or institutions who disagreed with the prevailing opinion, even if it was ineffective, biased, or inaccurate, were censored. For example, in the late twentieth-century antialcohol and antidrug movement, public school drug and alcohol education programs were forbidden to teach about the responsible use of alcohol, even for potential future use in adulthood. Abstinence was the only message allowed by federal mandate, beginning in the late 1980s. Any other educational messages threatened the elimination of governmental funding to the school. Few scholarly works in the United States even examined, or advocated, the benefits of alcohol consumption from the early 1980s until the early 1990s. For a researcher to investigate or advocate moderate drinking could lead to denial of a federally funded grant, being ostracized by one's colleagues, or even being branded as a "spokesperson of the beverage industry," resulting in the loss of credibility as an objective scholar (Engs 1991a, 1992b).

Some individuals have even lost their jobs due to nonpolitically correct health opinions. Surgeon General Jocelyn Elders (b. 1933) was fired from her position in the late twentieth-century movement because, in reference to safe sex as a means to curb the spread of the HIV/AIDS epidemic, she stated, as quoted in *U.S. News and World Report*, December 19, 1994, that "masturbation is a part of human sexuality and a part of something that perhaps should be taught." One of the reasons Surgeon General William Hammond (1828–1900) was fired from his job at the end of the first movement was because he argued that calomel, a popular but dangerous mercury-based compound, was poisonous and should not be used in medicine. He also was ostracized from the American Medical Association for these remarks (Blustein 1991, 84–91).

During both the ebb and the surge of a cycle, statements that opposed the viewpoints of the group in power have been subject to suppression. This has been found, for example, with data concerning both the damaging and beneficial effects of alcohol. During the ebb in temperance sentiments from approximately the late 1930s through the 1960s, the harmful effects of alcohol were rarely mentioned. In the surge of the late twentieth century antialcohol and antidrug movement, language in federal guidelines suggested there was no safe threshold of alcohol consumption, a view also espoused by reform organizations in the first and second movements. In the mid-1980s, leaders from the National Institute of Drug Abuse told librarians, educators, and researchers to purge all material that suggested responsible use of alcohol and other substances (Engs and Fors 1988; Musto 1996).[16]

In all three movements, hyperbole has been common. Terms such as "crisis," "epidemic," and "explosion" have been used to describe health-related issues. As will be seen in subsequent chapters, the effects of alcohol, tobacco, drugs, certain sexual behaviors, specific foods, and other substances or activities have all been overstated as to the harm caused to the individual or to society. This hysteria about an activity on the part of reformers has served to alarm the public, which in turn has sanctioned restrictive social control in an attempt to eliminate the behavior. In the third movement, an upcoming epidemic of crack babies born to cocaine-addicted mothers was proclaimed by antidrug activists in the late 1980s. Reformers advocated sentencing these women to mandatory treatment. However, the crack-baby epidemic never materialized.[17] Alarmist rhetoric often came as the behavior or disease was actually on the wane. In the third movement, after the use of drugs had decreased continuously for five years, the *Christian Science Monitor*, April 26, 1985, quoted "one expert" who remarked that there was an "epidemic" of drug abuse.

The Domino, Stepping-Stone, or Gateway Theory

Burnham (1993, 5–7) has noted that an association between smoking, drinking, gambling, and other "bad habits" has been observed since colonial times. However, the correlation between a cluster of activities sometimes became confused with causality in each of the three movements. Causality is where one behavior statistically predicts the engagement in another.[18]

This domino, stepping-stone, or gateway theory, in which one behavior was thought to lead to other activities, has become a justification for the elimination of various activities in each Clean Living Movement. During the first movement, health reformers, including Sylvester Graham and William Alcott, suggested that ingesting "stimulants," such as meat, alcohol, or spices, would precipitate impure thoughts and "self-abuse," and lead to "debility" among youth. Reformers in the second Clean Living Movement claimed that cigarette smoking among boys led to poor classroom performance, alcohol consumption, cocaine use, and engagement in "vice" (prostitution). During the third movement, cigarette smoking purportedly led to marijuana and alcohol, which in turn led to "harder" drug use and sexual activity among teenagers. In the second movement, this perceived causality led to saloons being closed because patronizing them was thought to lead not only to alcoholism but also to prostitution and the disintegration of the family. It was also a justification for the Eighteenth Amendment (Prohibition) to the constitution. In the late twentieth-century movement, it was a justification for the strict prohibition of cigarette sales in 1997 to individuals under age eighteen.[19]

Purity, Family Values, and Women's Rights

In all three movements, campaigns against some aspects of sexuality, concerns about the disintegration of the family, and agitation for women's rights arose. Reformers in the first Clean Living Movement were most concerned about preventing masturbation in youth. Near the end of this movement, agitation for women's rights and the elimination of "ardent spirits" emerged. During the progressive era cycle, the Women's Christian Temperance Union (WCTU) advocated not only for the elimination of alcohol and tobacco, but also for "purity"—sexual abstinence outside of marriage—and suffrage for women. However, in certain instances different factions within these movements worked against each other. For example, some women associated with suffrage and temperance also favored birth control and eugenic measures. In the late twentieth-century cycle, the women's liberation movement agitated to allow women to engage in traditional male-dominated professions, receive equal pay for equal work, and the right to terminate an unwanted pregnancy. Opposed to this more liberal movement was a conservative movement against pregnancy termination and any form of nonmarital sexuality, and for a return to the traditional family. At one point during this era, a coalition formed between these wings, opposing pornography.[20]

Fear of Dangerous Classes and Undercurrents of Nativism and Eugenics

In all three movements, fear of foreign immigrants and other "dangerous classes"—minority groups, poor people, and rebellious youth—was an underlying factor in campaigns against activities engaged in by these individuals.[21] If a behavior was found among the upper and upper-middle classes, it was generally not considered alarming. As will be discussed in subsequent chapters, the use of medicinal opiates by upper-middle-class white women or the use of hallucinogens by eccentric artists at the turn of the century was largely ignored. During this same period, when opium smoking by Chinese, cocaine use by southern blacks, and heavy alcohol use by Irish and other immigrants was seen as creeping into the white middle class, measures were taken against these substances. Tuberculosis developed romantic overtones when it afflicted poets, such as Shelley and Keats. However, when it affected crowded urban immigrant slums at the turn of the century or the homeless and people with HIV/AIDS today, it became unglamourous and dangerous. In the late twentieth-century movement, baby-boomer youth threatened the status quo by engaging in behaviors which, for the most part, had been confined to the lower classes or the rich and eccentric. This included unmarried sex, cohabitation, out-of-wedlock births, heavy alcohol consumption, and marijuana and other drug use. These activities frightened the middle class, who reacted to the fear of this rapid social change, as they had in previous movements, by enacting measures to control these immoral and "dangerous" behaviors.

"Nativism"—pro-traditional rural Protestant values—and eugenic concerns for healthy offspring have been underlying factors in health reforms, particularly during the first two movements. Native-born white Protestant Americans of Anglo-Saxon stock feared the Roman Catholic "alien menace" from Ireland and southern and eastern Europe. These Nativists blamed immigrants for many diseases, crime, and other social problems. There was a belief that drunkenness, tuberculosis, and poverty could be passed down to succeeding generations, leading to more poverty and disease among these "undesirables" due to inheritance of acquired characteristics (Lamarckian theory). The desire for healthy offspring and for keeping the "race from being polluted" led to eugenic reforms that were prominent, in particular, during the second movement. This eugenic anxiety led to immigration restrictions and sterilization of criminals, the mentally disabled, and the "insane."[22]

Some Other Commonalities

Socioeconomic Class

For the most part, health-reform crusades have been launched and adopted by the educated, the middle class, or those with aspirations to become middle class, as will be seen in the following chapters. The middle class, for the most part, has also been more healthy than the poor. During the first movement, religious evangelizers realized that they could not "save souls" until people were free from disease and drunkenness. Thus, they began reform efforts to clean up the cities and reduce the various health problems in the slums. The tuberculosis crusaders of the second movement also realized the association of urban slums, poverty, and TB and made some effort, not only for slum reform but also for personal hygiene and other health reforms to eliminate this disease. Middle-class Americans readily adopted abstinence from alcohol and tobacco. It was poorer people that frequented saloons and smoked. In the third Clean Living Movement, middle-class Americans began to exercise, ceased smoking, and switched to low-fat diets. This change in lifestyle from the mid-1970s through the 1990s resulted in a decreased death rate from heart disease and cancer among the middle class.[23]

Wars

Real wars (as opposed to health-reform wars) have played an important role in halting reform movements and have tended to make crusades for various health-related issues, such as temperance, appear irrelevant (Walters 1978, x). The Civil War and World War I halted the momentum of the first and the second Clean Living Movements, respectively. In the aftermath of wars there has been an increase in the use of mood-altering substances among soldiers, which may have been caused by exposure through medicine, commercial interests, and social pressure. After the Revolutionary War, there was an increase in alcohol consumption, which peaked in 1830. It began to decrease after this time and continued to do so until after the Civil War. Following this war came an increase in tobacco use and also morphine addiction among war veterans. Following both World War I and World War II, cigarette smoking spiraled upward. Alcohol use increased after World War II and did not peak until 1980. Following the Vietnam War, an upsurge in the use of many mood-altering substances, including illicit drugs, occurred, which also peaked around 1980.[24]

Orthodox versus Alternative Medicine

In all three movements, certain segments of the population rebelled against traditional or orthodox medicine. During the first movement, several systems, including hydrotherapy, homeopathy, and botanical medicine, became popular. During the second movement, Christian Science and New-Thought religions, which were also medical systems because they sought to cure diseases, reached their pinnacle. During the third movement, New Age, alternative, or complemental health systems began to be practiced by a large percentage of the population.[25]

SUMMARY

This chapter discussed the emergence of health-reform movements as an aspect of Great Awakenings. It presented an overview of the similarities between the three Clean Living Movements that have emerged approximately every eighty years during the past two hundred. The chapter addressed the phases common to individual health crusades, which together make up the whole movement era. Typical characteristics of health reformers, the tendency for reformers to demonize and militarize health problems and people who do not agree with them, and the censorship of factual information either during the surge or repose of a cycle were mentioned. Undercurrents of religious revivalism, nativism, feminism, and eugenics that help precipitate and foster health-reform movements were briefly explored. The rise of alternative-cure systems, campaigns for virginity and traditional values, and the gateway theory of a behavior were alluded to as common components of Clean Living Movements. Details of many of these aspects will be elaborated upon in subsequent chapters.

NOTES

1. Several works discuss in detail these cycles of religious awakenings and their ensuing political and socioeconomic changes. See, in particular, McLoughlin (1978) and Fogel (1995). Strauss and Howe (1998), in their recent popular work, discuss four subcycles—turnings—within the overall 80- to 110-year awakening cycles. The first turning of the cycle is the "high," which tends to be a postsocietal crisis boom era when things are going well and there is a high degree of optimism. The second, the "awakening," begins a rebellion against tradition and reform for perceived problems in the society. The third turning, the "unraveling," is when health reform and other crusades come to a peak and there is a feeling of hopelessness. The "crisis," or fourth turning, is a period of profound social crisis such as war or deep depression that dramatically shakes the pillars of society. Based upon this schematic, the health-reform movements discussed in this book have emerged in the awakening stages. They peak and begin to ebb in the unraveling.

2. Health-reform movements have attempted to clean up society; hence the name Clean Living Movement. Lucy Gaston, the progressive era antitobacco reformer, had children sign "clean life" pledges in which they agreed to abstain from tobacco (Warfield 1930, 244). Bernarr Macfadden of this same period was sometimes called a crusader for clean living (Greene 1986, 242). Clean Living Movements have been called by different names by various authors, including the New Temperance, Neo-Prohibition, or Neo-Puritan movements.

3. After the Revolutionary period at the end of the first Great Awakening, some individuals, including physicians Benjamin Rush and Anthony Benezet, were concerned about drunkenness, tobacco, and gluttony. These individuals recommended exercise, diet changes, and moderation in the use of "ardent spirits." However, there were no organized crusades to change health behaviors as have been found in the subsequent three health-reform movements.

4. In this work, "temperance" refers to antialcohol sentiments. At the beginning of a temperance cycle, the term usually means moderation or responsible use of alcohol. As the movement progresses, the term will evolve to mean abstinence or even prohibition. "Smoking" refers to the use of cigarettes, "drinking" denotes the ingestion of an alcoholic beverage, and "alcohol" refers to beverage alcohol unless otherwise noted. Mood-altering drugs refer to any psychotropic agent, including coffee, tea, alcohol, tobacco, cannabis, cocaine, heroin, and so on.

5. See Chapters 3, 8, and 13 for details concerning the temperance and antitobacco movements in each of the three movements.

6. An example of the popularization of a health issue that led to successively increasing coercive measures was the antismoking crusade of the third Clean Living Movement. The dangers of smoking were mentioned in the medical and then the popular literature. Sociologists Troyer and Markel (1983, 61–62) list the steps in which "cigarette smoking has come to be seen as deviant, both by the public and by official proscription." The progression is as follows: (1) Medical research claimed smoking was harmful, (2) the public began to believe cigarettes were harmful, (3) the public stigmatized cigarette smoking, (4) official action was taken against cigarettes, and (5) official action was taken against individual smokers "after a majority of the public defined smoking as undesirable." I would like to add another step, which began to emerge in the mid-1990s: (6) litigation against cigarette manufactures to recoup medical-related expenses from the result of smoking.

7. Opinions vary as to the number of antialcohol movements in American history. Most authors, including David Musto (1996), Robin Room (1987), David Pitman (1980), Dwight Heath (1989), and myself (Engs 1992a) suggest three major temperance and/or prohibition movements, which are part of the three Clean Living Movements discussed in this work. Jack Blocker (1989), however, suggests five movements, divided into the following periods: 1784–1840, 1840–1860, 1860–1892, 1892–1933, and 1933–1980. See Chapters 3, 8, and 13 for more details concerning the three antialcohol movements.

8. For details concerning modern interpretations of antialcohol cycles and their phases, evolution, and characteristics, see Blocker (1989), Engs (1997), Gusfield (1986), Musto (1996), and Levine (1984).

9. See Burnham (1993) for details about the influence of commercial entities and the use of the media, political maneuvering, and advertisements to change attitudes toward a variety of behaviors related to health.

10. Several popular works published from the beginning to the peak of the third Clean Living Movement discussed manifestations of and criticized America's obsession with vice and sin, puritanical repression of pleasure, rhetoric against perceived health dangers, and moral crusades against pleasurable

behaviors. See, for example, works by Peele (1989), Shaw (1996), Sullum (1998), and Wagner (1997). An example of this underlying antipleasure sentiment in the United States is the prohibition of heroin for any medical use, including long-term paid relief for terminally ill patients. Ethan Nadlemann, director of a drug-advocacy think tank, remarked in the August 12, 1998 *Associated Press Report* that "there's been a de facto self-censoring of any discussion of this. There's a reluctance to *keep people on drugs they might like*" (italics added).

11. Chapters 2, 7, and 12 will discuss further details about the development of new religions as part of Clean Living Movements and their embracing of health as part of religious belief.

12. The June 22, 1992 *Los Angeles Times* reported that the U.S. Surgeon General, leaders of the American Medical Association, and schoolchildren paraded through downtown Chicago to protest Joe Camel as a "merchant of death," an act that is symbolic of the demonization of tobacco, the tobacco industry, and its advertising. It is interesting to note that in the second movement Lucy Gaston, the anticigarette reformer, also held parades in the Chicago area with children to "stamp out the cigarette evil" (Gray 1909, 315). In subsequent chapters, other examples of demonization will be presented for many substances and activities that are the subject of health reforms.

13. For more discussion concerning scapegoating and demonization in terms of alcohol, see Levine (1984, 109–112). Numerous examples of demonization and the scapegoating of alcohol from the first movement can be found in various issues of the *Temperance Almanac* published in Massachusetts and New York State between 1834 and 1842. In the second movement, many works were published by the Women's Christians Temperance Union and the Anti-Saloon League illustrating this process. Information on the demonization of tobacco and the tobacco industry can be found in Sullum (1998). More information about demonization and scapegoating for various health-related issues will be discussed in subsequent chapters.

14. See, in particular, Chapter 5 in Snowball (1991) concerning the use of war metaphors against immoral behaviors by the late twentieth-century Christian Right's Moral Majority movement.

15. See Allsop (1961) for details concerning Chicago bootleggers and their battles with federal officials.

16. In 1976, the National Institute of Alcohol Abuse, immediately before the surge of the late twentieth-century antialcohol movement, published a pamphlet, *Drinking Etiquette for Those Who Drink and Those Who Don't*, which discussed methods for responsible drinking and hosting and the pros and cons of alcohol consumption. It was one of the many objective publications eliminated by the Health and Human Services publishing office in the mid-1980s because it was not stridently antialcohol. *High Times*, a drug advocacy publication, in an article entitled "Fed Dope Bureau Censors Drug Info" (1984), discussed NIDA's advocacy of censoring "outdated" materials even if they were based upon scientific studies. This article mentioned that material the agency wanted "purged" could not be old because "the government hasn't allowed any research with any of these drugs since the 1960s, so the information can't possibly be out of date." This purging was a method to eliminate publications that were not strictly opposed to drugs or alcohol. For further

information concerning the suppression of information, either in favor of or against the use of certain substance or behaviors in all three cycles, see also Musto (1996, 78–83) and Levine (1984, 109–112).

17. The September 10, 1989 issue of the *San Diego Union-Tribune* remarked, "America is paying a terrible price for our failure to prevent a tragedy of truly epidemic dimensions—substance abuse by pregnant women," and "We are experiencing a crack baby explosion." Ten years later, the May 3, 1998 *Tampa Tribune* reported that the nation did not experience an epidemic of crack babies. A healthcare worker was quoted as stating, "Media hype that talked about a 'lost generation' was misleading."

18. During the end of the twentieth-century antialcohol, antitobacco, and antidrug movements, a multitude of studies from the 1970s to the present have shown a high correlation between smoking, drinking, the use of other mood-altering substances, and/or other socially unacceptable behaviors or diseases (see, for example, Anderson and Dahlberg 1992; Engs and Teijlingen 1997; Engs and Hanson 2000; Johnson et al. 1987; and Torabi et al. 1993). However, the results are mixed in terms of smoking or drinking as predictors or "causes" of behaviors. Positive statistical correlation between these behaviors may be due to the fact that certain individuals are more prone to engage in "risky" or non–socially approved behaviors because of rebellion against authority, the "establishment," or parents; as a symbol of independence or "outsider" status; or as reactance—the act of engaging in a behavior because a person is told not to do it and/or because it is illegal (O'Donnell and Clayton 1982; Yamaguchi and Kandel 1984; and Engs and Hanson 1989, 2000).

19. An example of the gateway hypothesis in the second Clean Living Movement is a quote from W. S. Osborn, superintendent of the State Hospital for Inebriates in Iowa, found in an article by H. S. Gray (1909, 300): "[Cigarette smoking in] undeveloped youth often paves the way to and rapidly enters upon a course of drug and liquor taking as well as crime through this harmful form of tobacco addiction." Gray (1909, 294) attempts to enlighten educators concerning association and causality. He suggests "the problem of determining to what extent cigarette smoking is the cause and to what extent the effect of a bad physical, mental, and moral condition in a boy is a difficult one. The cigarette habit is partly cause and partly effect in the same person." In the third movement, an example of the gateway hypothesis is suggested in the *Christian Science Monitor's* April 26, 1995 report on a White House conference on drugs. It quotes a Mr. Browne, who contends, "The most effective ways to help youths was to stop the use of gateway drugs—alcohol and marijuana. A can of beer or a marijuana cigarette might seem relatively harmless, but they quickly lead to other things." Not everyone agreed with this. The *Los Angeles Times* of January 8, 1989 quotes a letter writer who suggests that alcohol and tobacco were not gateway drugs but rather "together account for 99% of all deaths attributed to drugs in the United States. All of the illegal drugs combined account for the rest." By the early 1990s, cigarette smoking was considered to be the major gateway drug among youth by health reformers.

20. These issues are discussed in Chapters 3 and 4 for the first movement. See Chapters 8 and 9 for the second, and Chapters 12, 14, and 15 for the third Clean Living Movement for discussions concerning the antagonism between

more conservative and liberal movements in terms of sexuality-related issues such as sex education, obscenity, women's reproductive rights, change in family structure, and hereditarian concerns. The August 26, 1985 issue of the *New York Times*, in an article entitled "Joining Hands in the Fight Against Pornography," discusses Andrea Dworkin, a member of the National Organization for Women (NOW) supporting Jerry Falwell of the right-wing concerning "harm in pornography."

21. For more information concerning middle-class fear of the "dangerous classes," including immigrants, as a factor in the precipitation of health reforms in all three movements, see Epstein (1981), Gienapp (1987), Gusfield (1986), Pivar (1973), Tyrrell (1979), and Walters (1978).

22. The nativistic and heredity/eugenic movements and their importance in health reforms are discussed in Chapters 5, 6, 9, 10, and 15. For more information concerning eugenics, see, in particular, Bajema (1976), Dowbiggin (1997), Haller (1963), Kevles (1985), Larson (1995), Paul (1995), and Pickens (1968). See also the sources cited in note 21.

23. A summary of a report from the Department of Health and Human Services in the July 30, 1998 *Milwaukee Journal Sentinel* notes, "Americans' health seems to be getting better, but low-income families or those less educated aren't benefiting as much."

24. For statistics concerning the ebb and flow of tobacco and alcohol consumption, see, in particular, Rorabaugh (1976, 232–233) and Heimann (1960, 248–249). During both World War I and World War II, cigarettes were passed out to soldiers, as will be discussed in more detail in Chapter 8.

25. See Chapters 2 and 6 for the first movement, Chapters 7 and 11 for the second, and Chapter 12 for information regarding the third movement. In all three time periods, dissatisfaction with traditional medicine and the emergence of alternative medical practices occurred, launching alternative practices and clashes with orthodox medicine.

PART I

The First Clean Living Movement, 1830–1860

The vegetarians, phrenologists, water-cure doctors, and anti-tobacco, anti-corset and temperance people were so often crossing paths, they began to look like participants in a single reform movement.
Ronald Numbers, *Prophetess of Health: Ellen G. White* (1976)

Arising after the War of 1812, antebellum reform crested in the 1830s and 1840s, declined in the 1850s, and seemed almost quaint by the 1870s.
Ronald G. Walters, *American Reformers 1815–1860* (1978)

Hereafter, we may presume that the anti-tobacco flag will be nailed to the temperance mast, and that both causes will rise or fall together.
Dwight Baldwin, *Prize Essay: Evils of Tobacco as They Affect Body, Mind and Morals* (1855)

The Jacksonian era, sometimes called the era of the common man or the Antebellum Reform era, underlied the first Clean Living Movement. This health-reform era extended from the late 1820s until the Civil War. During this approximately thirty-five-year span, many crusades for health and social reforms emerged. Several sociological, economic, and political explanations can be given for the reform enthusiasm of this era, and the reader is encouraged to explore the great body of literature that addresses this period.[1] A major contribution to this reformist zeal was burgeoning popular distrust and disillusionment with practicing physicians, clergymen, and politicians. This sentiment, in turn, led to the rise of health, religious, and political sects that celebrated the virtues of the common man and sought to bring America to a golden age free of crime, poverty, and disease.

Before health-reform agitation began, an upsurge in religious revivalism arose, often called the second Great Awakening. Historian Ronald Walters (1978, 24) suggested, "It was evangelical Protestantism that provided most of the ideological and organizational foundation for antebellum reform." Out of this religious fervor, feelings of pietism and the "perfectibility of man" led to efforts to eliminate the evils of society. New religions, temperance, personal hygiene, diet reform, and botanic cures appeared early in this reform era, while hydrotherapy, eugenics, women's rights, and sanitation and public health became more prominent nearer the end of this period.

At the end of this first Clean Living Movement, the burning issues of the period, such as women's rights, temperance, and diet, began to wane. However, they smoldered just beneath the surface of the culture. Part I discuss the health-related crusades of the first Clean Living Movement. Many of these same reform issues erupted again approximately eighty years later in the progressive era and again in the millennial era at the end of the twentieth century.

NOTE

1. See Schlesinger (1950), Sellers (1958), and Remini (1989) for some general information about the Jacksonian age. About 5,000 titles concerning this time period are found in Remini and Miles (1979). Several authors have discussed the health and social-reform movements of this antebellum era and have suggested different time periods for when it began. Within the whole movement, different health reforms emerged at different times in the approximately three to four decades before the Civil War. Walters (1978) suggests that the movement began after the War of 1812 and ended prior to the Civil War in about 1860. Whorton (1988, 56), Nissenbaum (1980), and Rosenberg (1987, 227–229) suggest its range was from approximately 1830 until the Civil War. For other remarks concerning health and social reforms of this age, see Cayleff (1988, 84), Davis (1967, 2–10), Numbers (1976, 70), Reid (1982, 22–48), and Remini (1989, 76–98).

2

Millennialism, New Religions, and Health Reform

> A Word of Wisdom. . . . Strong drinks are not for the belly. . . .
> Tobacco is not for the body, neither for the belly, and is not good
> for man. . . . Hot drinks are not for the body or belly. . . . Flesh also
> of beasts and fowls of the air . . . are to be used sparingly . . . and
> only in times of winter. . . . All grain is ordained for the use of man
> . . . to be the staff of life.
>
> Joseph Smith, Doctrine and Covenants[1] (1974)

> Tobacco is a poison of the most deceitful and malignant kind. . . .
> Tea and coffee are stimulating [and] . . . the whole system under
> the influence of these stimulants often becomes intoxicated. . . .
> Indulging in eating too frequently, and in too large quantities, over-
> taxes the digestive organs. . . . Strict habits of cleanliness should be
> observed. . . . The body, which God calls his temple, should be
> preserved in as healthy a condition as possible.
>
> Ellen G. White, Spiritual Gifts (1864)

A wave of Protestant revivalism, the second Great Awakening, swept
through the United States from about 1800 to the mid-1830s. This evangelical fever occurred primarily in the Northeast, and, in particular,
western New York. Out of this ferment arose deeply religious individuals with a passion for perfectionism. In addition, two new religious sects, the Mormons and the Seventh-Day Adventists, evolved.
The new religions incorporated healthy lifestyles as part of religious
belief. Converts to the more traditional groups translated their new
religious enthusiasm into health-reform crusades.

REVIVALISM AND HEALTH REFORM

In the second Great Awakening, a frenzied effort emerged to convert the "unchurched" in an attempt to usher in the millennium, the second coming of Christ, and a thousand-year reign of Christianity. At the core of the second Great Awakening was a renunciation of the "old" Calvinist preoccupation with human helplessness before a vengeful God. They renounced the fatalistic acceptance that considered illness as "God's will" (Cross 1965; Sweet 1984). According to some historians, this change in attitude resulted in a belief in an egalitarian society with emphasis on the ability of the average person to seek his or her own salvation though positive action and the ability of the "common folk" to think for themselves.[2] Whorton (1988, 56–57) suggests that disease was now seen as an avoidable evil. To escape disease, the individual had to take positive action to prevent it, just as a person needed to take measures to eliminate sin from his or her life for spiritual salvation.

Emerging from this revivalist enthusiasm was also a perfectionist impulse. This is the belief that with God's grace the common man could speed the coming of the millennium by improving not only himself or herself, but also society on earth in general. Rosenberg (1976, 12), in *No Other Gods,* which addresses reform movements of the nineteenth century, suggests that health reform was a continuation of this religious fervor. Health and salvation became intertwined because the soul could not be saved if the body was harmed or forced to dwell in a filthy environment.

The first Clean Living Movement was rooted in these revivals and heralded by clergy. Charles Grandison Finney (1792–1875), a Presbyterian preacher and lawyer, was one the most influential evangelists of his era, presenting spirited revivals in the villages of the Northeast, and in particular upstate New York, in 1824–1832. He is often considered the father of modern evangelism. Abstinence from "ardent spirits" was part of Finney's message. Indeed, in the Rochester, New York, revival of 1831, in order to be saved one had to sign a temperance pledge. As part of salvation, Finney considered the care of the body, "the temple of God" (I Corinthians 6:19), a holy duty. Anything that harmed this "temple," including alcohol, tobacco, coffee, and tea, would prevent salvation and indirectly short-circuit the millennium (Johnson 1978, 113–114; Hardman 1987, 361).

Finney's revivalist methods during the late 1820s were not always acceptable to the more staid religious leaders of the day, however. Besides Finney, conservative ministers, such as Lyman Beecher, also advocated temperance and health reform. Beecher (1846), a Congregational minister from Connecticut, published a book in 1826 entitled *Six Sermons on . . . Intemperance*. This thirty-one-page booklet discussed intoxication as "a national sin," advised abstinence from "ardent spirits," and proposed legislation to "banish strong drink as a lawful article of commerce." These sermons were quickly accepted by most Presbyterian and congregationalists as well as by health reformers during the late 1820s (Fletcher 1943, 336; Nissenbaum 1980, 72; Rosell 1984, 136–137). Other clergy during this era advocated or published works with health-reform advice, including John Wesley, the founder of the Methodist Church, who published a book entitled *Primitive Physick*, and Sylvester Graham, a Presbyterian minister, who began preaching in 1831 about human physiology and diet.

In 1835, after the peak of his revivalist career, Charles Finney became a professor at the new Oberlin College Theological School, which had been founded two years before. Prospective students, called "colonists," were required to sign a covenant that required them to eat only plain, healthy food and renounce all evil habits, such as smoking and chewing tobacco and "strong drink," including coffee and tea (Fletcher 1943, 319–327; Hardman 1987, 361). Diet as part of moral reform, however, became stricter at Oberlin in 1840. The elective meat table was eliminated and Graham's vegetarian diet was required for all. After ten months of spartan existence, students and faculty members protested and a more varied diet was reinstated. During Finney's peak years, he enlisted thousands of northerners and New Yorkers into revivals and reform work. He undoubtedly had an influence, even if indirect, on individuals who were instrumental in founding the new religious groups in the Northeast in which health reform became doctrine (Fletcher 1943, 329–333; Hambrick-Stowe 1996, 111–112).

SOME NEW RELIGIOUS SECTS

The religious fervor of the second Great Awakening reached its peak in 1826. The center of revivalism underwent a gradual transfer westward from New England into western New York. From this area, sometimes called the "burned-over region" because of its many fiery sermons, several "alternative" religious groups emerged (Cross 1965, 13). Converts to the new religions were "self-educated people, surprisingly literate, and manifesting a thirst for knowledge" (Hatch 1984, 124). They strove to create a totally new order, rather than improve the old one as temperance and health reformers sought to do. In the subsequent awakenings, new religions also attempted this.

A few of the new sects that emerged from the evangelical ferment embraced health reform as a necessary part of salvation. These groups shared the belief that the body was "the temple of God," and anything that harmed the body also harmed the spirit. Health-reform issues such as antialcohol and antitobacco stances and vegetarianism were incorporated into some of these nascent sects as a matter of faith. And like the Branch Davidians of the early 1990s, some of these newly formed mid-nineteenth-century groups were persecuted. Members were killed for behaviors that supported their belief system. Some of the groups lived communally and had sexual practices that deviated from mainstream culture.

The Mormons and Adventists, in particular, were influenced by the health-reform aspect of this first Clean Living Movement. Indeed, these two sects became the epitome of Christian physiology by incorporating temperance, diet, exercise, and other health issues into their scriptures and beliefs. A large number of Methodist and Baptist congregations, in which many Midwestern and Southern revivalists had their roots, kept temperance as part of their faith and frowned upon tobacco. Vegetarianism and sentiments against other "stimulants," such as coffee and tea, were generally not incorporated into these religions when the first Clean Living Movement began to lose momentum on the eve of the Civil War.

THE CHURCH OF JESUS CHRIST OF LATTER-DAY SAINTS (MORMONS)

The founder and prophet of this new religious group was Joseph Smith. His writings comprise the theological foundation for the group.

Joseph Smith

Joseph Smith (1805–1844), born in Sharon, Vermont, grew up in western New York during the intense religious revivals of the region. As a teenager in 1820 he claimed to have found "golden plates" containing a history of Native Americans and directions for bringing back the "ancient order of things." He established his church in 1830 and announced periodic revelations on widely divergent matters, including health-reform issues.

Smith and his growing band of followers moved to Ohio, Missouri, and Nauvoo, Illinois, to escape persecution due to rumored practices of polygamy and group solidarity that posed a political and economic threat in the emerging "western" communities (Foster 1981, 242). Political problems and increasing hostility toward their lifestyle led to Smith's death by mob action in 1844. The mantle of leadership went to Brigham Young, and the majority of Smith's followers went on to found Salt Lake City.[3]

Health Reformers' Influences on Early Church Teachings as Expressed in the Word of Wisdom

Smith, like others of his day, had misgivings and mistrust concerning regular or orthodox physicians. In Smith's case, he and other family members suffered at the hand of these regular "heroic" physicians. A brother died in 1823 due to complications of calomel poisoning, a popular mercury-based drug of the day. As orthodox medicine began to be challenged by botanic medicine in the Northeast during the 1820s and 1830s, Smith, along with other individuals in the budding Mormon community, began to use herbal treatments (N. L. Smith 1979, 39). Divett (1979, 23) implies that, with two Thompsonians among Smith's closest advisers, it is not surprising that he became an advocate of botanic medicine and other health ideals. It is likely they influenced his advice about health as reflected in the "Word of Wisdom," the primary health guidelines of the church.[4] Indeed, N. Lee Smith (1979, 41) states that "the wording of the Word of Wisdom frequently parallels that of health-reform tenets." Thomas Alexander, a Mormon historian, in the autumn 1981 *Dialogue,* suggests that antitobacco and antialcohol sentiments were, in addition, based upon the influence of evangelical Protestant sentiments against liquor and tobacco, as evidenced by a diary from an early elder of this era. Beside the Word of Wisdom, other health-reform guidelines are found in the *Doctrine and Covenants* (D&C) (Smith 1974, 88:124), such as advice to "keep clean" and to go to bed and rise early.

Both the domestic health and medical texts written by physicians warned against excessive consumption of meat, hot drinks, alcohol, tobacco, or other substances that were considered stimulants. However, not all religions discouraged the same items. In addition to these substances, standard texts for physicians also advocated exercise, adequate sleep, and cleanliness, which corresponds with Mormon health beliefs.[5]

The Word of Wisdom originally was considered "advice" in the church's early years. Underlying the advice was a sense of moderation. For example, believers were advised to eat meat in moderation, not necessarily be vegetarians. Even wine in moderation was more or less acceptable. After Young led the pioneers into Utah, vineyards and wine presses were established in the Virgin River Basin. Wine manufactured there was used for tithes, bartering, and the Sacraments. Surplus wine was sold to the "Gentiles," what LDS members called non-Mormons (Larson 1946, 347–350). It was not until the early twentieth century that the Word of Wisdom was accorded the status of revelation and was prescribed as mandatory in order to remain a "Mormon in good standing." This occurred after polygamy was banned in the

1890s. Shipps (1985, 156, 128) suggests that this revelation may have been a means of keeping the religion easily identifiable from other religious groups.

Common "Health" Sense

Hansen (1981, 41) suggests that the Word of Wisdom could be considered commonsense "health promotion" in the mid-nineteenth century. During this era, high mortality resulted from infectious disease in the population as a whole, including the Mormons. Since disease was considered caused by overstimulation of the body, avoiding anything stimulating could be considered a practical health measure based upon the teachings of the time (Bush 1992, 42–51).

Early Mormon leaders were concerned about other common health-reform issues of the day. This included exercise, the "cursed corset," and long skirts that dragged on filthy streets. Comfortable practical clothing was recommended (Underwood 1986, 50). In the early 1830s, ball playing, dancing, and other forms of sport and exercise were frowned upon by the church. This may have been because many converts came from religious backgrounds that proscribed these types of activities as evil. However, by 1844 "wrestling, running, climbing, dancing, or anything that has tendency to circulate the blood is not injurious, but is considered beneficial to the human system" if pursued in moderation (Underwood 1986, 53). In denouncing the social evils of the day, the Latter-Day Saints were little different from other reform and religious groups. The other new religion to develop health reform in this era was the Seventh-Day Adventists.

THE MILLERITES AND SEVENTH-DAY ADVENTISTS

Similarities exist between Mormons and Seventh-Day Adventists in regard to health reform. The public sometimes confused the two religious groups in their early years. Both incorporated many of the ideals of health reform, including diet and temperance, into scriptural or church teachings. Both groups believed in a prophet who received revelations or visions on a variety of matters including health. They both practiced divine healing and "priestly" or "elder" blessings for illness. Both groups are indigenous to the United States and their leaders felt their respective group was called to restore the "ancient order of the church." They both originated in the eastern part of the country and the center of their denominations moved west with the western expansion. The Seventh-Day Adventists, however, were incorporated thirty years after the Mormons, when health reform was no longer an important issue among most Americans.

Early Adventist Leaders and the Beginnings of Health Reform

The founder of the group that eventually became the Seventh-Day Adventists, and some smaller Adventist groups, was William Miller. In 1831, Miller, a retired army captain and farmer, after an intense study of the bible, calculated that the earth would terminate around 1843 with the second coming of Christ. During the late 1830s, Miller presided over many popular tent revival meetings and won numerous converts. He taught that anyone who consumed alcohol would be wholly unprepared for the Second Coming and gained many converts from followers who were temperance enthusiasts (Numbers 1976, 37–38). This set the stage for antialcohol sentiments among later Adventists.

At the peak of the "Millerite" movement (as the press called Miller's followers), a number of believers waited expectantly for the Second Coming or "Advent." Because Christ, however, did not return on the first date, Miller and his followers set a second date, October 22, 1844. The uneventful passing of this day led to what became known as the "Great Disappointment" among Adventists. Some Millerites left the ranks after this date. Others met in 1845 to sort out the problem. Among those who persisted after the failure of Miller's prophecy were three individuals who shaped the group into what became the Seventh-Day Adventists: Ellen G. White, her husband James White, and Joseph Bates. These individuals also were largely responsible for including health reform as part of religious teachings.[6] They introduced several doctrinal changes, including, Saturday, rather than Sunday, as being the Sabbath. In 1863, the "Sabbatarian Adventists" incorporated as the Seventh-Day Adventists church (Numbers 1976, 44; Butler 1974, 178–179).

Ellen G. Harmon White

Ellen G. Harmon White (1827–1915), born near Portland, Maine, was the prophet and a founder of this new denomination. As a girl she was involved in an accident that left her in ill health for several years and with a permanent facial scar. White was brought up in a devout Methodist household and became involved with Millerism as an adolescent. In late 1844, she began to have "visions" on a variety of subjects. One of these led her to travel and minister among "the scattered flock" of Millerites. During these travels she met James White (1821–1881), an itinerant Millerite preacher, whom she married in 1846. This young minister did not use alcohol or tobacco, or consume coffee, tea, or meat, and was influential in the health beliefs of the group during its early beginnings (Numbers 1976, 14, 38).

In 1848, Ellen White began to receive the first of her many visions on healthful living. Although she spoke out against various stimulants, alcohol was not specified. This was likely because it was considered such an "obvious evil," or so little abused by members, inasmuch as many Adventists had been temperance supporters, that it did not need to be mentioned. As part of the development of the nascent sect, the Whites launched a succession of periodicals, cumulating in a small magazine called *The Advent Review and Sabbath Herald* in 1851, which is still published today. This journal contained many articles, including those by Ellen White, and chronicles the progress of health reform among the early Adventists (Numbers 1976, 212).

The Influence of Hydrotherapists on Adventist Health Teachings

Hydropathy, or "water cure," was a major treatment philosophy during mid-nineteenth-century America. Reid (1982, 79–83), in *A Sound of Trumpets*, a history of the Seventh-Day Adventists, suggests that the hydropathic movement asserted a direct influence on Adventist teachings about disease prevention and cure. After the Whites spent time in 1864 at "Our Home," James Jackson, a hydrotherapist's Danville, New York, water cure institution, hydrotherapy became popular among the Adventists. Leaders of the church decided to open their own hydrotherapy treatment center for Sabbatarians, as they did not like the card playing and dancing offered at Jackson's center. As a result, the Western Health Reform Institute was established in Battle Creek, Michigan, in 1866.

By the end of the nineteenth century, this center combined the ingredients of a European health spa and a twentieth-century Mayo Clinic. The health food and cereal industries had their beginnings at the sanitarium. John Kellogg, a physician, became head of this institution. He modified Jackson's "granula," the cereal that was served at Danville. It became "granola," which was similar to modern Grapenuts. The cereal was introduced for patients, but it became so popular that Kellogg made it available to the health-minded public. His brother, W. K. Kellogg, launched the ready-to-eat cereal business with some of these recipes (Reid 1982, 145).

Health Reform and Its Influence on Ellen White's Visions and Adventism

As health reform began to wane in the general population in the 1850s, it was kept alive among the Adventists. As early as 1848, James and Ellen White opposed tobacco publicly, along with coffee and tea. However, tobacco's use was condemned as an economic waste and not specifically a health issue (Numbers 1976, 38). In 1854, Ellen White received a second vision on health, including diet and cleanliness, which compared to Grahamism. After this vision, the Whites, in 1855, wrote a major article in the *Review and Herald* deploring tobacco. The article marked the beginning of a crusade that ultimately drove tobacco use from the ranks of the small but rapidly growing Adventist group. Tobacco use began to be seen as a violation of the physical laws of health and was considered to be a moral violation similar to the use of alcohol (Reid 1982, 56).

These growing sentiments on health issues during the 1840s and 1850s led to a major vision in June 1863. This included most of the health-reform issues of the time. In this revelation, Ellen White learned that the Seventh-Day Adventists were instructed to give up meat and other stimulating foods. They were to shun alcohol and tobacco, and avoid drug-dispensing doctors. When sick, they were expected to rely solely on nature's remedies, including fresh air, sunshine, exercise, proper diet, and water. The Adventist sisters were instructed to give up fashionable dresses in turn for shorter skirts and pantaloons similar to the "bloomer" outfit. Masturbation and excessive sex were also to be curbed. Good health became a moral issue. If people violated the laws of health by being intemperate in food and drink, they brought on disease. In addition, White received a vision to the effect that a person's moral and spiritual nature was largely affected by his or her physical condition and that "all [were] required to do what they can to preserve healthy bodies and sound minds" (White 1864, 124, 140, 148; Numbers 1976, x).

After Ellen White's 1863 vision, healthful living to prevent disease became a major issue in the church. The strong biblical emphasis in Adventist publications broadened to include health. While the Bible provided moral direction and some specific information regarding healthful living, most of the reform content came from the visions of White. A healthy lifestyle was so important to the church that, in 1866, the Whites launched another publication, the *Health Reformer*, to spread information concerning health (Reid 1982, 120, 129).

Influences of Reformers on Ellen White's Health Writings, as expressed in *Spiritual Gifts*

Ellen White's health writings, which shaped the direction and content of Adventist health reform, addressed three general areas: (1) the theory of disease and its causes, (2) reform in diet, and (3) protective health practices. This outline first appeared in 1864 as part of her major work, *Spiritual Gifts Volume 4*, in an essay simply called "Health" (White 1864, 120–151). These ideas were all similar to the health reformers of this era, including advice from the botanic physicians, home medical-treatment books, Sylvester Graham, and the other Christian physiologists to be discussed in the next chapter.

Perhaps the most influential health reformer, in terms of writings and directly influencing White and the Adventists, was Larkin B. Coles (1803–1872). Coles, a Millerite convert and physician, wrote *Philosophy of Health* (1854), a popular health book. His book addressed the traditional arguments of the health reformers, such as fresh air, exercise, a vegetarian diet, the avoidance of stimulants, dress reform, sexual purity, and drugless medicine. His moralistic view of health reform, as seen in his elevation of hygienic laws to equality with the Ten Commandments, was similar to that of other reformers, such as William Alcott, who emphasized the moral obligation to preserve health (Numbers 1976, 59–61).

Although White claimed no influence from Dr. Coles or the other health reformers, many of her health proclamations in *Spiritual Gifts* came almost directly from his work (Numbers 1976, xi, 61). These early Adventists, from a current perspective, can be seen as a bona fide religious group based upon holistic health. They embraced all the tenets of the contemporary health movement, including an interconnection among body, mind, and spirit, along with proscriptions against tobacco and other substances and encouragement of a healthy lifestyle.

OTHER MILLENNIUM RELIGIOUS GROUPS

Several other religious sects arose during the second Great Awakening but did not embrace health reform to the extent of the Mormons or Adventists. The Oneidas, founded by Humphrey Noyes, were a communal enterprise. They advocated an alternative sexual lifestyle with eugenic practices and will be discussed in Chapter 5. The Spiritualists, Campbellites (Disciples of Christ), and other religious groups were founded in this era, but were not noted for health reform. Christian Science, founded by Mary Baker Eddy, which embraced health-reform efforts, has some roots at the end of this first movement. However, since it did not become incorporated as a church until the end of the nineteenth century, it will be discussed in Chapter 7 as part of the second Clean Living Movement.

SUMMARY

During the second Great Awakening, religious fervor spawned a reformist impulse. If the body was the temple of God, it must be kept pure and undefiled by alcohol, stimulants, and other harmful substances or activities. Only perfection of the body would bring on the millennium, a golden age free from crime and disease. These beliefs led to crusades against alcohol and the promotion of other health-reform issues. Out of this religious awakening, as occurred in subsequent awakenings, new religious denominations were founded. When health reform sentiment began to wane in the general population during the mid-1840s, the newly formed Mormons and Seventh-Day Adventists incorporated health-reform activities into church doctrine that are still practiced to this day.

NOTES

1. Among Latter-Day Saints, this work is considered scripture, containing the revelations of God to Joseph Smith, his prophet, about a variety of issues, including healthful living.

2. Many works have been devoted to the second Great Awakening and its influence on social reform during the antebellum era. The religious ferment of the time was not just limited to revivals and the numerous reform crusades they generated. Permanent divisions occurred in established churches. Evangelicalism emerged in response to social change. People became inner directed in response to social dislocation and turned to evangelical movements, which in response accelerated social change. A rebellion by the "common people" against educated clergy, physicians, and politicians resulted in a self-help movement with regard to religion, medicine, and politics. See Gordon-McCutchan (1981), Johnson (1978, 109), Carwardine (1978, 4), Kselman (1983, 80–83), Hudson (1974, 7–8), Hardman (1987), Cross (1965), Fletcher (1943), and Sweet (1984) for further readings on the religious aspects of this reform era.

3. A wealth of information abounds on Joseph Smith, Brigham Young, and the development of the early Mormon church. Besides those cited in this chapter, see also Hill (1983) and Bushman (1984).

4. Numerous works have considered the origins of the Word of Wisdom (Smith 1974, 1–21) in Mormon scripture and lifestyle. See Bush (1981, 1992) for a detailed exploration of hypotheses pertaining to the influences from both botanic and orthodox medicine. Arrington (1959) and McCue (1981) discuss other aspects of these writings. The classic study of this topic is Peterson (1972).

5. "Domestic medicine" texts were written by regular orthodox physicians with medical degrees during the early nineteenth century. These works were often reprinted several times through the mid-nineteenth century. As stated by Shadrach Ricketson in *Means of Preserving Health and Preventing Disease* (1806, v), his text was "designed not merely for physicians, but for the information of others." A very popular book, *Domestic Medicine*, was published by William Buchan (1838). For further information on the numerous medical and popular texts of the time, see Francesco Cordasco (1985). This work contains a listing of all health- and medical-related works of the nineteenth century. Many Americans were undoubtedly familiar with some of these, since they likely used them for home doctoring.

6. The best secondary sources for the history of health reform and its incorporation into Seventh-Day Adventist teachings are Numbers (1976), Reid (1982), and Gaustand (1974). Numbers, in particular has many references to original manuscripts that are sometimes difficult to obtain. See White (1958, 1938, 1864) for her proclamations concerning health.

3

Temperance, Tobacco, and Women's Rights

Intemperance is the sin of our land.
> Lyman Beecher, *Six Sermons on the Nature, Occasions, Signs, and Evils on the Remedy of Intemperance* (1846)

How great an evil in this country, is the use of alcoholic and narcotic substances. . . . The use of alcohol and tobacco tends powerfully to debilitate the constitution; and the complaints which they generate descend hereditarily to posterity.
> Edward Hitchcock, *Journal of Health* (1830)

Banish Intemperance, and you banish vice and poverty from the land.
> *Temperance Family Almanac* (1835)

Smoking has everywhere . . . become a tremendous evil. . . . [We need] to induce the rising generation to turn the current of public opinion against it. . . . Smoking is indecent, filthy, and rude, and to many individuals highly offensive.
> William Alcott, *The Young Man's Guide* (1835)

In Europe, two divergent drinking attitudes, beverage preferences, and patterns of alcohol use developed in antiquity. The Mediterranean daily use of wine by all segments of the population contrasted episodic drinking of grain-based beverages and ambivalence toward alcohol in northern and eastern European cultures. The Roman expansion brought the urban wine-drinking patterns to north-central western Europe. During the early middle ages, when Roman power waned in that region, northern Germanic tribes migrated to these areas. Britain and other former Roman provinces developed a "blended pattern," in which both grain-based beverages and wine were consumed. The Nordic cultures, untouched by Roman influence, retained their episodic drinking practices, and the ancient Mediterranean areas continued daily wine drinking as part of the diet (Engs 1991b, 1995, 227–230).[1]

British immigrants, whose culture became dominant in North America, transported their drinking traditions into what is now the United States and Canada. Southern European colonists brought their Romanized patterns to South America, thus establishing conflicting drinking attitudes and patterns in the New World. Consumption patterns by Roman Catholic immigrants pouring into the United States during the nineteenth century—which differed from those of the native-born Protestant establishment—set the stage for cultural clashes regarding drinking in the United States (Engs 1995, 227–228; Wiseman 1997, 12–16).[2]

THE TEMPERANCE MOVEMENT

A major factor contributing to the emergence of the antialcohol temperance movement in the Jacksonian era was the second Great Awakening and its resulting fervor to "perfect the world." A primary focus of this agitation was the elimination of drunkenness and other problems among intemperate laborers and immigrants.[3] "Along with Abolition and Nativism, Temperance formed one of a trio of major movements during the 1840s and 1850s" (Gusfield 1986, 5–6).

Antialcohol sentiment stirred before the other health-reform crusades during the first Clean Living Movement. "The entire health-reform movement had in a way developed from the temperance drive" (Reid 1982, 45). Robert Fletcher (1943, 336), a historian specializing in Oberlin College, has suggested that "the temperance movement was the parent of the 'physiological reform' movement. If it was sinful to drink liquors harmful to the physical body, it followed it was sinful to eat harmful foods, take poisonous drugs, wear tight inadequate clothing or neglect exercise, bathing, or nutrition." Most of the health reformers in the first movement were first involved with temperance reform.

The Colonial Period and Its Attitudes toward Alcohol

In the late seventeenth century, alcohol, "a good creature of God" (Rush 1812), was considered an indispensable food, beverage, medicine, and commodity. Drinking, but not drunkenness, was accepted. By the end of the eighteenth century, the general positive attitude toward alcohol, primarily spirits, found throughout most of the colonial period began to change. This shift in attitude was attributed to many reasons, including the need for sober laborers to operate machinery arising from the industrial revolution. Anthony Benezet, a wealthy Philadelphia Quaker businessman, in 1775 had recommended total abstinence from spirits for these practical reasons (Levine 1978, 145–147; Fehlandt 1904, 19–22; Krout 1925, 64–66; Rorabaugh 1979, 35–37).

A few years later in 1785, response to the perceived increase in drunkenness resulted in a tract by another Quaker and the "Father of American Medicine," Benjamin Rush. *His Inquiry into the Effects of Ardent Spirits on the Human Body and Mind* (1812) suggested that "ardent spirits" could have negative health and social consequences. Rush censured distilled spirits but saw merit in the beneficial effects of fermented beverages, such as hard cider, wine, and beers. Later temperance leaders acknowledged their indebtedness to Rush by reprinting his tract as part of their moral suasion messages. However, the abstinence-from-spirits message was largely ignored by Americans (Levine 1978, 147–151; Fehlandt 1904, 19–35; Tyler 1944, 315).

Phases of the Temperance Movement

The mid-nineteenth-century temperance movement had several stages. Various authors have given different time spans for these stages.[4] The evolution of the temperance movement can also be classified by the typical phases of health-reform cycles. These, as discussed, include complacency and the acceptance of drinking, moral suasion (social pressures against drinking), coercion (social sanctions to reduce or prevent drinking), and backlash (noncompliance or repeal of negative social sanctions).

Complacency Phase: Moderate Drinking and
Beginnings of Concern, 1810–1826

In the early nineteenth century, water supplies were often polluted, milk was inconsistently available, and coffee and tea were extremely expensive. Most Americans regarded alcohol as a necessary companion to every mood and season. Refusal to drink was considered a breach of social etiquette, particularly among males. However, a change in drinking patterns evolved, which began to alarm some Americans. Rather than drinking small amounts frequently throughout the day or occasional overindulgence leading to intoxication with companions, an increase in solitary bouts of "spree" drinking emerged. This pattern led to the disintegration of the family. Concern about this change led to the beginnings of a temperance movement in local communities. The first temperance groups were local organizations associated with churches or benevolent societies in upstate New York and

New England, and lasted only a few years. These societies accepted temperance—moderate drinking—but had little influence outside their geographic area (Blocker 1989, 9–11; Rorabaugh 1979, 19–21, 150, 163, 169, 189; Tyrrell 1979, 34–36; Rohrer 1990, 229; Krout 1925, 77–78).[5]

In 1810, a number of evangelical Calvinist ministers associated with a new Andover seminary in Massachusetts began to meet and write articles concerned with abstinence from spirits, to be used by their clergymen for sermons. Many of their members joined with the Massachusetts Society for the Suppression of Intemperance (MSSI), formed in 1812, to combat drunkenness. The MSSI was spearheaded by more liberal Congregational and Unitarian clergy. It enjoined employers not to furnish ardent spirit to their laborers. Moderation, rather than abstention, was advocated. This elitist society reached its peak of influence in 1818, but by 1820 the organization had virtually ceased to operate, leaving no significant mark upon later temperance development (Tyrrell 1979, 33–42; Blocker 1989, 11–12; Fehlandt 1904, 39–45). Concurrent with this more urban organization, abstinence-oriented sentiment began to develop in churches in rural eastern and western frontier communities. The association of ministers of Litchfield, Connecticut, voted in 1812 to exclude ardent spirits from meetings and to discourage parishioners from consuming liquor, after evangelist Lyman Beecher admonished the group. On the western frontier, the Bethany Tract Society, formed in Livingston County, Kentucky, in 1817, required its members to abstain from ardent spirits and to encourage others to do so (Cherrington 1920, 72–78; Rohrer 1990, 229, 233–235).[6]

These first temperance societies, both in urban and rural areas, had little effect outside their regions. Their appeal to abstinence through speeches and pamphlets brought little public response. In fact, alcohol consumption increased during this period and did not begin to decrease until after 1830.[7] Although many of these early groups dissipated, some of their evangelical methods, such as the public pledge, public meetings, and tract distribution, were adopted by national organizations, such as the American Temperance Society (ATS), in the next phase of the temperance movement (Rohrer 1990, 234–235; Krout 1925, 113–114).

Moral Suasion Phase: Promoting Abstinence from
Ardent Spirits, 1826–1840

The temperance movement began to evolve rapidly during the 1820s and 1830s as it became popularized among the middle classes. The moral-suasion (social pressure and education) aspect of the cycle began to be seen on a more national level, rather than predominantly among small local or state groups. As aristocratic dominance gave way, the more evangelical middle class began to hold sway. Out of the second Great Awakening, abstinence became a necessary part of conversion and salvation rather than mere personal choice. Intemperance began to be seen as an enemy of organized religion, spawned by Satan and viewed as sinful. The "drunkard was beyond the reach of God's saving grace," and the nondrinking man a model of community respectability (Gusfield 1986, 44–45; Krout 1925, 114–115).[8]

The Clergy's Role in a Campaign for Abstinence from Ardent Spirits. One of the most influential clergy to push for abstinence from spirits was Lyman Beecher. Beecher (1775–1863), born in Guilford, Connecticut, studied at Yale University, where he was ordained a Presbyterian minister. He became concerned with the "evils arising from the use of liquor among the clergy" and preached six sermons against intemperance before his Litchfield, Connecticut congregation in 1825. These sermons, published the next year for general circulation (Beecher 1846), became widely read. They condemned daily use of spirits, recommended formation of voluntary associations pledged to total abstinence from spirits, and advised all denominations to condemn the liquor traffic (Krout 1925, 105–108; Daniels 1878, 62–90).

The first response to Beecher's powerful appeal came from Massachusetts. In 1826, the American Society for the Promotion of Temperance, better known as the American Temperance Society, was founded in Boston by several evangelical ministers. The ATS took a stance on "total abstinence from the use of ardent spirits as a beverage." Beecher's position, by implication, supported moderate use of wine and beer. The society adopted techniques from the revivalist movement and made direct appeals to the masses. Its ambitious clergy began a national crusade for total abstinence from spirits and the shutting down of distilleries and taverns. Itinerant agents were sent out, in a manner similar to revivalists, to organize societies and preach against intemperance (Blocker 1989, 12–19; Krout 1925, 108–112). Under the influence of the ATS, several thousand affiliates were organized in most states by 1833 (Cherrington 1920, 111). Societies in some of the larger communities began to publish temperance almanacs, which not only suggested the best planting and harvesting dates, but also offered information regarding temperance issues. For example in 1833, the New Haven, Connecticut, *Temperance Almanac*, published the "eight signs of a hard drinker" and symptoms of intemperance. This was similar to "signs of a drug user" in antidrug publications of the late twentieth-century Clean Living Movement.

The Push for "Teetotalism" or Abstinence from All Alcohol. In 1834, some temperance literature began to suggest abstinence from wine in addition to ardent spirits. Between 1835 and the early 1840s, the temperance movement went from a stand of abstinence from liquor to total abstinence from all alcoholic beverages. Only pure water was recommended for drinking, and temperance advocates became known as the "pure-water army."[9] Critics began to decry alcohol as the root of most physical and social problems. During this time period, Beecher and other reformers worked to eliminate the notion that moderate drinking was acceptable. In 1836, a large faction of temperance reformers pressed the American Temperance Union, which had formed out of the ATS, to adopt a "teetotal" pledge, binding signers to abstain from *any* alcohol, including beer, hard cider, and wine. This teetotalism stance caused resistance from more moderate members and affiliates, resulting in conflicts among various factions of the movement (Cherrington 1920, 119; Blocker 1989, 23–24). Gerrit Smith, an abolitionist, suggested, based upon new knowledge in the nineteenth century, that the biblical view of wine was now rendered obsolete. This was curiously similar to the position of some antialcohol advocates in the late twentieth-century movement, who argued that if alcohol had just recently been discovered, it would be illegal because of its potential danger (Engs 1991a, 26).

Some Americans did not agree with the reformers' point of view or remained opposed to the movement. Although there were temperance societies in the South, as the movement became more and more linked with abolition the Southern groups pursued independent courses. Immigrant groups, such as Germans and particularly Irish Catholics, for whom drinking was an essential part of their culture, were hostile to the movement.[10] The increasing importance of immigrants in the liquor business, which reflected the declining status of the trade brought about by two decades of temperance agitation among "respectable native born" classes, caused prohibition agitation to emerge by the late 1840s (Blocker 1989, 46–47; Tyrrell 1979, 297–299, 321).

Washingtonians. In 1840, a group of working-class Baltimoreans, influenced by the distress of the depression of 1837–1842, formed the Washington Temperance Society. This group strove primarily to reach drunkards and campaigned against the consumption of any alcoholic beverage. The group also recruited women and children as members and stressed alcohol's role in destroying families. With the formation of this society, the Temperance Movement became more democratized and nonsectarian. The nonsectarian Washingtonians engaged in emotionalism and public confession, and conducted festivals, dramas, and songs to recruit members, as described by the 1842 *Temperance Almanac of the Massachusetts Temperance Union*. They gave testimony to their own careers as drunkards and demanded similar confessions from those who attended their gatherings, an emotionally charged practice older temperance reformers found vulgar. Despite their flair for entertainment, the Washingtonians only lasted a few years due to the fact that once the pledge was taken there was little else to offer. In its wake, during the mid-1840s, many other nonsectarian abstinence organizations were established with similar formats (Daniels 1878, 95–98; Walters 1978, 131–132; Blocker 1989, 39–48). Symbolic of the democratization of temperance was the fact that the newer Washingtonians were dominated by lay Methodists and Baptists. This contrasted with older temperance societies that had been controlled by upper-middle-class Presbyterian and Congregational clergy (Tyrrell 1982, 135).

Coercive Phase: Legislation to Prevent All Alcohol
Sales and Consumption, 1840–1860

The primary political effect of the Temperance Movement from the late 1830s to late 1840s was agitation for more social and legal sanctions against alcohol on the state level. These activities reflected the beginning of the coercive phase of the movement. In 1837, Massachusetts gave counties the right to refuse the issuance of liquor licenses. Tennessee made retail sale of ardent spirits an offense punishable by fine. In the next two years, four states passed local-option laws regarding dispensing of liquor licenses. However, in the 1840s some of these laws were repealed (Cherrington 1920, 119–124).

Closely connected to the temperance movement was a growing hostility to German and Irish immigrants among Nativists (native-born Americans of Protestant stock) who made up the bulk of temperance leaders and members (see Chapter 9). Riotous "tippling" among the foreign-born in many communities was seen as mocking the reformers' social values. The Nativists, in reaction, began to enact laws to eradicate public drinking and disorderly behavior, including laws to prevent the sale and distribution of alcohol (Tyrrell 1979, 297–300; Gienapp 1987, 45, 97–98). Maine was the first state in the union to adopt statewide prohibition. As early as 1837, Neil Dow, a respected prosperous merchant who later became Portland's mayor, was a leader in temperance reform. He organized the Maine Temperance Union, which was based on total abstinence. Dow was author of what became known as the "Maine law" in 1846 to control alcohol distribution. In 1851, it was amended "so as to confiscate all liquors stored for sale by private parties," and the sale of all alcoholic beverages was prohibited, as were "drinking-houses and tippling-shops." Fines and imprisonment were levied for breaking the law, and "the liquor business" was outlawed (Daniels 1878, 20, 21–22).

Modeled after the Maine law, twelve other states north of the Mason–Dixon line passed restrictive laws concerning the sale of spirits during the 1850s. However, opposition was prevalent everywhere, making enforcement difficult. By the Civil War, most states had repealed such laws, and the temperance movement subsided in the late 1850s, the backlash phase of the movement. State prohibition experiments did not occur again until the 1880s, during the inception of the second Clean Living Movement.

TOBACCO AND OTHER STIMULANTS

Besides alcohol, substances such as tobacco, tea, and coffee were considered harmful in awakening "evil traits." Men were considered to become debilitated by alcohol and tobacco, and women were believed injured by coffee and tea. Along with temperance reform, antitobacco sentiment arose during the first Clean Living Movement. However, antitobacco agitation did not reach a coercive stage in which prohibition measures were enacted, as was the case during the latter two Clean Living Movements. Most reformers in the antebellum period who spoke out against alcohol simultaneously attacked tobacco and other substances.

Tobacco

Tobacco has always been part of American cultures. It was smoked in pipes by Native Americans for medical and ceremonial purposes and introduced by European explorers around the world at the beginning of the sixteenth century. Even though tobacco use ran into opposition and some Old World cultures prohibited it, its consumption increased. Early colonists, including women and children, smoked tobacco in clay pipes. During the mid-eighteenth century, snuff became popular among the wealthy. In the early nineteenth century, there was a decline in use of snuff and tea, as chewing tobacco and coffee replaced these primarily British habits (Robert 1949, 99–104; Fairholt 1859, 13–42).

Use in the Antebellum Era

Chewing became the dominant form of tobacco use during the first half of the nineteenth century. Unlike snuff and pipe smoking, chewing originated among mid-nineteenth-century Americans. It was symbolic of the rise of the common man, inasmuch as the habit had originally been found among laborers and sailors. However, Europeans considered chewing to be a particularly disgusting American form of tobacco vice. Although few women used tobacco in this era, those who did preferred snuff (Robert 1949, 102–103; Gibbons 1865, 31; Shew 1855, 7–13).

Cigars formed the bridge between the calumet and clay pipes of colonial times and the twentieth-century briar pipe and cigarette. Imported "Spanish" or "Havana" *segars* came to the republic under John Quincy Adams's presidency in the mid-1820s. Tobacco consumption increased in the late 1840s when the cigar was popularized during the Mexican–American War. The gold rush and the prosperous early 1850s also increased tobacco use. Cigar consumption continued to increase over the nineteenth century, reaching a peak in 1920 (Heimann 1960, 91–92; Robert 1949, 91–95, 101).

Russell Trall (1855, 4–5), a hydropathic physician, commented that by the mid-1840s in some urban areas children were smoking cigars and women had begun to smoke cigarettes, which were considered more feminine than cigars. By the early 1850s, most saloons, eating houses, public places, and public conveyances such as stages and railroad cars were filled with the smoke or spittle of the "all-pervading narcotic." Trall, similar to reformers of the last two decades of the twentieth century, considered this situation a serious health menace.

Antitobacco Movement, 1830–1860

In colonial Massachusetts, few laws were enacted against tobacco. In 1798, Benjamin Rush, the Quaker physician concerned over the evils of tobacco, published "Observations Upon the Influence of the Habitual Use of Tobacco Upon Health, Morals and Property," as described by Robert (1949, 106–107). Rush considered tobacco an expensive habit that led to idleness, uncleanliness, poor manners, and intemperance. However, antitobacco agitation did not begin until the 1830s, when it arose in tandem with the antiliquor crusade in the aftermath of the second Great Awakening (Robert 1949, 106–107; Baldwin 1855, 15–16).

From the 1830s until the Civil War, health reformers operated on the thesis that tobacco was a deadly poison. In an effort to encourage individuals to quit, or not start its use, reformers portrayed the disgusting figures of tobacco chewers as intemperate, physically ill, and morally depraved. In 1849, as the result of reformers' increasing concern over tobacco, and in conscious imitation of temperance efforts, the American Anti-tobacco Society was organized (Alcott 1835, 183–185; Trall 1855, 10–20; Numbers 1976, 40).

Many reformers and physicians of the day discussed the health consequences of tobacco. Edward Hitchcock (1830, 314), of Amherst College, considered tobacco and alcohol to be dangerous substances even when used moderately; he believed they caused moral deterioration and inherited weakness. Alcott (1835, 183–185) regarded the use of tobacco as evil for similar reasons. Caleb Ticknor (1972, 110–111), a physician, deemed tobacco "the most deadly, most noxious poison," and considered it addictive. Larkin Coles (1855, 7, 58, 64, 88), a Seventh-Day Adventist minister and physician, suggested tobacco did far more damage than alcohol to the health and welfare of Americans. Joel Shew (1855, 6–13), a hydropathic physician, published a tract listing eighty-seven diseases caused by tobacco, the first being insanity and the last cancer. He considered chewing to be the most harmful form of intake.

Like the gateway theory of drugs during the late twentieth-century movement, in which the use of tobacco was claimed to lead to marijuana, alcohol, and "harder drugs," tobacco use was implicated in the first movement as leading to intemperance and other immoral behaviors. This was also found in the second movement. It was suggested that "while the use of tobacco continues, intemperance will continue to curse the world" (Baldwin 1855, 14–15). Catherine Beecher (1856, 182) suggested that "tobacco destroys more than alcohol, because so many more use it, and so many are led to opium and alcohol by its influence" (see also Robert 1949, 107–111).

The antitobacco movement, like most other health-reform issues of the first Clean Living era, waned by the beginning of the Civil War.[11] During and immediately after the war there was an increase in tobacco use, from smoking cigars and newly introduced cigarettes (Robert 1949, 112; Fiske 1869, 8).

Other Stimulants

Tea and coffee were important parts of the diet and social activity of more affluent early Americans. However, reformers from the 1830s through the 1850s considered these substances to increase sexual appetites, retard digestion, and drain the "vital energy," leading to poor health or earlier death. The September 1829 *Journal of Health* considered coffee too stimulating and advised the "feeble, nervous, dyspepsia and others prone to weakness" to avoid it, along with chocolate. Cooking spices or condiments such as mustard, vinegar, ginger, cloves, cinnamon, and Native-American red peppers were also thought to stimulate the appetite to an unnatural degree. Salt was considered particularly onerous by some reformers (Graham 1837, 57–58; 1839, 352, 611–616; Alcott 1833, 52–55; Fowler 1841, 36–37; Beecher 1856, 97; Trall 1854, 47).

Not all health advocates of the day condemned coffee, tea, or spices. In 1836, Ticknor (1972, 106) suggested, "Those, therefore, who class tea and coffee, in their effects, with ardent spirits, are hurried away by a mistaken, though well meant zeal; and it becomes them to pause in their course, and consider whether or not their notions are incompatible with every day's observation, and the dictates of common sense." Except for a few newly formed religious groups at the time, such as the Mormons and Seventh-Day Adventists, these admonishments against the use of stimulants were largely ignored. Over the past 150 years, spices, in particular, have become integrated into the diet by various immigrant groups, which in turn has led to "American" foods such as pizza, hot dogs, and chow mein.

Opium and Patent Medicines

Cultivation of the opium poppy has been traced back to the Middle East during the fourth millennium B.C. The main method of taking opium, from antiquity until the late nineteenth century in the west, was to mix it with wine or other alcoholic beverages. This mixture, *laudanum*, was used for medicinal purposes. Most individuals who became addicted to opium did so through medical use, either prescribed by "regular" physicians (as opposed to botanic ones) or from patent medicines (Booth 1996, 15, 26, 51; Courtwright 1982a, 42–43).

Admonishments Against Abuse of Medical Opiate Use

In the first decade of the nineteenth century, one physician, Shadrach Ricketson (1806, 274–275), suggested that opium could be abused, and warned against its overuse in medicines. However, his advice was largely ignored. Over the first third of the nineteenth century an increase in the use of opium in patent medicines emerged. These cures were proffered without specific information as to their composition. Many contained opium in sufficient quantities to establish dependency in a short time if used regularly. Most of these nostrums were used for coughs, dysentery, diarrhea, upper respiratory infections, and cardiovascular and pulmonary diseases, especially tuberculosis. Mothers and nurses also increasingly used opium to hush crying infants, and it was widely used to relieve symptoms in the cholera epidemics of 1832 and 1847. There was an increase in addiction due to these uses which generated new concern over opiate abuse. By 1830, the premise that opiates were harmless began to be increasingly challenged by health reformers (Courtwright 1982a, 41–49; Booth 1996, 63; Dai 1937, 34).

Recreational Use of Opium

Taking opium for pleasure was considered a quaint pastime or an eccentric vice in the late eighteenth century, and it was not until the early nineteenth century that the euphoric use of opium became increasingly popular among European romantic writers. A primary influence in the increased recreational use of opiates was an 1821 work by Thomas De Quincy, a British author, called *Confessions of an English*

Opium-Eater. In the United States, opium was used by Edgar Allen Poe and other intellectuals, but it was not considered a problem among the general population. Around 1832, high-society ladies began to take opiates to steady nerves and enhance their wit (Booth 1996, 34–49; Dai 1937, 33–34; Courtwright 1982a, 41).

The social dangers of opium were not addressed until the early 1850s. Nathan Allen (1853, 32–35, 71), a physician, discussed the opium trade in China and argued that it was "a great curse destroying property, health and morals, and consigning the soul to eternal death." Opium began to be seen as extremely addictive and was considered ten times worse than ardent spirits. In the mid-1850s, the development of the hypodermic needle increased the use of morphine, particularly after the Civil War, when opium addiction became known as the "soldier's" or "army disease" as a result of its use by both armies to alleviate pain and dysentery (Dai 1937, 35; Booth 1996, 73).[12] However, there was no organized crusade against opium or its use in patent medicines in the first Clean Living Movement. Agitation against it died with most other health aspects of this antebellum era.

WOMEN'S RIGHTS AND HEALTH REFORM

The women's rights movement was intimately entwined with temperance and health-reform agitation. It began to bud during the end of the first Clean Living Movement, and blossomed during the second movement with the passing of both women's suffrage and the Eighteenth Amendment. Much has been written about the women's rights movement in the Jacksonian era; therefore, it will only be briefly mentioned as it relates to health-related reforms during the first Clean Living Movement.

Nineteenth-century women were subjected to drunken husbands, ill health, and tight corsets. Middle-class women were often seen as sickly, dependent, and ornamental. Like abolition, which became a means for the elimination of slavery, the temperance and health-reform movement became a means to advance women. The changing socioeconomic order at the end of the eighteenth century resulted in a decline of domestic industry and agriculture. A woman's prime responsibility in life began to be seen as being a good wife and mother and the moral and spiritual fountainhead of the family. Several authors have suggested that this "cult of domesticity" confined them to the home and church and to subjection by their fathers and husbands. Middle-class women, however, began to see slavery in the South as a metaphor for their own plight and desire for greater freedom (Morantz 1977, 78–79; Tyrrell 1982, 129–131; Epstein 1981, 69, 73–82; Walters 1978, 104–106).

Women and Temperance

Women were inconspicuous but deeply involved in temperance agitation from the time of the American Temperance Society crusades of 1826–1836, when they formed a number of local ladies temperance groups. Temperance was a critical link between traditional religious and charitable work of women in church and secular reform. Women also participated in male-led societies and comprised from 35 to 60 percent of these groups in the 1830s. Within the movement, their prime responsibility was to exert positive moral influence in the home and social settings. It was the daughters of these temperance workers who formed the Women's Christian Temperance Union in the next generation (Tyrrell 1982, 128–133; Dannenbaum 1981, 236–237).

Some women between 1835 and 1840 actively joined campaigns to refuse licenses to retailers in northeastern states and became more militant. Many became involved in the Washingtonian societies—which developed auxiliaries for women called Martha Washingtonian societies—and undertook to provide food and used clothing for reformed inebriates and their families. However, when temperance agitation shifted from moral suasion to prohibition in the late 1840s, women began to lose their role in the movement and felt useless and powerless. Since they generally were not allowed to speak publicly or take leadership roles, they began to form their own temperance organizations and started to advocate for the rights of women to speak publicly, have control over their property, and vote (Bordin 1981, 4–5; Dannenbaum 1981, 238–240; Tyrrell 1982, 134, 144–145; Walters 1978, 107–108).

By the late 1840s, a close link developed between women's rights and female temperance activism. Several leaders of the first women's right convention at Seneca Falls, New York, in 1848, including Amelia Bloomer, Elizabeth Cady Stanton, and Susan B. Anthony, had been active in both the temperance and abolition movements during the 1840s. Other women, including Mary Gove Nichols and Lydia Folger Fowler, not only were involved with temperance, but also began to lecture on female physiology and became involved with health reform (Morantz 1977, 73; Dannenbaum 1981, 238–240; Tyrrell 1982, 146; Walters 1978, 105–107).

Women and Health Reform

Women health reformers, like their male counterparts, were concerned about the health of women in their traditional roles as wives and mothers. This concern spread beyond the family, because health reformers shared a widespread belief in the inheritance of acquired traits that could lead to further "degeneration" of the human race (see

Chapter 5). Victorian modesty prevented many women from going to male physicians for gynecological problems or attending lectures presented by males who discussed female anatomy and physiology. The desire for female physicians and lecturers was a major force that pushed women into the health movement. In addition, regular physicians, as opposed to botanic and alternative practitioners (discussed in Chapter 5) were not effective in treating most "female" and other illnesses, while specific treatments, such as hydrotherapy, were found helpful. Health reform contributed to women's rights, because many women who became involved in various self-help, prevention, and alternative-cure aspects of the first Clean Living Movement became healthier. Their improved lot, in turn, led women to assume more authority within the family and engage in more activities outside the home (Whorton 1982, 105–107; Morantz 1977, 86–90).

Women Health Reformers

Women health reformers were prominent during this era. Three symbolized the linking of various health reforms. Mary Sargent Gove Nichols (1810–1884) symbolized the link between "Grahamism" and hydrotherapy. She lectured in female physiology, and opened a vegetarian boarding school and a hydrotherapy training center. Lydia Folger Fowler (1822–1879) represented the link between temperance, health reform, and women's rights. She lectured on phrenology and female hygiene, and became the first woman to hold a medical professorship. Elizabeth Blackwell (1821–1910), born in England, was the first woman to receive a medical degree in the United States. She expounded on the laws of health and strongly advocated exercise and a proper diet. Her writings also reflected the sentiments of the developing hereditarian (later called eugenic) reform movement (Whorton 1982, 107–108, 121; Lender 1984, 178; Blackwell 1852, 33).

Other female reformers, including Marie Louise Shew, wife of the editor of the *Water Cure Journal*, a popular health-reform publication, also lectured widely in New England and the West. The women health reformers instructed other women, through lectures and publications, in how to avoid illness by obeying the "laws of health" and physiology, which included proper diet, cleanliness, and exercise. Catharine Beecher in particular pushed for greater opportunities in physical education and sport as a primary means of increasing the health of women (Morantz 1977, 75–78; Vertinsky 1979, 38–49).

Self-help and the prevention of disease among both men and women became a moral imperative to reformers (see Chapter 4). About one-fourth of the members of the American Physiology Society, founded by Sylvester Graham and William Alcott in 1837, were women. The society advocated holistic reforms, including clothing, exercise, fresh air, diet, and temperance. In addition, it promoted women as lecturers. Most important, health reform offered countless women a means of coping with an undependable environment amid rapidly changing antebellum America. The movement generated journals and domestic tracts that offered friendly advice to women in remote areas. Lectures, study groups, and water-cure centers became means for women to discontinue their isolation. A sense of sisterhood developed from these activities, as suggested by frequent use of the term in various writings of the era (Morantz 1977, 77–81; Numbers 1976, 57–58).

Dress Reform

Dress reform became a principal element in health reform for women. Health advocates, including regular and alternative physicians and other reformers, condemned women's dress. The fashion of the early and mid-nineteenth century included tight corsets, which prevented physical movement and damaged internal organs, and long, heavy skirts with many petticoats, which dragged on garbage-strewn and muddy streets. In addition, these outfits were believed to cause weakness and debility in women, which, in turn, could be transmitted to the next generation (Morantz 1977, 82; Numbers 1976, 132–133; Kesselman 1991, 497).

The dress-reform movement emerged from the interaction of three movements: the Oneida Community, health-reform, and the women's rights movements. The first women to become involved with dress reform were the women of the Oneida Community (see Chapter 6), who began to wear an outfit that consisted of knee-length skirts and pantaloons around 1849. In 1850, Elizabeth Smith Miller, daughter of abolitionist Gerrit Smith, who lived near the Oneida Community, visited her cousin Elizabeth Cady Stanton in Seneca Falls, New York, wearing the outfit. Stanton started wearing the costume, and, in response, her neighbor and friend, Amelia Bloomer, soon decided to "lay aside her fetters and don the freedom suit" and began advocating dress reform in her temperance and women's rights magazine, the *Lily* (Numbers 1976, 132–133; Robertson 1970, 274; Kesselman 1991, 496–498).

Amelia Jenks Bloomer

Amelia Jenks Bloomer (1818–1894), born in Homer, New York, was both a temperance leader and women's rights activist. After marrying Dexter Bloomer, she settled in Seneca Falls and began publishing the

Lily in 1849. This tract increasingly discussed women's rights, marriage laws, and dress reform. Because she popularized the outfit, the press began calling it the "bloomer" costume. Bloomer, like many other women's rights advocates, wore this reform dress and it became associated with the women's rights movement (Whitman 1985, 89–91).

In 1850, the year Bloomer began to champion the reform dress, the hydropathic *Water Cure Journal* began calling for a simpler women's costume compatible with exercise in the open air and physical labor. The "American costume," also a knee-length skirt and pants, began to be worn at hydrotherapy centers. It was developed by Harriot Austin, cofounder of the water-cure center in Danville, New York. Some women at these centers also cut their hair short to facilitate easy drying due to their frequent bathing (Numbers 1976, 133; Kesselman 1991, 497–498).

The National Dress Reform Association was formed in 1851 to advocate more practical and comfortable dress for women to free them from the "slavery" of confining costumes. Because of negative reactions the outfit elicited from the public, many feminists began thinking that the outfit took away from the important messages of woman suffrage and temperance. After a decade, most feminists abandoned the outfit (Kesselman 1991, 495, 506). By the 1860s, dress reformers had become isolated, not only from the organized women's rights movement but also from much of the water-cure community as well. As a result, the push for dress reform faded. However, more practical shorter skirts that did not drag on the ground and less lacing were adopted by pioneer women in the westward expansion, including Mormons and Seventh-Day Adventists, whose leaders had been influenced by the health movement (Kesselman 1991, 495, 506; Numbers 1976, 131–134; Underwood 1986, 50).

SUMMARY

In summary, a feature of the first Clean Living Movement was the intertwining of temperance with other health-reform crusades. Temperance appears to have predated many other issues and, in its wake, concerns about tobacco, patent medicines, and narcotics arose. Temperance spawned concerns for women's rights, including the right to wear healthier clothing and improved physiological health (to be discussed in the next chapter). The lasting legacy of the temperance movement was an overall decrease in alcohol consumption and the beginning of concern for women's health and other social problems. The overlapping of temperance activism and other submovements in the overall health-reform era was echoed in subsequent health-reform cycles. By the time of the Civil War, the temperance and other movements had begun to wane.

NOTES

1. For detailed information concerning the origins of drinking patterns and attitudes in antiquity and the lingering norm of these ancient cultures in modern times, see Engs (1995, 2000).

2. Hundreds of works have discussed the antialcohol (temperance, anti-saloon, prohibition, anti–drunk driving, minimum drinking age laws, etc.) social movements in the United States over the past 200 years. Selected secondary sources for this chapter include contemporary works by Blocker (1989), Gusfield (1986), Lender (1984), Lender and Martin (1987), Levine (1978), Musto (1996), Nissenbaum (1980), Pittman and Snyder (1962), Rorabaugh (1979), Rumbarger (1989), and Tyrrell (1979), and earlier works by Cherrington (1920), Daniels (1878), Fehlandt (1904), and Krout (1925).

3. The term "temperance" was coined early in the 1820s to denote moderate use of alcohol. As the movement developed, by the late 1840s it came to mean total abstinence from all fermented beverages. Throughout most of the twentieth century, temperance has generally been used synonymously with no drinking or prohibition in the United States.

4. Authors over the years have given different time spans for different temperance-related activities. August Fehlandt (1904, 11–12), writing from the perspective of the growing prohibition movement at the turn of the twentieth century, divided the temperance movement into four periods: moderation, 1785–1826; abstinence from ardent spirits, 1826–1836; teetotalism, 1836–1851; and outright prohibition, 1851–1856. Ernest Cherrington (1920), following the implementation of national prohibition, suggested that the first stage of the movement, "moderation," began around 1810 with the advent of some local temperance societies. In contrast, Ian Tyrrell (1982, 129), writing at the beginning of the current third movement, suggested three stages of the temperance movement: the "evangelical" period, from 1826 to 1840; "popularization" through the Washingtonians and other self-help groups during the 1840s; and the "political and prohibitionist campaigns" of the 1850s. These authors, however, primarily focused on the reform aspect of the movement and did not mention backlash eras.

5. Several authors over the past century have discussed reasons for the development of this temperance movement. Krout (1925), immediately after passage of national Prohibition, suggested that the movement was merely one of the many early nineteenth-century reforms arising from rapid social change, as did Walters (1978) at the beginning of the late twentieth-century movement. Gusfield (1962) argued that the movement emerged because the "old order" felt threatened by the rise of the common man. Tyrrell (1979) also accepts this idea and, along with Blocker (1989), implied that it was a reaction of the middle class to serious social problems related to drinking. Rorabaugh (1979) and Lender and Martin (1987) have inferred that the temperance movement, beside being a reaction to profound cultural changes, was also due to concerns about problems caused by increased intemperance. Rohrer (1990) has argued that the origins of the temperance movement lay in a search for perfection among lower-class evangelicals.

6. Cherrington (1920, 71–73) suggested that other church denominations made resolutions against intemperance and "strong drink" during this decade. These included the Eastern Conference of the United Brethren Church and the General Convention of the Universalist Church in 1814, and the African Methodist Church in 1816.

7. Rorabaugh (1979, 232) calculated per capita consumption of all beverages to be about 3.9 gallons in 1830. For spirits alone, the *Temperance Almanac of the Massachusetts Temperance Union* of 1834 suggested "5 gallons each for every man, woman, and child."

8. "Drunkard," "inebriate," or "intemperate" were the terms used in this era for what we would now call "alcoholics" or "problem drinkers." "Tippling" is overdrinking to intoxication.

9. See the New York *Temperance Almanac* for 1836 and 1838, and the *Temperance Almanac of the Massachusetts Temperance Union* for 1841, 1844, and 1845 for articles which demonstrate the evolution of sentiments from temperance to abstinence.

10. Some Irish Catholic immigrants became involved with the movement. Temperance publications by 1841 had begun to discuss the work of Father Theobald Mathews of Ireland, who came to the United States in 1849 for a "pledge signing tour" to encourage abstinence among his countrymen. During his tour, he administered the pledge to about 600,000 Irish–Americans, as noted in the 1841 *Temperance Almanac of the Massachusetts Temperance Union*. Although some Nativist groups were suspicious of his motives, the tremendous political power of the temperance movement was suggested by the fact that Mathews was invited by President Tyler to speak in Congress. By that point in American history, the only other foreigner who had received the same honor was Lafayette (Cherrington 1920, 132; Lender 1984, 32; Tyrrell 1979, 299).

11. During the 1860s, antitobacco essays were written by some individuals, including John Griscom, a public-health reformer, and Henry Gibbons, a medical professor, who based their writings upon earlier health reformers' writings. Griscom (1868, 15, 35) discussed cancer, insanity, and other health problems, including "opium-eating" resulting from tobacco use. Gibbons (1865, 18–20) suggested that the use of tobacco was a violation of "the laws of health," a sin against users' "progeny," and a cause of insanity, based upon the 1843 annual report of the Massachusetts General Hospital. However, there also was a satire of an antismoking essay by John Fiske (1869), a lawyer, entitled *Tobacco and Alcohol: It Does Pay to Smoke; the Coming Man Will Drink Wine*, which suggested that health reformers were perceived as a bit quaint and as "do-gooders" by many.

12. Dai (1937) points out that, beside the Civil War, after World War I there was a rise in morphine addicts. This was also true for the Vietnam War, when there was concern about opiate addiction from heroin in returning soldiers.

4

Christian Physiology, Diet, and Sexuality

> The millennium, the near approach of which is by many so confidently predicted, can never reasonably be expected to arrive, until those laws which God has implanted in the physical nature of man are, equally with his moral laws, universally known and obeyed.
> Third Annual Report,
> American Physiological Association (1839)

> The young man who has fallen into the habit of self-pollution will, almost of a certainty be found greatly attached to hot and exciting food and drink. He will not be apt to relish plain water, or·good bread and fruits,—I mean as a means of meeting and satisfying the natural demands of the system.
> William A. Alcott, *The Physiology of Marriage* (1972a)

> Health—The poor man's riches; the rich man's bliss.
> Masthead of *Journal of Health* (1829–1833)

Promotion of personal hygiene, vegetarian diets, and admonishments against some forms of sexuality emerged during this era. Health education became a moral crusade. This health reform campaign, called the "Christian physiology" or "body" reform movement, was a major component of the first Clean Living Movement. Although it was strongest in Boston and New York City, it had followers throughout New England and was national in scope.

THE CHRISTIAN PHYSIOLOGISTS

Many health reformers of the era became known as Christian physiologists because they turned health reform into a moral crusade and because they had strong religious beliefs. Reformers, such as Sylvester Graham, had generally been involved with the temperance movement subsequent to the physiological campaigns.[1] The whole movement was called the body-reform movement by Ronald Walters (1978, 146). Reformers believed that if the laws of health were not obeyed, then disease and debility followed as punishment. Leaders of physiological reform were convinced that they were part of the process by which God was restoring the purity of the "ancient order of things" and would bring the nation back to a "gilded age" of better health. Their aim was to make America a godly, sober, and healthy place (Hatch 1984, 121; Whorton 1975, 467).

The Progenitors of the First Clean Living Movement

The two most influential individuals during the first Clean Living Movement were Sylvester Graham and William A. Alcott. Graham and Alcott differed on a few minor points, but, they shared consensus on major ideas. Many of their suggestions were identical to the recommendations found in conventional medical literature. It was common sense to advise people not to overeat, for women not to wear tightly laced corsets, and for all to take exercise and fresh air daily. Both orthodox and botanic medical texts called for moderation in drinking and eating. What set the health reformers apart from other writers was a call for total abstinence from alcohol and other stimulants and reliance upon moral and biblical beliefs as the basis of scientific arguments for this abstinence. Alcott and Graham together turned health reform into a moral crusade (Whorton 1988, 61).

William Alcott

William Andrus Alcott (1798–1859), a Connecticut native and cousin of transcendentalist Bronson Alcott (father of Louisa May Alcott), became equally well known, and was a far more prolific writer than either relative during the nineteenth century. He began to teach school at age eighteen; however, declining health, probably tuberculosis, inspired him to read medical books and enter Yale Medical School. Although he established a practice, he soon left medicine after finding that abstinence from alcohol and a near-vegetarian diet helped restore him to health. Alcott began to write on educational subjects. In 1831, he moved to Boston to edit an educational magazine and a periodical for children. In 1834, Alcott (1844) first published as a book a series of his children's articles, called *The House I Live In*. This book was designed to provide physiological and anatomical information for youngsters. Alcott also wrote many advice and how-to manuals, including the popular, *The Young Man's Guide* (1833). He championed health instruction in schools and is considered one of the fathers of the school health program (Walters 1978, 152–153; Whorton 1982, 51–53; 1988, 57–59).

Much of Alcott's advice concerning exercise, diet, and tobacco would be considered acceptable today. However, at least by current standards, he would not be considered wholly enlightened in regard to personal hygiene and bathing. He wrote, "There are those who are so attentive to this subject as to wash their whole bodies in water, either cold or warm, every day of the year; and never to wear the same clothes, during the day, that they have slept in the previous night. . . . I consider this extreme" (Alcott 1833, 88).

Sylvester Graham

Although Alcott was well known for his lectures and many works, he was overshadowed by the person whose name became synonymous with "body reform" during the first Clean Living Movement, namely Sylvester Graham (1794–1851). "Grahamism" became synonymous with health reform among both followers and detractors alike. Even today he is the only health crusader of the era whose name is commonly known—through his Graham cracker. He was born in West Suffield, Connecticut, and, like a number of other reformers, was a sickly child. After some schooling and teaching, he entered the Presbyterian ministry in New Jersey in 1829, where he acquired a reputation as a powerful and successful evangelist, especially in addressing his favorite topic, temperance.[2]

In June 1830, Graham was engaged by the Pennsylvania Society for Discouraging the Use of Ardent Spirits to lecture for the Philadelphia Temperance Society. In reflecting about temperance, he realized that, besides alcohol, other voluntary habits could be just as destructive. He soon resigned from the society and started lecturing on his own about correct physiology, diet, and morality in a lecture, "The Science of Human Life" (Graham 1839, iii–iv). Graham gained a following among the educated and middle class in major eastern cities who were tired of heroic medicine and its purging, blistering, and bleeding. In addition to writing and lecturing, Graham and his followers opened boardinghouses in New York and other eastern cities in which cold baths, unbolted wheaten bread, vegetarian diets, hard beds, and exercise were required of all boarders. These boardinghouses became gathering places for various other reformers, including feminists, temperance workers, and abolitionists (Blake 1974, 41; Sokolow 1983, 144–153).

Graham's ideas were not new. They derived from the same basic medical doctrines to which both regular and botanic physicians of the day subscribed. What was new about Graham was the way he turned health reform into a moral crusade. As Grahamism began to be associated with the monomaniacal and ascetic personality of its founder, it lost adherents who were once sympathetic to its message. Graham became an extremist in all aspects of the body, including sexuality. His influence started to wane in 1838; but unlike Alcott, who wrote for much of his life, Graham went into a bitter retirement and died at a relatively early age (Blake 1974, 41; Sokolow 1983, 144–153).

Other Health Reformers

Besides Alcott and Graham, other physiological reformers proved to be influential during the first Clean Living Movement. Horace Mann (1796–1859) is best remembered as a champion of public schools during his tenure as secretary to the Massachusetts State Board of Education. He also was an eloquent spokesman on temperance and personal hygiene. Inspired by Alcott, he urged the state board in 1842 to require instruction in "physiology" in all the public schools, which became a reality in 1850 and is still a base of modern school health instruction (Numbers 1976, 58–59).

Another reformer, Edward Hitchcock, an Amherst College professor of chemistry, wrote the book *Dyspepsia Forestalled and Resisted* (1831) which offered advice on avoiding the "disease" of heartburn and lassitude. Besides the usual diet and temperance themes, he strongly promoted regular exercise. The transcendentalists, including Amos Bronson Alcott, Ralph Waldo Emerson, William Ellery Channing, Henry David Thoreau, and Margaret Fuller, were concerned with exercise, play, recreation, and other personal health issues. Like other health reformers of this era, these philosophers shared an abiding faith in the integrity and "perfectibility of man," believed the physical body provided the home for the spiritual body and needed proper care, and subscribed to "the laws of health" (Park 1977, 34–49).

The Influence of Texts and Journals on the Christian Physiologists

Health-promotion ideas advanced by reformers had been around before the 1820s. However, it was not until the second Great Awakening that it was turned into a moral crusade. The ideas for this reform movement were based upon many earlier works. Besides the popular reprints of John Wesley and Benjamin Rush, many physicians addressed personal hygiene and disease prevention in the early nineteenth century. These early works included those by Shadrach Ricketson (1806), James Thatcher (1826), and William Buchan (1838), and the translation of a work by the noted French physician François Broussais and Swiss physician Simon André Tissot (1832). Graham and Alcott may have been aware of the *Journal of Health* in the late 1820s and Samuel Thomson's botanic writings in the early 1820s. The medical texts, for the most part, presented a commonsense regime that nearly all readers could agree to in theory, if not always in practice. Moderation was the underlying theme of most authors.[3]

A typical text of the time was that of Ricketson, a New York physician. In his *Means of Preserving Health and Preventing Diseases* (1806, v), he discusses many of the health ideas promoted by the later reformers. These include advice about fresh air and climate, drink, food, sleep, cleanliness, exercise, and clothing. On the cover he states that the book was "designed not merely for physicians, but for the information of others." A prime goal of his book was to educate nonphysicians. James Thacher (1754–1844) expressed similar sentiments. He was particularly interested in fresh air and exercise and thought that "exercise should be ranked as among the most powerful agents which we can employ for the preservation of life and health" (Thacher 1826, 77).

In the area of sexuality, Simon André Tissot's (1728–1797) *Treatise on the Diseases Produced by Onanism*, was translated in 1832. In his opinion, the sexual vices of "whoring and adultery" could bring on diseases because of sexual excess. These included "the clap" (gonorrhea) and "the pox" (syphilis). Tissot expanded the idea of sexual excess to masturbation, suggesting that excess from the "secret vice" was equally powerful in causing disease. However, like many authors of the day, he relied on citing authorities rather than empirical evidence (Money 1985, 53–55).

At the peak of the physiological-reform movement, more moderate health writers similar to critics in the succeeding two health-reform cycles were not at all kind to the health activists. The physician Caleb Ticknor (1804–1840), in the preface to his *Philosophy of Living* (1972, iv), decried the fanaticism and "madness" of his time in regard to abstention from all alcohol and meat and consumption only of cold water and vegetables. Because of the extremism, he predicted a backlash against this rigid philosophy due to the "laws of nature." The decline of Grahamism about ten years later appeared to support his prediction.

Both Graham and Alcott, like some other reformers, were reluctant to give credit to their sources. Graham claimed that he developed his regime and philosophy on his own (Graham 1839, v). However, it is likely both reformers were acquainted with some of the works just mentioned, or similar works published during the first few decades of the nineteenth century. Graham's basic philosophy of "stimulation" is thought to be taken from François Broussais. Broussais suggested that all disease resulted from excessive stimulation of some body tissue, leading to irritation and inflammation. Stimulation in this era became a term loaded with physiological, moral, and sexual meaning (Graham 1837, 18; Sokolow 1983, 62–63; Nissenbaum 1980).

A means of popularizing health among the middle class was through the *Journal of Health*, first published in 1829 by "an association of Philadelphia physicians." Many articles were published that were similar to what Graham began to espouse.[4] However, the journal only lasted until 1833. This was likely due to the fact that the physician editors underestimated the increasing hostile reaction to orthodox medicine as botanic and alternative medicine began to gain a foothold among the American populace. This journal likely influenced various reformers of the day.

Health Reform Institutions Formed by Reformers

The American Physiology Association (APA), formed by Alcott, Graham, and early converts to body reform in 1837, existed for only three years. However, this organization influenced other aspects of the first Clean Living Movement. Its mission was a full-fledged crusade for radical reform. Its purpose was to acquire and diffuse practical information on human physiology to promote health and longevity. Leaders of the APA espoused the revivalist theme of the 1820s that God had united the human soul with the body and it was everyone's duty to study that structure in order to learn how to be healthy. It was considered a sin to ignore the body and the laws of health, on grounds that the millennium would not come until these laws were obeyed (Hambrick-Stowe 1996, 111; Blake 1974, 42–43).

The association organized the nation's first health-food store to supply Graham bread, fresh fruits, and vegetables grown in "virgin, unfertilized soil," and supported the establishment of physiological boarding-houses. When Grahamism began to diminish after 1840, some of the most enthusiastic Christian physiologists would not give up the cause. In 1850, the American Vegetarian Society was formed, with William Alcott as president. Other reformers of the day attended the society's annual meeting in 1853, included Amelia Bloomer and Susan B. Anthony (Fletcher 1943, 331; Greene 1986, 53; Whorton 1982, 59; 1988, 52).

DIET AND OTHER HEALTH ISSUES

The basic teachings of the Christian physiologists can be divided into six areas, including diet; abstinence from ardent spirits; abstinence from other stimulants such as coffee and tea; exercise and fresh air; clothing, bathing, and cleanliness; and sexuality. The morality of health-reform physiology is most evident in its pronouncements on diet and sex (Whorton 1988, 62).

Diet: Food, Spices, and Drink

The diet recommended by the Christian physiologists was similar to the "pyramid diet" introduced in the early 1990s at the peak of the most recent Clean Living Movement. This was primarily a vegetarian diet with little meat. In fact, Grahamism meant vegetarianism. The health reformers of the mid-nineteenth century were most agitated by the hazards of "flesh food." They considered meat to lead to stimulation of the stomach, which in turn led to disease, debility, and, by implication, excessive sex (Graham 1837, 18).

Graham and Alcott believed that anything that potentially harmed the body should be avoided in the diet. This included most meats, salt and salt pork, gravies, fried foods, butter, and pastries. Good cheese could be taken in small quantities. A proper diet, in their opinion, included wheat bread and other grains, vegetables, fruits, nuts, and perhaps an occasional custard made with eggs. Butter was especially objectionable. They believed meals should not be taken any more frequently than every six hours and never before retiring. Tea, coffee, wine, cider, beer, spices, and other stimulants, including tobacco, were forbidden because they were considered highly stimulating to the body. Only pure water, they believed, should be drunk, and all alcohol was forbidden. One of Graham's favorite themes was breadmaking. He considered coarse bread the mainstay of good health and believed it would cure both diarrhea and constipation (Graham 1837, 57–58; 1839, 616; Alcott 1833, 52–55).

Clothing, Sleep, Bathing and Cleanliness, Fresh Air, and Exercise

Graham considered clothing a necessary evil in cold climates. He suggested it should offer as little restriction as possible in order to free the body for unrestricted movement. Tight-fitting corsets, stays, or garters were frowned upon as being injurious to the body. In his opinion, clothing should be adequate but not too warm or tight. Dress, as discussed in Chapter 3, became a reform movement in itself as part of the feminist movement (*Defense* 1835, 190–191; Graham 1839, 637).

Seven hours of sleep a day, preferably from 10 P.M. to 5 A.M., was recommended. Fresh air and good ventilation of the bedroom, along with a hard bed, were also considered desirable for good sleep. Reformers eschewed feather beds—comforters—because they "retained impurities cast off by the skin" and led to diseases and room odors. Reformers recommended that bedding and nightclothes be aired daily. From a modern viewpoint, these materials likely retained dust mites, lice, and scabies because they were washed infrequently, thus leading to diseases. Alcott viewed early rising as a mark of industry and a boon to longevity. Each hour of sleep before midnight he judged to be worth two after that time (Alcott 1833, 39–45; Graham 1839, 623–625; *Defense* 1835, 185–187).

Reformers considered it essential to keep the skin clean and healthy so it could perform its function of ridding the body of impurities. Graham urged a daily sponge bath just after arising, followed by a brisk rubdown with a towel as coarse as the body could bear. Both Alcott and Graham deemed it best to bathe in cold water. Good grooming and clean clothing were considered components of healthful living (Alcott 1833, 72–73; *Defense* 1835, 190; Graham 1837, 629).

Both Graham and Alcott were concerned about the lack of fresh air in theaters and other areas crowded with people, and considered this a source of disease. Alcott was particularly concerned with overheated, underventilated schoolhouses, which he thought dulled children's minds and damaged their bodies. Fresh air and exercise also were seen as important to adults' good health. However, dancing in the evening was opposed on grounds that going out into the cold or damp night air predisposed the body to disorders and "mischief." Alcott viewed physical exercise for growing children as a way to improve society, out of the belief that strong and healthy children were more likely to become healthy adults (Alcott 1833, 171–174, 191–192; *Defense* 1835, 91, 181, 193).

Exercise also was promoted for girls and women. Catherine Beecher is credited with writing a book on calisthenics—a modification of French and English exercises—for young ladies in 1856. This marked the beginning of popular interest in calisthenics, first espoused for girls and ultimately both sexes. In the 1850s, when the exercise movement was accelerating, Elizabeth Blackwell published a tract, *Popular and Practical Science: The Laws of Life* (1852), specifically for women. She discussed the importance of exercise for women and the "laws of health" to prevent debility, disease, and "degeneracy of the race." She considered the first law of health to be the "law of exercise" and considered this the foundation of good health. Like other reformers of the day, Blackwell considered the body to be the temple of the soul and in addressing both aspects favored "an education that allows . . . no antagonism or injury to either." Like her male predecessors, Blackwell believed neglect of these laws leads to disease and debility (Blackwell 1852, 34, 38, 47, 155; Greene 1986, 91).

As Grahamism and temperance sentiments declined, enthusiasm for physical activity increased. Physical fitness, along with eugenics, were two movements that gained momentum near the end of the first movement and culminated in the second (Numbers 1976, 59).[5]

SEXUALITY

A strong undercurrent in the first Clean Living Movement was deep concern about "animal passions," or sexuality. Fear of animal passions underlies the health reformer's promotion of abstinence and restraint in many areas of life. To the body reformers, it made perfect physiological sense that stimulations fraught with danger for the soul could be equally dangerous to the body. Thus, the health-reform regime was built around denial of any stimulation. As pointed out by Whorton (1988, 62), this philosophy was the antithesis of the "Playboy" philosophy, "If it feels good, do it." Anything stimulating should be avoided on grounds it stimulates sexual appetites, thus leading to debility.

Smith-Rosenberg (1980) suggested that restraint of sexual passions and promotion of sexual purity were initially a male reform movement manifested by fears of male sexuality. This is particularly found in Alcott's and Graham's works. Graham (1848), in his *A Lecture to Young Men on Chastity*, originally published in 1834, discussed three types of sexual activity: marital, pre- and extramarital, and masturbation. He explained how stimulation associated with each leads to avowed physical injury. These activities were placed on a hierarchy, with marital sex being the least injurious and masturbation the most, based on their degree of stimulation. Nissenbaum (1980, x, 4–9), in his work concerning Grahamism and sexuality, implied that Graham's work was different from older sex manuals because it was based on "scientific" and physiological, rather than biblical, argument. In addition, it focused upon the problems of masturbation and marital excess, rather than "fornication."

Marital Sex

Within marriage, Graham (1848, 78), in particular, thought there was a danger of sexual excess, which could cause disease and debility. He stated that the "mere fact that a man is married to one woman, and is perfectly faithful to her, will by no means prevent the evils which flow from venereal excesses." He went on to write that even in the marital bedchamber, sexual contact produces "the most intense excitement" and a "violent paroxysm" that racks the body with the "tremendous violence of a tornado" (pp. 49–50).[6]

Graham conceded that a certain amount of contact was necessary for procreation, but any more than once a month was considered pathological. Once a month was granted as permissible to the young and robust. Older and more "delicate" lovers would have to get by on less if they wished to maintain physiological health (Graham 1848, 82–83). Alcott (1972a, 118–119) also endorsed once-a-month sexual intercourse, but was a bit more lenient. He compared sex to eating and drinking: Gluttons in food and drink would not experience as much pleasure as a more temperate person who imbibed more moderately.

Women and Sexuality

The stereotypical view of women of this era was one of sexless passivity, piety, and domesticity. However, McCall's (1989, 1994) recent analysis of *Godey's Ladies Book*, a popular magazine for women from about 1830 to the Civil War, has not supported the twentieth-century stereotype of passive and sexless women during this era. Neither did 104 bestselling novels of the era. Male reformers of the first Clean Living Movement may have been instrumental in developing this myth. Until the beginning of the nineteenth century, sex was considered a natural and pleasurable activity for both men and women. Alcott (1972a, 118) displayed an ambivalence regarding women. Though he denied that normal women ordinarily felt sexual desire, his discussion of actual behavior indicated that women did, indeed, feel such desire at some times.

Fornication, Venereal Diseases, and Obscene Material

In Graham's hierarchy of sexual vices, the second most sinful depravity was sex outside the marriage bond, namely, fornication. Graham reasoned that the more immoral the activity, the more harmful it was to the body. Since illicit sex was more exciting because it was forbidden, it followed that it would cause more injury and disorders to the genital organs and the body as a whole. Alcott (1972a, 99, 207) considered fornication an utter sin. Contracting a venereal (sexually transmitted) disease out of wedlock was a "heaven appointed penalty" and "an almost direct punishment of the crime." This was similar to attitudes found in the 1980s and 1990s toward gay men and fornicating heterosexuals who had contracted HIV/AIDS.

Syphilis was considered punishment for visiting prostitutes, which also had dire consequences for the next generation. Alcott (1972a, 106, 207–208) believed one of the worst things a man could do was to bring this disease home to his wife, and possibly to unborn children. In his view, sexually transmitted diseases such as syphilis arose "from dens of prostitution," because the laws of health, including cleanliness, had been grossly neglected.

Social Errors and Obscene Material

The health reformers were concerned with an assortment of activities that could lead to moral corruption and disease. For example, Alcott (1833, 156–158) thought the theater was "a school of vice" because of its "lewd songs or dances" that increased passions, perverted tastes, and corrupted the morals of youth. He was also concerned about "obscene pictures and books" and "certain paintings and engravings," all of which, in his opinion, could lead to fornication, masturbation, and other evils (p. 309).

The Crimes of Abortion and Artificial Birth Control

The Christian physiologists were against most means of pregnancy control. Alcott (1972a, 181–184), for example, categorically opposed abortion and any mechanical means of birth control, including chemical preparations. He called these "crimes without name." He also condemned physicians who assisted in these efforts. This sentiment was echoed in the Christian Right and other groups during the late twentieth-century Clean Living Movement.

Alcott (1972a, 180) was also opposed to publications that advocated pregnancy contol. For example, he condemned a physician who twenty years before had published a "widely circulated book," the object of which was to "teach people, both in married life and elsewhere, the art of gratifying the sexual appetite without the necessity of progeny." Alcott may have been referring to the 1839 translation of a work by Jean Dubois, a French physician, entitled *Marriage: Physiology Discussed* (1974). Dubois recommended several methods for preventing conception. Today only one of them is considered a reliable method, namely, "the 'kundum,' a sheath of fine silk to be placed over the penis" (Dubois 1974, 92).

Alcott (1972a, 181, 121) preached that overindulgence in sex could prevent conception. He based this upon the observation that "prostitutes rarely conceive." Of course, sterility among prostitutes was probably due to gonorrhea or other sexually transmitted diseases. Alcott also suggested that young couples who overindulged in sex during the early years of their marriages often did not have children. He suggested that if they were more temperate in their sexual lives, they would be more likely to conceive.

Onanism: The Great Evils of the "Secret Vice" or "Self-Pollution"

The most evil form of sexual indulgence, according to Christian physiologists, was Onanism, or masturbation.[7] In Graham's chain of reasoning, "self-pollution" was considered the most morally disgusting habit. He reasoned that it was the most stimulating, as it did not require someone else's cooperation, could be started earlier in life, and could be engaged in more frequently. Therefore, it was considered to "inflame the brain more than natural arousal" and was likely to result in insanity among "depraved young men." Likewise, Alcott viewed masturbation as the most damaging form of sexual indulgence. It was "the greatest moral sin" of the time and "one of the worse scourges ever inflicted on the civilized world." However, he did caution that "it does not thence follow that fornication is not a great evil" (Alcott 1972a, 68, 98–99). Masturbation among females was thought to inflict disease on the next generation, as it was an acquired habit (Alcott 1835, 312–315, 320).

An anonymous work on masturbation in 1844, along with that of Alcott, both cite a Dr. Woodward, the superintendent of a Massachusetts insane asylum, who claimed that masturbation brought on insanity. Woodward came to this conclusion because many inmates in his asylum were known to engage in the practice. These sources were likely the origins of the myth that masturbation causes insanity. To cure masturbation, Graham recommended the usual bland diet without meat, spirits, spices, or the like.

Homosexuality

Homosexuality per se, sometimes called sodomy, was rarely discussed in this era. The word *homosexuality* was not coined until the 1890s. However, hints of it were found among the Christian physiologists' writings. Bullough and Voght (1973, 143–155) suggest that the "secret vice" was also a euphemism for homosexuality during the early and mid-nineteenth century. Masturbation may also have been thought to be its cause. This is hinted at by Jean Dubois (1974, 13), who stated that "the contempt which single men so often boast of for female society, is indeed in nine cases out of ten, the effect of *Onanism.*"

The anonymous author of *Important Facts for Young Men* (1844), which illustrated the destructive effects of masturbation, posited that if "the mind was accustomed to seek pleasure" in a certain way, such as through self-pollution, then the "union of the sexes has no attraction." This author gave an example of a young man who had "contracted the habit of Onanism in his childhood" This "frightful habit . . . prevented him the development of any desire for the other sex. Even when thirty years old, he had never been excited by the sight of a female. . . . He had earlier studied drawing [and] . . . the beautiful forms of men, . . . finally inspired him with an extraordinary emotion—a vague passion, for which he could not account." This anonymous author suggested that he did not think this man was a "sodomist," as he was "not excited by the sight of any man" (*Important Facts* 1844, 28–29).

SUMMARY

The Christian physiologists of the first Clean Living Movement had a lasting influence in the United States beyond the mid-nineteenth century in terms of hygiene, diet, exercise, and sexuality. During the nineteenth century, average alcohol and meat consumption declined, the use of fruits and vegetables increased, and personal hygiene improved. These reformers also helped popularize exercise, athletics, and sport. Negative feelings about sexuality, including rebuke of activities such as masturbation and nocturnal emissions as causing disease and debility, have also survived among some groups through the twentieth century. In addition, the recurring themes of vegetarianism, abstention from alcohol and tobacco, exercise, and fertility control reemerged as crusades in the later two Clean Living Movements.

NOTES

1. Robert S. Fletcher (1943, 336), a historian of Oberlin College, noted, "Historically the temperance movement was the parent of the 'physiological reform' movement. If it was sinful to drink liquors harmful to the physical body, it followed it was sinful to eat harmful foods, take poisonous drugs, wear tight inadequate clothing or neglect exercise, bathing or ventilation." It was also sinful to have "excessive" sex.

2. Besides Graham's own writings, a number of works have addressed his dietary and moral crusade. See, in particular, *A Defense of the Graham System of Living* (1835), Cole (1975), Craig (1991), Nissenbaum (1980), Money (1985), and Sokolow (1983).

3. See Cordasco (1985) for a listing of numerous health and medical works during this era.

4. *The Journal of Health*, in its first two years of publication, discussed a number of topics that Graham later espoused. For example, in the first two volumes, there were articles 126 on temperance, 108 on diet and food, 74 on consumption of pure water, 67 on hygiene and personal cleanliness, 57 on exercise or physical education, 30 on early rising and sleeping, 29 on bathing, 20 on tobacco, and 12 on clothing and dress reform. The remaining items concerned a variety of other health issues (Index, *Journal of Health* 1829, 385–390; 1830, 387–391).

5. See Chapter 7 for more information concerning the exercise movement.

6. The diseases believed to result from sexual intemperance—intercourse more than once a month—included languor, lassitude, muscular relaxation, general debility, loss of appetite, indigestion, faintness, and a "sinking at the pit of the stomach," along with feebleness of the circulation and headache. Even if people "pursue their indulgences for a number of years, without seem-

ing to be affected by them they sooner or later reape the transgressions." They were likely to succumb to "wasting infirmity and protracted and loathsome disease, and early and extreme dotage." Consumption, weak eyes, disorders of the stomach, a predisposition to insanity, and epilepsy were also common, in Graham's opinion (1848, 78–82).

7. Onanism stems from a Bible verse (Genesis 38: 9–10). Onan was killed by God for "spilling his seed on the ground."

5

Inherited Realities, Phrenology, and Groups with Quasi-Eugenic Undercurrents

Let the unmarried choose *healthy* companions or none.
Orson Fowler, *Love and Parentage* (1847b)

Whose heart does not beat high at the bare possibility of becoming the progenitor of a world, as it were, of pure holy, healthy, and greatly elevated beings—a race worthy of emerging from the fall—and enstamping [*sic*] on it a species of immortality.
William Alcott, *The Physiology of Marriage* (1972a)

We believe the time will come when involuntary and random propagation will cease, and when scientific combination will be applied to human generation as freely and successfully as it is to that of other animals.
John Humphrey Noyes, *Male Continence* (1872)

Health reformers during the peak of the first Clean Living Movement began raising the social implications of inherited or acquired (Lamarckian) characteristics, such as tendencies toward drunkenness, consumption, and general debility. They became concerned that humankind increasingly had degenerated since antiquity and that a Christian millennium of perfect, healthy humans might be forestalled if the laws of health were ignored. Obeying these laws began to include, by the late 1840s, selection of the right marriage partner and not just Grahamism. One way of selecting the most genetically compatible partner was through phrenology, or the study of human character through the shape and attributes of one's head. Some religious and other groups incorporated hereditarian thought, either consciously or unconsciously, into their belief system as a way to expedite the millennium. As the first

Clean Living Movement waned, the hereditarian movement—which would be called the eugenics movement by the turn of the century—began to evolve.

THE LAWS OF INHERITANCE AND THE "DEGENERATION OF THE RACE"

Up through the first few decades of the nineteenth century, both the educated and uneducated generally held to the axiom that "like begat like." Besides physical characteristics, it was also assumed that certain tendencies or predispositions, as well as diseases including consumption, insanity, heart disease, and gout, were inherited. Acute infections, such as influenza, smallpox, and cholera, were not considered hereditary. Natural endowment, environmental stress, inadequate or improper diet, and climate were seen as strong factors that interacted to produce health or disease. However, Rosenberg (1976, 34) points out that the transmission of certain traits, including antisocial behaviors, became a social concern in the third and fourth decades of the nineteenth century. This was the case even though the basic body of knowledge, which legitimated such ideological thought, had not changed.

Inheriting Acquired Characteristics

In the 1830s, some reformers suggested that certain practices, such as the use of alcohol and tobacco, and certain behaviors could produce constitutional weaknesses in offspring, which, in turn, could be passed to successive generations. Writing in 1830, Edward Hitchcock, professor of chemistry at Amherst College, for example, stated, "The use of alcohol and tobacco tends powerfully to debilitate the constitution; and the complaints, which they generate, descend hereditarily to posterity" (pp. 312–313). Caleb Ticknor (1972, 309), a physician, in 1836 wrote, "The natural constitution is not alone transmitted to posterity; acquired characters, and peculiarities, and diseases, are by the same law hereditary, and descend, under favorable circumstances, to the remotest generations." Alcott (1972b, 92–93) in 1855 posited that behaviors and acquired traits, such as tendencies toward lack of exercise, drunkenness, and promiscuity, could cause disease and debility to the "third and fourth generation."

However, some reformers suggested that a person could escape a hereditary predisposition for a disease if he or she obeyed the laws of health. For example, if a man prone to gout avoided meat, alcohol, and a sedentary or dissipated life, he could avoid getting the disease. But a man with a normal metabolism who led a sedentary or dissipated life could fall victim to the disease and more likely pass it on to his children. Others contended the "constitution of the offspring" could be improved, if a person had a propensity toward such constitutional weaknesses, by marrying a healthy mate (Buchan 1838, 28; Graham 1839, 109–110).

The Degeneration of the Race Since the Fall of Man

Beginning in the late 1830s, health reformers expressed growing concern with what they considered the degeneration of the human race since antiquity. In response, many of them looked longingly to a time of peace, joy, and tranquility when Christ would rule during a 1,000-year period, the millennium. For example, Sylvester Graham (1839, 364, 373) writes, "God created our first parents perfectly beautiful." These first humans, along with the other ancients, had a balance between mind and body and were handsome, healthy, and intelligent. Graham decries the "little real bodily symmetry and comeliness to be found among the present generations of the human race" and suggests that as humans became more civilized, they became less beautiful and more diseased due to neglect of the body and improper diet. Later health reformers agreed and expressed concern with "racial degeneration."

Elizabeth Blackwell (1852, 16–17), suggested "evidence" that the ancients enjoyed perfect health when she wrote, "Who ever imagined Adam suffering from dyspepsia, or Eve in a fit of hysterics. The thought shocks us—our Eden becomes a hospital." This perfect health was also thought to be tied to the ancients' physical beauty. Like Graham, Blackwell suggests that as humans crowded together in cities, "vice, misery, and disease increased" and "the lofty ideal of perfect health in the past [has] become almost lost under the existing evil" (pp. 10–12). The results of these evils, which included licentiousness, intemperance, and neglect of the body, led to "a physical degeneration of the race which is strikingly exhibited in the external appearance of any assembly of individuals" and an increase in insanity, disorders of the stomach such as dyspepsia (heartburn), nervous diseases (anxiety), and diseases of the generative system (Blackwell 1852, 25–26, 28–30). Bringing on the millennium, according to this thinking, would restore the perfect health and beauty of the ancients, the elimination of diseases, and the problems of society.

PHRENOLOGY

These concerns about physical beauty and health, body symmetry, and inherited degeneracy became embodied in the developing pseudoscience of phrenology, the study of the conformation of the skull as indicative of mental faculties and character traits. Phrenology became instrumental in popularizing hereditarian ideas and became entwined with other health-reform issues during the peak of the first Clean Living Movement. Health advocates tended to endorse phrenology, while phrenology enthusiasts urged the need for hereditary improvement through proper diet, temperance, and "hygienic marriages."

The Development of Phrenology

Phrenology was developed by Franz Joseph Gall (1758–1828), a late eighteenth-century Viennese physician. As conceived by Gall, phrenology had five principles: (1) The brain is the "organ" of the mind; (2) the mind is made up of thirty-seven separate organs, each corresponding to a distinct mental faculty; (3) each faculty is found in a definite region of the surface of the brain; (4) the relative strength of any "propensity," or personality trait, for a mental faculty is determined by the its size; and (5) the correspondence between the outer surface of the skull and the matching organ on the brain surface beneath is sufficiently close to enable a knowledgeable practitioner to determine the temperament and the character of the person (L. Fowler 1844, 37–41).

Phrenology was brought to the United States by John Gasper Spurzheim (1775–1832), a physician and popular lecturer who argued that propensities could be strengthened or inhibited. To Gall's basic precepts, American phrenologists, in the spirit of perfection and self-improvement, added several more principles: (1) Each and every faculty is susceptible to improvement, (2) the developmental direction of the different faculties of the mind depends on education and circumstances, and (3) perfection of mind and character depends upon the full and harmonious action of the faculties and their proper training and direction (L. Fowler 1848, 21–22).

The various organs of the mind were believed to be found in various locations of the brain. The relative strength of any propensity could be determined by carefully measuring and examining the outer surface of the head which corresponded to the organ lying beneath it. For example, the organs which governed "animal" or "domestic" propensities were located in the back and lower part of the head, while those of intellect and reason occupied the frontal regions.

Phrenology, as a legitimate field, came into its own in the United States during the 1820s and became popular among the middle class. By 1840, phrenology as a discipline began to split into two directions, one for serious scientists and the other for practical phrenologists focused on giving character readings and addressing such intangibles as human happiness. The split eroded the discipline's scientific respectability, but increased its constituency in the late 1840s and 1850s (Walters 1978, 158). The practical phrenologists, who conducted "head readings" and asserted that various faculties and their actions could scientifically influence such human activities as career choices and mate choices, severely damaged phrenology's reputation among America's physicians and academicians (Wrobel 1987, 125).

The Fowlers

The popularity of phrenology in the United States during the 1840s and 1850s was in large measure due to the work of Orson Squire Fowler (1809–1887), his brother Lorenzo Niles Fowler (1811–1896), and his sister-in-law Lydia Folger Fowler (1822–1879). These three individuals authored numerous publications and lectures on phrenology, anatomy, physiology, hygiene, marriage, eugenics, temperance, and other reform issues. The Fowler brothers were born and raised in Cohocton, New York. Orson Fowler went to Amherst to prepare for the ministry, where he was introduced to phrenology in the early 1830s. He believed phrenology was reinforced by Graham's physiology and that the two systems were most effectively employed in combination. This became the basis of many works published by the Fowlers. Lorenzo Fowler joined his brother in efforts to proselytize phrenology though writings and lecture tours. In 1835, the Fowler brothers set up headquarters in New York City. Various publications by them rapidly spread interest in phrenology to all segments of society (Mott 1957, 447–448; Nissenbaum 1980, 148, 156).

In 1852, the Fowler brothers were joined by brother-in-law Samuel Wells, a phrenologist and hydropath, who, since 1845, had become associated with them in publishing the *Water Cure Journal*. The threesome formed the Fowlers and Wells publishing house. Wells later became a founder of the American Vegetarian Society in 1850 and the American Anti-Tobacco Society. Besides phrenology, the company also printed works on temperance and health-reform issues. It kept Sylvester Graham's *The Science of Human Life* on its list into the 1880s. At their peak in the 1850s, operating from their New York City headquarters at Clinton Hall, the brothers created a phrenological empire that included health, religion, and political and eugenic reform (Mott 1957, 447–448, 441; Nissenbaum 1980, 148, 156; Walters 1978, 161).

Phrenology and Health Reform

The Fowler brothers helped broadcast various health-reform issues to thousands of American families who subscribed to their *American*

Phrenological Journal. They published numerous guides, manuals, and books on all aspects of mental and physical health, and embraced most of the health reforms of the first Clean Living Movement. Advertisements for books and manuals in the 1850 issue of the *Phrenological Almanac* reflect their wide interests in reform issues.[1]

The phrenology literature of the 1840s and 1850s relied heavily on the principles of Grahamism to promote health. The Fowlers' writings included long sections on anatomy, physiology, vegetarianism, and concerns over sexuality. For example, two years after publication of Graham's *The Science of Human Life* (1839), Orson Fowler (1841, 36–37) advised readers that anything that "excites the body . . . such as tea, coffee, flesh" should be avoided because they stimulate sexual urges. To subdue sexual feelings, a person was encouraged to avoid these items and consume only "water, breadstuffs and vegetables" and engage in physical exercise. Strong admonitions were made against wearing corsets with tight lacing, because "the practice radically deranges the temperaments" (L. Fowler 1844, 51).

Incorporation of health issues into phrenology was not one-sided. Many health reformers alluded to phrenology, but apparently were not overly enthusiastic about adopting its scientific merits. Through the waning years of the first Clean Living Movement, many health reformers interacted with the Fowler brothers, who published or reprinted their works. The Fowlers's headquarters became a lodestone for reformers and reform issues of the day. At the organizational meeting of the American Vegetarian Society in 1850, for example, William Alcott, Sylvester Graham, Joel Shew, and Russel Trall were present. Although the phrenologists advocated health reform and helped spread its ideas to middle-class Americans, they went a step further and set the foundations for "inherited realities" that evolved into the "science" of eugenics (Numbers 1976, 70).

INHERITED REALITIES: THE ORIGINS OF EUGENICS

During the mid-nineteenth century, health reformers began to emphasize the importance of inherited realities in marriage-partner selection, avoidance of certain activities during gestation, and a healthy environment in early childhood to ensure the development of moral, intelligent children instrumental in bettering the human race. The Fowler brothers waxed prolifically on heredity reform and it is estimated their publications reached millions of Americans. Readers were instructed how to evaluate their phrenological organs in order to choose the most compatible marriage partners and to determine the sort of children they would bring into the world (Aspiz 1987, 149; Sokolow 1983, 156–157).

Phrenology and Eugenic Thought

Phrenology, hereditary, and health reform became intertwined at the peak of the first Clean Living Movement. Health advocates tended to endorse phrenology, while phrenology publicists urged the need for hereditary improvement through proper diet and hygienic marriages. However, unlike some other aspects of the first Clean Living Movement, such as Grahamism and temperance, which peaked during the late 1840s and 1850s, respectively, heredity reform—termed "eugenics" in 1883—began to accelerate in the mid-1840s as the first Clean Living Movement waned.[2]

Inherited Realities

The term "inherited realities" began appearing in some writings in the mid-1830s. In 1836, Caleb Ticknor (1972, 311) hinted at eugenics, mentioning that "consumption, scrofula, insanity, and many other diseases are hereditary." He questioned a couple's right to marry if both branches of their family were affected with hereditary diseases, even if there was no objection to their union.

By the late 1850s, phrenologists and other authors began recommending inherited realities regarding marriage selection. Lorenzo Fowler (1850b, 176–177), for example, writes, "We take great pains to improve the breed of horses and sheep. Is it not absurd for any one to advance the opinion, that it is too delicate a subject to improve the human race." He argued that if people with a hereditary disease marry "with the intention to becoming parents, they should pay strict attention to the laws of physiology, and marry those only who are particularly well fortified in those qualities in which they are deficient—those having a strong and well-balanced constitution, a good stock of vitality, and an active and energetic mind."

Hereditary Reform to Improve the Race and Bring on the Millennium

As hereditary and millennium ideas became increasingly linked in the 1840s, the eugenics movement began to take form.[3] Increasing concern with heredity may have been spawned from observation that health-reform efforts during the 1830s and 1840s had not eradicated the problems of disease and poverty, nor ushered in the millennium. If eliminating alcohol, other "stimulants," and meat from the diet did not decrease the problems of drunkenness and the slums, then perhaps the problem was caused by heredity, and nothing could eradicate social problems other than hygienic marriages among healthy couples. Several reformers began to suggest eugenic marriages.

William Alcott (1972a, 94–96) recommended eugenic marriages as a way to bring on the millennium. He suggested that once the rules of health were universally adopted, each generation would be sturdier and longer lived than the previous one until the original long life expectancy found in the Garden of Eden was regained. Blackwell suggested that the teaching of physiology, hygiene, and exercise was needed to prevent "hereditary diseases," and to halt the present racial degeneracy (Blackwell 1852, 28, 31). Adopting health reform and eugenic marriages was a compelling argument for these reformers inasmuch as it made these issues not only an individual choice, but also a solemn responsibility to one's descendants. These ideals reassured parents of some control over their offspring's well-being (Whorton 1988, 66).

Contracting Eugenic Marriages

Rosenberg (1976, 42) has observed that a recurring theme of the *American Journal of Phrenology* in its first ten volumes, beginning in 1838, was the need to contract eugenic marriages and to take every precaution during gestation and early childhood to ensure the development of healthy, moral, and intelligent children. Marriage was not recommended for very young, delicate females, individuals disposed to hereditary diseases, or "partners too nearly allied in blood" or with great differences in age, because they were all likely to produce imperfect offspring (L. Fowler 1850b, 188–189).

As early as 1841, Orson Fowler, in *Fowler on Matrimony* (pp. 25–27) gave suggestions for selecting the best marriage partner. He recommended that special care be taken to blend and harmonize the best qualities of each partner. He advised that a mate should have a good physical organization, a strong constitution, and a "well balanced head," with uniformity of character. He warned against marrying if either party were subject to dyspepsia, liver complaints, indigestion, ennui, hypochondria, sour stomach, heartburn, or melancholia. In particular, Fowler (pp. 22–25) gave young men advice for choosing a wife. He warned that if a person marries for "amativeness"—sexuality— then as the beauty of his mate fades, so will enjoyment. He suggested that "an amply developed chest is a sure sign of a naturally strong constitution, which implies a strong hold on life whereas a small waist is an invariable sign of small and weak vital organs, of a delicate and sickly parentage, and, of all things being equal, of sickly offspring and a short life."

"A Spiritual Banquet of Love" and Avoiding
Too Much Sex to Create Perfect Children

It was believed that offspring took on the physical and mental qualities of their parents at the time of conception through a mechanism of
"biological magnetism" (O. Fowler 1847b, 25, 102). Lorenzo Fowler
(1850b, 191–192) suggested that "in exact proportion as the parents
are perfectly organized, physically and mentally, and in the full exercise of all the faculties of their mind and body, so will be their offspring; and, that imperfections will be the result, in precise proportion
as the parents are imperfect." Because of the concern of transmission
of characteristics at "generation," reformers offered suggestions for
conceiving perfect children through the timing and frequency of sexual
intercourse and the encouragement of a positive mental state. The
mental condition of the mother, in particular, at conception and before
birth was considered very important. It was recommended that the
mother stay away from situations in which she might experience anxiety or trauma, less she conceive and bear a mentally or physically de-
formed child.

Orson Fowler (1847b, 80–81, 102, 134, 138–140) maintained that desirable hereditary traits could be bestowed and superior offspring conceived only by married lovers engaging in a "spiritual banquet of love."
He considered it most important for the female to have an orgasm in
order to effect the most successful transmission of positive characteristics. As with Graham and Alcott, he did not recommend frequent
sexual intercourse. Fowler held that individuals should save their
sexual passions and "vital energy" for marriage and release them in
an ecstatic intercourse for conception—but only when the female was
feeling these passions. Concern prevailed among reformers over a
couple having too much sex early in their marriage, which could waste
"vital fluids" and cause deformity among offspring. Early in the day
was considered the best time to have sexual intercourse for propagation (Alcott 1972a, 122–123).

A COMMUNE AND A SECT WITH
EUGENIC UNDERCURRENTS

Eugenic reforms, in one way or the other, were found in a few developing sects and communal groups of this era. During the first half
of the nineteenth century there was a rise, and then decline, of various
communal societies, utopian experiments, and religious sects that
emerged in the aftermath of the second Great Awakening of the 1820s
and 1830s.[4] These groups were propelled by visions of an ideal or per-

fect life, which they sought to actualize within their membership. On the whole, the communal sects sought to create a new order, in contrast to the reformers, such as Sylvester Graham and the Fowler brothers, who strove to improve society as a whole during the first Clean Living Movement. Health and eugenic reforms were undercurrents in several of these groups.

As pointed out by contemporary historians Lawrence Foster (1991), Ronald Walters (1978, 73), and Lewis Perry (1983, 772), and even by Russell Trall (1972, 234–240), the mid-nineteenth-century hydropath, similarities emerged among three sects, two which developed and one which expanded, during this period; namely, the Mormons, Oneidas, and Shakers, respectively. Commonalities between these groups included revivalist ideals of "the perfection of mankind," belief that the millennium was at hand, and a desire to restore a biblical society on earth. In addition, each community followed the leadership of an individual who had intense religious experiences or visions, developed a highly successful economic base, endured over a long period of time despite public antagonism, and had sexual practices that deviated from the norm. The perfectionist impulse within these groups was interwoven with the goal of creating a perfect race by obeying the laws of health to ensure a strong and sturdy future generation. Mating of individuals with well-developed social, physical, spiritual, and intellectual traits was considered desirable. This concept was incubated in the Oneida community, in particular, in which "progressive" restrictions on human breeding within the group were imposed, and became an underlying theme in the developing Mormon community. The Shakers went to the opposite extreme by disavowing all sexual relations and striving for perfection (Perry 1983, 771–773; Walters 1978, 40–44; Kern 1981, 119).

The Oneida Community

The Onieda community fostered a eugenic marriage system. The founder of this group, John Humphrey Noyes (1811–1886), the son of a prosperous Vermont businessman, attended both Andover Seminary and Yale Divinity School but was refused ordination because of the belief that "conversion brought complete release from sin," which was incongruent with mainstream Protestant theology. Despite his failure to become ordained, he began to preach and gathered a group of followers. In 1838, after a disappointing love affair, he married one of his followers and settled in Putney, Vermont, with other like-minded perfectionists. This small group organized more formally in 1841, when they pooled their resources and instituted a primitive "Christian communism," in which property, and later marriage partners, were shared (Hudson 1965, 186–187; Walters 1978, 55–59; Noyes 1872, 10–11).

In 1846, when Noyes put into practice his theory of sharing marriage partners, which he termed "complex marriage," local Vermont citizens were outraged. To avoid the risk of being mobbed, the community disbanded and reestablished itself in Oneida, New York, in 1848, and became a prosperous business community (Hudson 1965, 186–189; Walters 1978, 55–59; Noyes 1872, 17). In 1848, Noyes published his widely read and condemned theory of sexuality, *Male Continence*. This tract outlined a formula for allowing a broad range of pleasurable sexual experiences while at the same time retaining semen for the sacred purpose of propagation. Noyes separated sexual intercourse into "two distinct acts, the social and the propagative" (Noyes 1872, 8, 19).

Within Noyes's community, the complex-marriage sexual system regarded each woman in the group as the wife of every man and every man as the husband of every woman. Sexual intercourse was encouraged as long as the woman consented and the man did not have an orgasm when sex was solely for "amative," but not reproductive, purposes. Social and pleasurable intercourse was clearly differentiated from procreation intercourse. Although Noyes's sexual practices violated Grahamite prohibitions over the frequency of intercourse, both the Christian Physiologists and the Oneidans believed they were restoring health and purifying the race by following the laws of health. Noyes, like other health reformers of the day, also condemned the use of alcohol, coffee, tea, tobacco, and meat (Hudson 1965, 187; Walters 1978, 57; Foster 1981, 235).

Complex marriage was a somewhat restrictive and organized system— not "free love," as might be imagined by outsiders. The system was instituted on religious grounds. The Oneidans considered themselves saints purified by religious experience and were committed to absolute fellowship among themselves. Up to about 1860, mutual consent between two people was generally all that was required for sexual intercourse. However, by 1860, all requests for intercourse had to be made through a third party and were recorded in a ledger. This led to a eugenic program with planned reproduction that Noyes called "Stirpiculture" (Foster 1981, 235, 239; Hudson 1965, 187).[5]

In 1869, a committee was formed to suggest scientific combinations of community members to become parents. Since Noyes believed moral traits were passed on to children, the men and women selected were expected to be the most spiritually advanced in the community, as well as physically healthy. Noyes believed, as did the health reformers, that extraordinary parents produced extraordinary children. Russell

Trall (1972, 237), a hydrotherapist, in *Physiology of Sex*, first published in 1881, summed up the eugenic practices of the Oneidas: "When children are desired, the best specimens of the flock—male and female—are to associate together for the purpose; but for purposes of personal enjoyment and mutual improvement, intercourse is to be promiscuous, or at least interchangeable" (Foster 1981, 239; Walters 1978, 58). When only certain individuals were allowed to have children, the resulting resentments and polarization within the group began to cause the disintegration of the Oneida communal marriage system. In 1880, the community disbanded and formed a joint stock company. The Oneida Company still exists today and manufactures tableware (Walters 1978, 56–60; Foster 1981, 239).

Mormons

The Mormons showed characteristics of a communal group in their quest for perfection and restoration of a biblical society among their members in contrast to reforming society as a whole (see Chapter 2 for discussion of the formation and health-reform aspects of the Latter-Day Saints). In addition, they had a marriage practice that in some cases appears to have had eugenic undertones.

The early Mormons, as Klaus Hanson (1981, 152–153) has suggested, did not share their contemporaries' concerns and fears of sexual excesses in marriage. They did not support a metaphysical dualism that elevated the soul above the body, spirit above flesh, as did the Grahamites. In Mormon theology, the dichotomy had been eliminated, and sex, in theory, did not represent the corruption of the flesh against the spirit. Sexuality was seen as a part of "man's eternal nature." This also meant there were no religious or moral sanctions against polygamous or "plural" marriages inasmuch as they were considered to be based upon scripture.

As part of their religious beliefs, the Latter-Day Saints felt it an obligation to produce many children in order to give "pre-existing spirits" a chance to be born. Plural marriages—technically, they practiced *polygyny* because only men were allowed more than one spouse—offered the opportunity to the husband to increase his progeny, his "kingdom," throughout eternity. Implicit in this belief was that honorable and righteous men and women were likely to produce more and better children than would marriage between individuals who were immoral and shiftless, because only worthy men were encouraged to marry. Men who were drunkards, idle, or extremely poor were consistently identified as being unfit for marriage. Polygyny allowed the worthy men to have many children (Bush 1976, 16–17; Perry 1983, 772).

Another Mormon religious belief held that "eternal marriage" between a man and a woman was an essential requirement for entry into the highest degree of glory, or "exaltation," in the "celestial kingdom," the highest heaven in Mormon theology. For a woman to obtain this glory she had to be married, or "sealed" for eternity to a man worthy of this success. Therefore, if there was an excess of righteous women over men eligible for this highest degree of heavenly glory, simple justice dictated that a worthy man take more than one wife to assure that all eligible women also attained this state (Hansen 1981, 168–169).[6]

Plural marriages were first publically announced in 1852 (Shipps 1985, 163). Foster (1981, 239) suggested that Mormons saw family life and the relationship between family and a larger kinship network as the ultimate basis for human progression, not only on earth, but also throughout eternity. Mormons empathically denied they were breaking up the family or failing to raise righteous and healthy children. They argued that "polygamy made it possible to bring up more children in the families of the best men" (Foster 1981, 239).

Lester Bush Jr. (1982, 236–237), a Mormon medical historian, has cited several passages with eugenic undertones from works examining the health of Mormons in the nineteenth century. Bush points out that the turn-of-the-century historian Hubert Howe Bancroft wrote that "only the better class of men, the healthy and wealthy, the strongest intellectually and physically" were polygamists. In addition, Mormons considered that by these men "becoming fathers to the largest number of children, the stock is improved." Bush quotes the editor of a 1924 issue of the *Journal of Heredity*, who suggested, "The fact that plural families were restricted by the Church authority to a select class of the population would explain the average superiority of the polygamous families." Producing fit offspring by allowing only certain men to have more than one wife so as to improve society by having more superior offspring could be considered a form of eugenic practice.

SUMMARY

Concern over inherited diseases, including acquired traits, improvement of society through obedience to the laws of health, and selection of the best marriage partners were found both among health reformers of the period and among several burgeoning sects and communal groups. Phrenology and its wide dissemination among the American middle class helped spread the hereditarian concept. As the first Clean Living Movement began to wane, increased attention focused on inherited realities that led to a eugenic reform movement near the turn of the twentieth century.

NOTES

1. The 1850 edition of *The Illustrated Phrenological Almanac* (L. Fowler 1850a) lists advertisements for the *Water Cure Journal* and booklets discussing temperance, tight lacing, teeth, the dangers of tea and coffee, the promotion of vegetarian diets, and good parenting and marriage. These tracts were written by a variety of health reformers of the day other than the Fowlers, including William Alcott.

2. The term "eugenics" was not coined until 1883 by Francis Galton (p. 24), although its concepts began to be discussed in the mid-1830s. Eugenics refers to selective marriage for the betterment of the human race. Its basic premise is that only fit parents, free from "disease, debility, insanity, and imbecilism," should reproduce. See Sokolow (1983, 156–157), Aspiz (1987), and Rosenberg (1976) for further reading concerning the beginnings of the eugenics movement in the mid-nineteenth century.

3. The eugenics movement peaked in the United States after World War I and is discussed in detail in Chapter 9.

4. It is estimated that several hundred communitarian groups developed from the end of the American Revolution to the beginning of the Civil War, with the greatest wave coming in the early 1840s. These groups included political, social, and religious experiments. Some were highly structured, while others were only loosely held together by certain belief systems. Most lasted only a few years, some for only a few months, and a few lasted for years (Perry 1983, 768–770; Walters 1978, 40). Walters suggests that more young people joined communities in this era than any other time in American history, except possibly the late 1960s at the inception of the late twentieth-century Clean Living Movement. See Robert S. Fogarty (1980) for more information and history concerning a variety of communitarian groups.

5. Attached to the Kinsey Library, Indiana University's copy of *Male Continence* (Noyes 1872) are the last four pages of an essay by a presumed follower of Noyes. It gives insight into how this system of complex marriage worked. The anonymous author of this essay suggests that "sexual meetings between the same parties in complex marriage seldom occurred oftener than once a month" (p. 10). The writer acknowledges that male continence was "a trying condition for the man and a severe test of his own control" (p. 11). In terms of a sexual liaison, the author of this essay writes, "From my own experience of those with whom I was familiar, that sexual interviews lasted generally an hour and a half. All night interviews were generally discouraged" (p. 10). The essayist acknowledges that male continence has not been found practicable in this age and suggests "some future generation may advance to this high plane of civilization required by such a mode of life and profit by the experience of the progressive committee"—the term Noyes, referred to as "Dr. Humphrey" by this anonymous author, calls "his devoted band of followers." The author concludes by suggesting, "We have shown that male continence is possible, practicable and safe under certain conditions. A future generation may profit by our experience" (p. 13).

6. Controversy exists over the percentage of Mormons who were engaged in polygamous marriages. Low estimates suggest no more than 5 percent of

married men had more than one wife, and these were primarily affluent individuals. Based upon the 1880 census, it is estimated that about 25 percent of males had more than one wife. During the mid-nineteenth century, about two-thirds of Mormon women were living in plural marriages in one small Utah community. Other studies have estimated about a third of Mormons lived in plural families (Pace 1982, 23–31; Bennion 1984, 27–42; Daynes 1991, 159, 186–193).

6

Nativism, Cholera, Public Health, and Cures

> Had it not been for intemperance, the cholera would probably not have visited the United States.
>
> *Temperance Almanac* (1833)

> Cleanliness is said to be next of kin to godliness.
>
> Old Saying

Beginning in the late 1820s, Roman Catholic Irish and German immigrants began to pour into America's eastern slums. In the summer of 1832, they brought Asiatic cholera, a disease with a high case fatality rate that quickly spread to other cities and was considered an illness of poor, immoral, and filthy people. Anti-Catholic biases against the immigrants, rooted in colonial times and fear that they would prevent the Protestant millennium, gave rise to the Nativist movement, which intertwined with temperance and other reform issues and inspired progressive legislation, such as state and local prohibition.

From 1832 until 1866, from the first to the last major cholera epidemic, a change in perception of the disease resulted. By the end of this period, cholera was not considered a moral failing among immigrants, but rather a problem that sanitation and public-health reform could prevent (Rosenberg 1987, 226–227). The public-health movement grew out of fear of immigrants breeding more drunkards, paupers, and insane people due to "hereditarian" beliefs and the fear that their diseases, especially cholera, would spill out of the slums into middle-class areas. Because regular, "orthodox" physicians were not always successful in treating most diseases, alternative treatments and cures arose in the Jacksonian spirit of "every person his own physician."

IMMIGRATION, NATIVISM, AND HEALTH REFORMS

Fear of Roman Catholics and other immigrants led to the rise of pro-"native American" or Nativist sentiments among many middle-class Protestants. Nativism became interwoven with temperance, hereditarian, and other health-reform efforts. The underlying theme of all of these movements was to bring the Protestant millennium to America, a golden age without poverty, intemperance, or disease.[1]

English Protestant Settlers' Fears of Roman Catholicism

Since the colonial period and the early days of the republic, fear, hostility, and hatred toward Roman Catholics had emanated from Protestant English colonists who settled in Virginia and Massachusetts. This had stemmed largely from attempted Catholic domination of Britain through war or political maneuvering, which had occurred in England within the memory of the settlers or their grandparents. Unlike Britain, which sublimated its religious fervor and adopted more liberal attitudes, the colonist "no-popery prejudices" deepened through sermons and written works in most of the American colonies (Billington 1974, 2–3, 10–11, 24–25).

The Rise of Nativism

The late 1820s saw the beginning of an influx of Irish Roman Catholic immigrants who settled in the slums of the eastern seaboard cities. The movement of many impoverished people into the poorest sections of the cities led to profound health and social problems over the ensuing years. The filthy slums, where most of the immigrants initially lived, bred cholera and other diseases. Few doctors and no effective public-health system made it difficult to control epidemics that infested these areas. Neither were there enough police to lock up the drunken brawlers in the streets. In 1846, two social upheavals in Europe—the potato famine in Ireland and economic and political unrest in Germany—unleashed a tide of migrants into these already crowded areas. Yet even before this huge wave of migrants, signs of trouble had surfaced. During the 1830s and 1840s, riots and bloodshed among immigrant groups and between immigrants and Nativists occurred at sporadical intervals in several cities (Billington 1974, 50–54, 457, 525–533; Van Dussen 1990, 21–36; Tyler 1944, 375–377; Rosenberg 1987, 135–137).

Beginning in the early 1840s, Nativists increasingly produced pamphlets and manifestos against immigrants, and Catholic immigrants in particular. These tracts claimed that most of the beggars, residents of public almshouses, and criminals were foreign-born and were becoming a blight upon the country because of their "intemperance, moral depravity, and sheer idleness." These writings reflected the fear that the refuse of Europe was being dumped on America. Immigration of the poorest was seen as a "papal plot" to ruin the United States as Catholic immigrant voters gained control over the ballot box. There was also fear that these immigrants would breed more paupers, drunkards, and criminals (Billington 1974, 525–533).

Increasing fear of Catholic immigrants and their perceived political power, in addition to rapid economic and social changes, inspired some nativists to form a secret society, commonly called the "Know Nothing Party."[2] This group evolved into a political force between 1853 and 1856. These Nativists hoped to stem the rising influence of the foreign-born in American economic and political life. The party opposed alcohol, immigrants, Catholics, and slavery; it was popular among the working class, old-line New England families, and the middle class in several Eastern and Midwestern states (Stewart 1976, 171; Billington 1974, i–ii; Rosenberg 1987, 135–137; Holt 1973, 309–331; Parmet 1966, 84–90).

As this party rose to power, it enacted progressive legislation—such as prohibition in many states—but it lacked the political leadership to sustain its prominence (Tracy 1988, 1–19; Holt 1973, 309–331; Gienapp 1985, 529–559). Some of the sentiments of this party—to bring America back to her Protestant roots and traditional values and a society free of crime and immorality—were echoed in the rhetoric of the Christian right political forces of the last two decades of the twentieth century.

FEAR OF IMMIGRANTS AS A FACTOR IN HEALTH REFORM

Beginning in the early 1840s, Nativism and various health-reform issues became increasingly interwoven. Irish immigrants, in particular, were decried for perpetuating an endless cycle of birth and death, poverty, intemperance, squalor, and disease. There was fear on the part of many Americans that the entire nation would be overrun with these "degenerates." Proponents of urban slum reform began raising the matter of "racial realities" as proposed by the phrenologists and other health reformers—certain races were seen to be more prone to health and social problems. They noted a disproportionate amount of insanity, criminality, alcoholism, and disease among Irish Catholic immigrants in the slums, compared to other groups (Rosenberg 1987, 55).[3]

Concern over the safety of the republic and its heritage as a result of lower-class immigration proliferated in both rural and urban areas. This fear cemented a bond between Nativists and temperance workers to do something about the perceived alcohol problem. Gienapp

(1987, 98) argued, "For both the Know Nothings and temperance crusaders, besotted Irish Catholics functioned as their primary negative reference group. However, for the Irish and German immigrants . . . drinking was an integral part of socializing [and] they were unwilling to give up their whiskey and lager beer to conform to American conception of proper social behavior." Nativists, reacting to immigrant drinking, enacted laws to eradicate public drinking and disorderly conduct and to exert social control over the immigrants' behavior. Neal Dow, creator of the Maine prohibition law of 1851, symbolized the connection between the two movements as a member of the Nativist society (Gienapp 1987, 45, 97–98).

CHOLERA'S INFLUENCES ON THE FIRST
CLEAN LIVING MOVEMENT

Infectious diseases were rampant in early and mid-nineteenth century America. Infant diarrhea, dysentery, diphtheria, scarlet fever, typhoid fever, tuberculosis, and malaria were common killers. Yellow fever and smallpox, the great epidemic diseases of the previous two centuries, were no longer a huge national problem. Yellow fever had disappeared from the North, and vaccination had curtailed smallpox. However, inadequate sanitation, unhealthy diets with few fruits and vegetables, and a lack of bathing resulted in many diseases. The expanding garbage-strewn slums of the eastern seaboard became an ideal environment for terrifying epidemics, one of which was Asiatic cholera in the summer of 1832.[4]

Charles Rosenberg (1987, 1–2), a medical historian, has suggested it was unlikely that a cholera epidemic had ever occurred outside the Far East until the early nineteenth century, when it began to spread throughout the world. Up to this time, most health historians had suggested that cholera was endemic to India, where it thrived in filth and want. The cholera epidemics of 1832 and 1849 were important motivating factors for health reform in the first Clean Living Movement. These two plagues played a key role in the banishment of cholera and other water- and food-borne diseases from North America. They also exerted an influence in overcoming centuries of governmental inertia and indifference with regard to the problems of public health and sanitation.

The Mid-Nineteenth-Century Cholera Epidemics

Rosenberg (1987) described the three nineteenth-century Asiatic cholera epidemics in depth in terms of religious and social thought and public-health reform. The first epidemic began at the onset of the first Clean Living Movement, and the last major epidemic after the movement had begun to wane. From 1832 until 1866, many changes altered society's view of health and disease. Evangelical fervor had been eroded by materialistic sentiments as well as by the outbreak of cholera, which was seen as a scourge of the sinful. Ministers in 1832 admonished their congregations to practice morality as a guarantor of health, and by 1866 their counterparts endorsed sanitary reform as a necessary prerequisite to moral improvement. By 1866, sanitary reformers could justify their program of clean streets and a pure water supply as a safeguard against certain epidemic diseases. This was based upon the findings of John Snow, a London physician, that cholera was spread through contaminated water supplies (Rosenberg 1987, 4–6).

As the first cholera epidemic raged in festering European cities, many Americans reasoned that the disease was unlikely to infect their homeland because they were a predominately rural, religious people. They believed the pestilence only attacked the filthy, indigent, and ignorant. Asiatic cholera first appeared in the New World around June 9, 1832, in Quebec "among the Canadian French, and wretched emigrants, chiefly from Ireland, who had, during the spring, been thrown in thousands upon the banks of the St. Lawrence. It quickly spread over the city, and affected many of the natives in comfortable circumstances" (Drake 1832b, 23). Many of these Irish immigrants who landed in Canada had no intention of staying, and so quickly crossed the border into the United States and made their way to the eastern slums. It was not known if cholera was initially imported by these individuals or by immigrants who came directly into New York City, where the first case in the United States was reported in late June (Rosenberg 1987, 25). The epidemic soon spread throughout most of the large cities and into rural areas.

Daniel Drake (1785–1852), a clinician, wrote a small book describing the history, prevention, and treatment of the disease. He noted that cholera mostly occurred around "navigable rivers, maritime towns, among armies, sought out the poor, the terrified, the afflicted, the badly lodged, clothed, and fed; the intemperate; the exposed; and the dwellers in damp and unventilated places" (Drake 1832b, 21, 25–30). Since cholera often started simultaneously in different areas of a town or city, most medical practitioners did not consider it to be contagious (Rosenberg 1987, 75–78).[5]

Cholera: "A Scourge of God to Cleanse the Earth"

Poverty and diseases such as cholera were considered moral—and not social—problems during the early nineteenth century. Rosenberg (1987, 55, 60, 62, 133–134) has suggested that there was "worthy" and "unworthy poverty." Cholera did not tend to attack the "prudent and industrious workingman," such as artisans, farmers, and mechanics who had made and sustained the republic. It was the "vicious poor, the drunkard, idler, prostitute and thief who were its proper victims."A high incidence of cholera was noted among urban "Negroes" and Irish immigrants. To many Americans, the epidemic was one of the alarming consequences of the unprecedented increase in immigration. Many middle-class Americans and clergymen considered the cholera epidemics of 1832 and 1849 to be a consequence of the "wickedness of man." The disease was seen as God's way of achieving moral purification and cleansing the earth of sinners. As quoted by Rosenberg (p. 44) from a religious periodical of the time, "a *scourge*, a *rod* in the hand of God." If a middle-class person succumbed to the disease, he or she died in suspicious circumstances and was thought to have had a secret transgression. The feeling that disease was a consequence of sin was similar to 1980s attitudes among some religious groups and individuals about homosexuals dying of AIDS.

Curing and Preventing Cholera

Rosenberg (1987, 68–70) pointed out that treatment of cholera by "regular" physicians was the usual bleeding, purging, and use of calomel, a poisonous mercury powder. Since these nostrums were unlikely to cure—and in many cases probably hastened the death of the victim—the public lacked confidence in medical treatment and began turning to increasingly popular "natural-pathic" cures. Some of these may have even been slightly effective. The Mormons, for instance, immersed the cholera victim in icy water, which had the desired effect of stopping the purging, vomiting, and cramping.

Sylvester Graham, Daniel Drake, and others offered a variety of regimes to prevent cholera. Graham believed that a main cause of the disease was from "over stimulation." To prevent the disease, abstention from stimulants such as meat and drink, adherence to a vegetarian diet with plenty of unbolted wheat bread, drinking pure water, and avoiding all excesses were recommended. In his 1833 tract, *A Lecture on Epidemic Diseases*, Graham claimed that those who followed his regime did not succumb to cholera. Daniel Drake (1832b, 21, 166–168) recommended some basic sanitation efforts. He suggested quarantines, sequestering inland towns, and eliminating filth and stagnant water. Other measures included cholera hospitals, medicines for the poor, retreating to the country, and avoidance of crowded rooms and seasonable vegetables. Drake was also one of the first to realize that cholera did not claim only the vicious, poverty-stricken, or drunkards, but had also stricken many in the "opposite of all these circumstances" as well. These suggested measures constituted the beginnings of the sanitation, or public-health, movement.

THE RISE OF PUBLIC-HEALTH REFORM

The cholera epidemic was a potent catalyst in public-health reform. Concerns about sanitation stirred about the same time as the physiological health-reform movement. Although these two movements were an outgrowth of pietism following the second Great Awakening and intertwined with temperance and other reform issues, the public-health and sanitation movement did not reach the peak of its agitation until the 1860s, well after Grahamism had faded.

In America's towns and cities, garbage, foul air and water, and human and other wastes abounded. Pigs as well as rats roamed freely in the streets, feeding on the accumulated refuse. Reformers began to write about the health perils of the city (Rosenberg 1987, 142–143; Blackwell 1852, 28–29). In England during this time, physicians and social reformers such as Edwin Chadwick and John Snow alerted their countrymen to the health dangers of cities through statistics and epidemiology, the new tools of medical science.[6] These techniques demonstrated that poor drainage, foul water, and crowded tenements shortened lives. Basing their practices upon these new methods, by 1849 many physicians had become convinced of the futility of traditional remedies for treating disease. Many diseases could not be cured but could be prevented through cleanliness and sanitation (Whorton 1982, 28–29; Rosenberg 1987, 142–146).

These new approaches to health became increasingly relevant to America. The nation was no longer predominantly rural, and the slums were overshadowing those of Europe. It became increasingly clear that cities bore responsibility in cleaning their streets, providing pure water supplies, and establishing better housing for the poor. In addition, personal cleanliness, healthy diets, and adequate ventilation were stressed in preventing and eliminating terrible diseases such as cholera. Dread of another devastating epidemic drove both physicians and the public to take an interest in the sanitary-reform movement developing in England. However, sanitary reforms did not take firm hold in America until about 1850 (Whorton 1982, 28–29; Rosenberg 1987, 142–146).

Bible Societies and Public-Health Reform

Rosenberg and Rosenberg (1968, 16–35) proposed that early sanitary reform in the 1830s and 1840s were not simply a reaction against unbearably filthy environments, but, more significantly, a positive continuation of religious commitments. In order for people to be saved they first needed to live in a clean environment and maintain healthy habits. Also contributing to the movement were nativistic fears of immigrant lawlessness and diseases spilling over from slums into middle-class areas and eugenic concerns of further racial degeneration because of ill health and intemperance. Physical health and living conditions, morality, and religion were all seen as a tightly knit series of causes and effects (Rosenberg 1976, 35–36, 114).

As early as 1810, Bible and missionary societies sought to reach the "heathens" in the cities. The organizations established urban missions and assigned volunteers to particular neighborhoods. Visitations to these areas exposed middle-class and wealthy Americans to the realities of squalor and vice in the slums resulting in the formation of benevolent organizations to prevent poverty. In the 1820s, volunteers saw moral failing as the root cause of squalor and insisted that religion, temperance, and thrift could prevent poverty (Walters 1978, 174–175).

Charles Finney's revivalism brought increased Protestant benevolence into impoverished urban areas in the early 1830s. Missionaries' untiring efforts contributed significantly to raising awareness about health conditions in the urban slums. These dedicated volunteers drew attention to social factors such as unhealthy food, poor housing, bad family life, and unemployment that kept people from escaping the slums. These missionaries formed organizations that became the forerunners of twentieth-century health and social-work institutions (Rosenberg and Rosenberg 1968; Walter 1978, 177–179).

Three individuals—two in New York City, John H. Griscom and Robert Hartley, and one in Boston, Lemmuel Shattuck—became important leaders of public-health reform in the United States. These individuals became involved in sanitation reform "as a result of their response to an intense Pietism widespread in their generation." As with other reformers during the first Clean Living Movement, religious fervor to bring on the millennium was a strong motivating factor (Rosenberg and Rosenberg 1968, 16).

John H. Griscom

John H. Griscom (1809–1874), born in New York City, was the son of a devout Quaker educator. Griscom graduated in 1832 from the University of Pennsylvania School of Medicine. In the late 1830s he became educated in physiology and hygiene out of concern that improving American health conditions hinged strongly on the dissemination of hygiene education. In his view, sickness was not a mysterious retribution from God, but rather the sum product of man's own ignorance of the laws of health; sin and ignorance were indistinguishable. If mankind were to properly utilize fresh air, pure water, and the intelligence granted them by God, disease would be far less frequent (Rosenberg 1976, 109–112). Griscom labored tirelessly in the 1840s to alert his fellow New Yorkers to the need for sanitary reform in the slums. He authored a classic of public health, *The Sanitary Condition of the Laboring Population of New York,* in 1845, based upon the testimony of missionaries of the New York City Tract Society.

Robert M. Hartley

Also active in New York City was a contemporary of Griscom, Robert M. Hartley (1796–1881), a pioneer in tenement and public-health reform. Born in England, Hartley came to the United States as a young child to the "burned-over" district of western New York State and experienced a conversion to evangelical Protestantism as a boy. Like his father, he went into the mercantile business. Soon after moving to New York City, Hartley became active in the Presbyterian Church, assuming leadership in the church's program of house missionary visits in the tenements, where he encountered appalling health conditions (Rosenberg 1976, 117).

Like many other health reformers of the day, Hartley's social activism was rooted in evangelistic pietism, which led to involvement in the temperance movement and then to other health issues. Because of the sickness and misery found in the slums by the tract distributors during home visitations, Hartley and other evangelicals realized that it was unlikely that the "souls of the poor could be saved while their bodies remained in such wretchedness." He began writing about these conditions and, in 1842, organized the New York Association for Improving the Condition of the Poor as an outgrowth of the tract society. This institution was considered America's first prototype social-welfare agency. The association established new medical dispensaries, helped distribute medicines, and opened a public bath and wash house. By 1862, the association's legislative efforts finally yielded a state law regulating the production and sale of milk (Rosenberg 1976, 117–121).

Lemmuel Shattuck

Lemmuel Shattuck (1793–1859), born in Ashby, Massachusetts, was a teacher, historian, book dealer, statistician, and legislator. Unlike other reformers, he was a layman, but had a keen interest in sanitary reform. He gathered, tabulated, and published Boston's vital statistics in 1841. As a result of his persistent criticism regarding the lack of sanitary progress, he was appointed chairman of a legislative committee to study health and sanitary problems in Massachusetts. This so-called "Shattuck Report" reviewed the serious health problems and filthy living conditions of Boston. Its recommendations included a design for a public-health organization, including a state health department and local boards of health in each town. Shattuck provided information for both the present and the future public-health needs of Massachusetts. The report also encouraged public health for the nation as a whole. The Shattuck Report was not fully appreciated for nearly twenty-five years, but it set the stage for twentieth-century public-health reform (Shattuck 1850).

The Demise of Cholera in North America: The First Public-Health Victory

The efforts of these reformers led to the elimination of cholera and other food- and water-borne diseases in the United States. Beginning in the early 1840s, indoor plumbing became increasingly common in both middle-class and upper-class American homes. Many early systems were private and it was not until the 1870s that sewer and water systems began being installed in smaller urban areas. This growth of indoor plumbing was also tied to increased interest in health reform and hygiene (Ogle 1993, 33–58). Purer water supplies and systematic sewage disposal were major factors in preventing "finger, flies, feces and foul water"-borne diseases, such as cholera.

Also contributing to the decline of cholera epidemics was emergence of local health boards. The New York City Metropolitan Board of Health was established in 1866. Sanitary measures quickly contained the spread of the cholera epidemic during this year. This board of health showed that cholera could be prevented—not with prayer and fasting, as had been suggested by religious and political leaders during the first two epidemics, but through concrete steps: disinfection, sanitation, and quarantine. Leaders in other cities called for the creation of health boards like those credited with saving New York. Preventive measures, and not the dubious "cures" of physicians, were seen as a way of improving the health of all Americans (Rosenberg 1976, 204–213).

HEROIC PHYSIC AND ALTERNATIVE CURES

Jacksonian concepts of democracy and the power of the common man led to the rejection of regular physicians. Because "heroic"—so called because of its drastic impact on the patient—or regular medicine was expensive and generally not very effective, natural and folk remedies evolved into a self-help movement of popular alternatives. These alternative methods were often associated with other health-reform ideas, such as hygiene, exercise, fresh air, vegetarian diets, and avoidance of stimulants. Several philosophies, including Thomsonism, homeopathy, and hydrotherapy, developed into popular treatment sects.[7]

Antagonism against Orthodox Medicine

Self-help and alternative treatment philosophies during the first Clean Living Movement emerged due to dissatisfaction with medical care from the regular or orthodox physicians. These practitioners relied on bleeding, blistering, purging, and calomel for almost every disease, including cholera. The average physician of the day often had little formal training. Many were illiterate or did not subscribe to medical journals to keep abreast of new developments. In addition, there was a lack of ethical standards within the profession. In France during the 1830s, statistical evaluation was being perfected and began to demonstrate that the traditional treatments were useless in most cases and injurious in many cases (Rosenberg 1987, 155–157; Whorton 1982, 23). American medical students who went to Paris during this era stopped using the ineffective treatments such as calomel. This brought conflict between old-line regular physicians and their younger colleagues who were more apt to let nature take her course. In addition, the body reformers, who emphasized prevention, challenged orthodox physicians to wrestle with questions of hygiene and to assume a more aggressive stance in health education and prevention (Whorton 1982, 22–23, 129–131).

Popular Medical Reform: Irregular and Unorthodox Cures

Rothstein (1988, 41) suggested that "in the 1820s opposition to heroic therapy coalesced into a social movement of broad public appeal." This popular movement became a major player in the first Clean Living Movement. As regular physicians lost influence, the way was cleared for many medical sects to emerge. The appearance of cholera in 1832, for which the medical profession had no valid remedies, pushed other alternative procedures into the forefront because they were often as successful, or more so, than orthodox medicine (Rothstein 1988, 41–42). New and perceived-safer treatment systems offered by these practitioners became entwined with the physiological reform movement. In addition, self-help or do-it-yourself home-remedy and recipe books became popular and accounted for much of the medical care among poorer Americans. An important part of the alternative therapy regime, and in particular hydrotherapy, was taken from William Alcott and Sylvester Graham (Bush 1981, 48).

Thomsonism

Samuel Thomson (1769–1843) was born in New Hampshire to a farming family. In 1806, he announced a divine call to the role of herb doctor and set about perfecting his system. Thomson's *New Guide to Health or Botanic Family Physician* (1831), first published in 1825, appealed to nonprofessional medical practitioners by confirming their mistrust of orthodox medicine which alienated "physick" from the ordinary person. Thomson also published an autobiography in which he reported how he came upon his various treatments (Thomson 1832, 16).

By emphasizing the use of herbs, Thomson's cures were brought within reach of the average American. The Thomsonian philosophy made every man his own physician, in the spirit of Jacksonian democracy. Advice in Thomson's text included descriptions of his six basic treatments, methods of preparing herbs, the value of internal and external heat, and the importance of perspiration as a treatment for practically all illnesses. One of his cures, using mint to cure indigestion, is still used today (Kenny 1990, 134; Thomson 1831, 38–82).

Thomson achieved national prominence, particularly in the South and the western frontier during the 1820s and 1830s. His medical treatment system attracted millions of Americans and influenced regular medicine indirectly for decades thereafter. Thomsonism gradually shifted from being a social movement of laymen to one dominated by professional healers. The popular appeal of Thomsonism had waned by the 1840s, and some botanic medications began to be integrated into the practices of many regular physicians. By the Civil War, botanic medicine was confined to more isolated and rural communities (Thomson 1825, 162–165; O'Hara 1989, 233; Rothstein 1988, 46–51).

Homeopathy

As Thomsonism and the botanic-cure movement waned, homeopathy rose to national prominence. It appealed primarily to those urban middle- and upper-class individuals who sought an alternative to the harsh treatments of regular medicine. In 1796, the founder of homeopathy, German physician Samuel Hahnemann (1755–1843), revived the Paracelsian doctrine of *similia similibus curantur*. This philosophy supposed that diseases or symptoms are curable by drugs that produce pathological effects on the body similar to those caused by the disease. According to Hahnemann, the effects of the drug could be heightened by giving infinitesimally small doses. In his writings, Hahnemann suggested that his dilutions caused a spiritual effect on the body's "vital forces" and brought the basic essence of health back to its natural state. Disease was considered an alteration in the inner workings of the human organism (Rosenberg 1987, 161; Hahnemann 1983, 1–31; Kaufman 1988, 99–101; Cordasco 1991, xvi–xvii).

Constantine Hering (1800–1880), considered the father of American homeopathy, cofounded a homeopathic medical college in Philadelphia in 1848, which still survives today as the Hahnemann University of the Medical Sciences. Homeopathy reached its peak during the early 1890s, but by 1925 had dramatically declined as allopathic medicine became the accepted doctrine. In the mid-1970s, interest in homeopathy began to increase as part of the late twentieth-century Clean Living Movement. Like other health-reform modalities during the mid-nineteenth century, homeopathy forced orthodox medicine to examine its harsh methods and to change its practices (Cordasco 1991, xix; Hahnemann 1983, 8; Kaufman 1988, 101–103, 123).

Hydropathy: The Water Cure

Hydropathy was developed in the 1820s by Austrian farmer Vincenz Priessnitz (1799–1851), who noticed that the use of cold water cured animals. He also used it to cure himself, and found it so successful he began to treat others. By 1836, Priessnitz had developed a thriving practice. American medical journals published accounts of the therapy throughout the 1830s, although the method, as outlined by Priessnitz, did not begin to be used in the United States until the beginning of the 1840s. Before this time, Americans had extolled the merits of several mineral springs and had always taken water with their meals, unlike Europeans (Legan 1971, 270–271; 1987, 80).

Hydropathy, like homeopathy and phrenology, was imported into the United States from Europe. In the spirit of the Jacksonian reform era, the practice underwent transformation and, like American phrenology, adopted Grahamite physiology and regimen. Water-cure therapy was more than just a healing art, because it offered a vision of human perfectibility. Its underlying principle was the advancement of individuals, and society as a whole, through health, as was the case among most reformers during the first Clean Living Movement. At the height of its appeal, from 1840 to 1870, more than 200 live-in hydropathic cure establishments were found throughout the United States (Legan 1987, 80; Walters 1978, 153; Nissenbaum 1980, 149–150; Cayleff 1988, 83).

Treatment at a hydropathic institute encompassed not only drinking and bathing in cold water, but also exercise and massage accompanied by sweating. Because of several treatments a day, women patients generally wore the American costume of a short skirt over pants and hair cut short for easy drying. This American costume, similar to the Bloomer outfit, was developed by Harriet N. Austin, codirector of the Dansville, New York, treatment center (Legan 1971, 268–269, 274–277).

Five individuals proved to be most responsible for the expansion and popularity of hydropathy in the United States: Joel Shew, James Jackson, Russell T. Trall, and Mary and Thomas Nichols.[8] All held "medical" degrees from either eclectic or regular medical colleges, were involved with lecturing, wrote texts and tracts, and established water-cure institutions. They integrated other health-reform issues of the day into hydropathy, including Grahamism, temperance, dress reform, and, to some extent, phrenology and eugenics.

Joel Shew

Joel Shew (1816–1855), born in Saratoga County, New York, was a regular physician who made at least two visits to Austria to study the Priessnitz system. In 1844, he opened the first water-cure institution in New York City. The clinic emphasized a Graham diet, including the elimination of alcohol, tobacco, and other stimulants and spices. Bathing, exercise, and massage were promoted. In December 1845, Shew launched *The Water-Cure Journal and Herald of Reforms*, which had a subscription list of 50,000 shortly after 1850. It became the literary vehicle of many mid-century health reformers and featured contributions by most of the well-known health leaders of the day (Numbers 1976, 64; Reid 1982, 80–81; Nissenbaum 1980, 149; Mott 1930, 441).[9]

Russell T. Trall

Russell T. Trall (1812–1877), a medical physician, began to practice in New York City in 1840. He came to water cure from the temperance movement. Trall opened the second water-cure establishment in America the same year as Shew and expanded the system to include a regimen of diet, exercise, and sleep. When the Nicholses abandoned their water-cure training institute, Trall opened his own hydropathic school in New York, which received its charter in 1857. This college, like that of the Nicholses, was open to both sexes. It quickly became the water-cure center of the United States, and Trall himself became the most known figure in the movement after Shew's death. One of the original faculty members at Trall's college was Lorenzo Fowler, a lecturer on phrenology and mental science, whose presence symbolized the close union between health reformers and phrenologists. A former student at this institute was John Harvey Kellogg, the most influential physician of the Adventist health program and brother of W. K. Kellogg of cereal fame, personifying the link between hydropathy,

Grahamism, and Seventh-Day Adventists (Numbers 1976, 67; Nissenbaum 1980, 149–151; Whorton 1982, 138–139).

Mary Gove Nichols and Thomas Low Nichols

Mary Sargent Neal Gove Nichols (1810–1884), born in Goffstown, New Hampshire, became a Quaker as a teenager. She ran a Graham boarding house and was one of the first female lecturers of anatomy and physiology in Boston. Even before she became a Grahamite, she practiced hydrotherapy on herself and daughter in the early 1830s. Both Whorton (1982, 137) and Walters (1978, 154) credit her for the merger of hydropathy and Grahamism. Overwork aggravated her consumption condition, and in 1844 she found water cure helpful in her own recuperation. In the spring of 1846, she opened a water-cure center in competition with Shew and Trall (Numbers 1976, 65; Blake 1962, 219–234; Malone 1957, 495).

In 1851, Mary and her second husband, Thomas Low Nichols, launched a water-cure school to meet the burgeoning demand for trained hydropaths. Thomas Low Nichols (1815–1901), born in Orford, New Hampshire, was both a regular physician and a journalist. He was a prominent author and lecturer, who also helped further the causes of water cure and other health reforms. Nichols was particularly concerned about prevention of disease through good living habits, as opposed to physician-directed cures and the surrendering of one's judgment and body. After three successful terms teaching budding hydrotherapists, the Nicholses lost interest in their educational venture and drifted in the direction of "free-love" and spiritualism (Malone 1957, 496; Cayleff 1988, 89; Legan 1987, 82).

James C. Jackson

James C. Jackson (1811–1895), born in Manlius, New York, and a graduate of an eclectic medical college in Syracuse, New York, was an active temperance and abolition speaker. After being a patient in 1847 at a water-cure center in New York, where his health was restored, he collaborated with Dr. Harriet Austin, an alumna of Mary Gove Nichols's hydropathic school. After several false starts, they established "Our Home," a very popular center frequented by many health reformers, in Dansville, New York. Jackson developed "granula," the pioneer dry breakfast cereal in 1863 which was copied in 1878 by John Harvey Kellogg and became known as "granola." He wrote numerous tracts and books concerning diet, temperance, tobacco use, and sexuality (Numbers 1976, 72–73; Nissenbaum 1980, 151–153).

Hydropathy, more than the other alternative therapies, integrated most of the other health reforms of the era. Like the other alternative medicines, it stressed self-responsibility for personal health care, including diet and exercise. Hydrotherapists can be viewed as early health educators, since they promoted prevention through altered living habits, as opposed to physician-directed cures.

SUMMARY

Sanitation reform was a positive continuation of Protestant religious commitments and not simply a reaction against unbearably filthy immigrant environments. Nativistic fears of immigrant diseases, including the deadly new Asiatic cholera, spilling into middle-class areas and eugenic concerns of further racial degeneration due to ill health and intemperance among this population led to reforms. Because regular, orthodox physicians were not always successful in treating most diseases, various alternative treatments and cures, including botanic medicine and hydropathy, which was linked to Grahamism and other reform issues, arose in this era of the common man.

NOTES

1. See the following sources for more information regarding connections between Protestant revivalism, anti-immigration, anti-Catholicism, temperance, and the rise of Nativist sentiments: Billington (1974, 527–528), Carwardine (1978, 18, 44–45, 50–53), Gienapp (1987, 45, 98), Johnson (1978, 128–136), and Rosenberg (1987, 135–142). See, in particular, the article by Robert Wernick (1996), which gives a thorough summary of the influences of Roman Catholic immigration on the rise of the Know Nothing Party.

2. In 1850, the secret Order of the Star-Spangled Banner was formed. It was taken over a few years later by the Order of United Americans. Only Protestant males, born and raised by Protestants, were allowed entry. This order began to establish a network of secret lodges in the East and Midwest. By early 1855, there may have been over a million members nationwide. New members to this secret society took an oath never to divulge to outsiders what went on inside. According to legend, they were instructed to reply to prying questions by saying, "I know nothing." As they began to gain political power and formed the American Party in 1854, they became known as the Know Nothing Party (Wernick 1996, 152).

3. The reason the lower classes, with different cultural values, were perceived as a threat to the dominant "civilized" social groups was that it was thought that these demographic factors were inherited.

4. A description of the filth of the urban areas in the 1830s comes from a summary of Graham's lectures by anonymous editors. "Should we stroll through the streets and alleys of our large cities, and visit the tenements of their inhabitants, we would be surprised to find that many of them were such

receptacles of filth. In passing through the various avenues of a city, the nostrils are offended with the putrid emanations from decayed animal matter, the noxious exhalations from decomposed vegetable substances, the insufferable effluvium of slaughter-houses, and the floating particles of matter that fill the air from innumerable manufactories. . . . The purity of the atmosphere being thus impaired, is it surprising that the small-pox, and the typhus and yellow fevers, whose very existence owe their origin to filth, should have become so prevalent among mankind?" (*Defense* 1835, 189–190).

5. In 1883, Robert Koch isolated the organism that causes cholera. This food- and water-borne disease was spread by unwashed hands, uncooked fruits and vegetables, and sewage-contaminated water supplies. It never became endemic in North America, because sanitation and public-health measures began to be instituted.

6. A classic study for students of epidemiology is still John Snow's (1849) *On the Mode of Communication of Cholera*. During the epidemic of 1854, Snow (1813–1858), a London physician, demonstrated that cholera was spread by contaminated water and unwashed hands. In his writings, he suggested its cause was not miasmic air, but rather "the emptying of sewers into the drinking water of the community." To prevent cholera, Snow recommends, "It would only be necessary for all persons attending or waiting on the patient to wash their hands carefully and frequently, never omitting to do so before touching food, and for everybody to avoid drinking, or using for culinary purposes, water into which drains and sewers empty themselves; or, if that cannot be accomplished, to have the water filtered and well boiled before it is used" (p. 30).

7. Numerous works have addressed the popular alternative and unorthodox medical movements during the mid-nineteenth century. See, in particular, Cayleff (1988), Dosch (1993), Gevitz (1988), Greene (1986), Kaufman (1988), Rosenberg (1976), Rothstein (1988), Walters (1978), and Whorton (1988). See Kett (1968) and Shyrock (1960) for information concerning the evolution of the regular medical profession during this era.

8. Not all contemporary authors agree on who were the most influential people responsible for introducing and expanding hydropathy in mid-nineteenth-century America. Legan (1987, 81) suggested the "Big Four" were Shew, Trall, and the Nicholses. Numbers (1976, 64) names Shew, Trall, and Mary Nichols, and Reid (1982, 80) suggested that Shew, Jackson, and Trall were the most important for the developing Seventh-Day Adventist health philosophy.

9. For most of its life during this era, it was published by Fowlers and Wells. During the height of the second Clean Living Movement in the progressive era, it merged with *Physical Culture*.

PART II

The Second Clean Living Movement, 1880–1920

> The first fifteen years of the twentieth century may sometime be remembered in America as the Age of Crusades. There were a superabundance of zeal, a sufficiency of good causes, unusual moral idealism, excessive confidence in mass movements, and leaders with rare gifts of popular appeal. The people were ready to cry "God wills it" and set out for world peace, prohibition. . . . It was a brave time in which to be alive.
>
> Gaius Glenn Atkins, *Religion in Our Times* (1932)

> The mania for prohibitions in one form or another is a country-wide disease. It is an affliction to which the busybodies of both sexes are particularly subject. The spread of this disease and the succumbing to it of our law-makers is the chief cause of lawlessness in this country to-day. An organized minority takes advantage of the indifference of the majority, and browbeats spineless legislators into writing into law prohibitions that are in defiance of the will of the majority.
>
> Utah's "No Smoking" Signs, *Literary Digest* (1923)

The third Great Awakening emerged approximately eighty years after the inception of the earlier nineteenth-century revitalization. This religious and populist awakening was driven by concerns similar to those of the Jacksonian and late twentieth-century reform eras. During the last three decades of the nineteenth century, rapid urbanization, immigration, and industrial expansion dramatically changed American society (Gould 1974, 1–5, 18; Hofstadter 1986, 1–2; De Witt 1968, 14–15).

In the wake of these profound changes, health and social problems began to mount. A perception of increased drunkenness, crime, and vice flowing out of the saloon in both large urban areas and smaller communities began to be considered a major health and social problem. Air pollution, the breakdown of sewage and garbage facilities in urban areas, and rising incidents of tuberculosis stirred concerns about the degeneration of health. Diseases resulting from adulterated food, patent medicines, tobacco, and narcotics became serious health issues among middle-class Americans.

By the last two decades of the nineteenth century, many "old-stock" Americans feared that their historic rural traditions were being destroyed by gigantic combinations of economic and political powers. They longed to bring America back to a mythical golden age and at the same time wanted to break with the past in a forward-looking philosophy, or progressivism (Pollack 1962, 2). These populist sentiments peaked in 1896 and became an important conduit for many programs embraced by the Progressive Movement and enacted into law during the first two decades of the twentieth century (Gould 1974, 19; Handy 1966, 3; Hofstadter 1959a, 4–5; Mann 1963, 2–3).[1]

The second Clean Living Movement peaked in the decade before and the decade after 1910. The numerous crusades that made up the movement embraced a variety of issues on local, state, and national levels. Similar to the Jacksonian and the late twentieth-century millennial reform eras, the populist–progressive period was made up of many single-issue crusades. In the 1870s, prohibition, suffrage, and "purity" agitation began before the main thrust of other health and social reforms. The anticigarette movement began in the early 1890s. The Eugenics Movement grew in intensity from the late 1870s and reached maturity during the first two decades of the twentieth century. Fundamentalism and nativistic (pro-traditional American culture) undercurrents were integral to some of these crusades. Physical culture, birth control, diet, and the concept of the "whole man" began to be emphasized, beginning in the mid-1890s. A crusade to regulate food, patent medicines, and the elimination of "narcotic addictions" arose in the first two decades of the twentieth century. Public-health reforms, such as sanitation, and crusades against specific diseases, such as tuberculosis, gained momentum during the first decade of the century. All these issues together cumulated in one of the most widespread reform eras in the history of the nation.

NOTE

1. The origins of the Populist and Progressive movements and the influences of populism upon progressivism are complex. Further reading on the various reform impulses spanning the period from approximately 1880 until 1920 can be found in numerous works. See, in particular, De Witt (1968), Ekrich (1974), Gould (1974), Hicks (1931), Hofstadter (1959a, 1986), Mann (1963), Pollack (1962, 1967), and Timberlake (1963).

7

Religious Zeal,
Physical Culture, and Diet

The last thirty years, though as dates go this is only an approxima-
tion, have witnessed a marked development of religious cults and
movements largely outside the lines of historic Catholicism and
Protestantism.

Gaius Glenn Atkins,
Modern Religious Cults and Movements (1923)

History . . . reveals that every great religious revival which has
swept over a whole country is usually followed by attempts at
social reformation.

Thomas M. Lindsay, *Contemporary Review* (1905)

In harmony of any kind involves weakness and suffering,—a loss
of control over the body. The depraved appetite for alcoholic drinks,
tobacco, tea, coffee, opium, is destroyed only by Mind's mastery
of the body.

Mary Baker Eddy,
Science and Health with Keys to the Scriptures (1906)

The demand of the public for better health, public and individual,
more bodily vigor and power, is on us, and surely it is for us to
recognize it in the Athletic Age.

Edward Hitchcock, Jr., *Outlook* (1895)

The third Great Awakening of religious enthusiasm stirred in the last
decades of the nineteenth century. The Social Gospel movement among
liberal religious groups and the fundamentalist movement among more
conservative Christians influenced health reforms. This revivalist en-

thusiasm encouraged new religious philosophies, alternative cures, and a "physical culture" movement. Some factions had eugenic and nativistic undertones or opposed the use of alcohol and tobacco. As was found in the Jacksonian and millennium period, a wave of health and social reforms resulted in its wake. Many reformers of the second Clean Living Movement had deep religious convictions which they funneled into health crusades. Accompanying this general revivalist enthusiasm was a growth in the YMCA and increased concern for diet and physical fitness. By the 1920s, religious enthusiasm was on the wane, along with most other health-reform crusades.

SOCIAL GOSPEL, NEW RELIGIONS, AND FUNDAMENTALISM

The religious awakening was composed of three factions: the Social Gospel movement, fundamentalist evangelical crusades, and the emergence of mental-healing faiths. In terms of health, Social Gospelists were concerned with urban conditions, temperance, and purity; evangelicals adamantly opposed alcohol; and new-thought religions shunned traditional medicine and advocated mental healing. "Muscular Christianity," "men's brotherhoods," and the increased involvement of the YMCA in physical culture, purity, and alcohol and tobacco reform developed as part of this movement.

The Social Gospel Movement

The Social Gospel movement, a religious social-reform movement prominent from about 1870 to 1920, reached its peak during the first two decades of the twentieth century.[1] This progressive crusade was found among mainstream Protestant religions (Methodists, Presbyterians, Episcopalians, Lutherans, Congregationalists, among others). Social gospelists as a whole were native born middle-class Americans of Anglo-Saxon heritage. Many were active in the Republican Party and were concerned with the many social problems spawned by massive immigration and rapid urbanization (Reichley 1992, 187; Atkins 1923, 156; Handy 1966, 3–4; Pittman and Snyder 1962, 109).

This Social Gospel movement was dedicated to the betterment of industrialized society through application of the biblical principles of charity and justice for workers. A shorter work week, child-labor laws, women's suffrage, temperance, and purity reform were championed by individuals associated with this religious revival. Churches and reform organizations aligned with religious groups exerted direct political action, which helped spur passage of legislation against gambling, lotteries, prostitution, alcohol, vice, and the saloon. The movement also included the growth of "Muscular Christianity," a form of social gospel that affirmed the compatibility of robust physical life with a Christian life of morality and service. The term was coined in 1851 by British writer Thomas Hughes, who developed the notion of a link between athletic involvement and moral development (Philips 1996, 121; Whorton 1982, 271; Haley 1978, 107–109, 214–215; Hopkins 1961, 7, 11–12; Handy 1966, 3–4).

Muscular Christianity: The Men's Movement and the YMCA

By the 1880s, women had become the mainstay of Protestantism and the church had allegedly become "feminized" by the Victorian "cult of domesticity." Ministers were beginning to be stereotyped as "sissy fellows," which church leaders perceived kept men away from the church. Men were joining fraternal lodges, such as the Masons, which offered ritual celebration of male virtues and the affirmation of a male-focused spirituality. Churches saw themselves competing with lodges for men's alliance and respect. Out of this concern came church-related brotherhoods and character-building programs within the YMCA, which personified the ideals of Muscular Christianity and manliness. In addition, men were becoming increasingly engaged in sedentary office positions which did not offer the same opportunity for exercise as farm or factory work. Alarmed by the prospect of a weakening of the old-stock middle class in contrast to more muscular immigrant laborers, many reformers hurried to endorse artificial exercise. Theodore Roosevelt became a model of the progressive mood for action and change, and coined the term for this more vigorous lifestyle as "the strenuous life" (Putney 1994a, 451–459; 1994b, 4–7, 59–60; 1991, 50, 58–59).

Church Brotherhood Movement. The church brotherhood movement was an effort to recruit men back into the church through creation of men-only societies. Foremost among these were the lay denominational brotherhood organizations that flourished within mainline Protestant churches from early 1880 until World War I (Putney 1994a, 459). One of the most noted crusades was the interdenominational Men and Religion Forward Movement (1911–1912), a nationwide evangelical campaign devoted to Christian idealism and human concerns. It was initiated by the YMCA and aided by various denominational brotherhoods. This crusade increased church attendance and membership and is considered by Clifford Putney (1994a, 466), a historian of Muscular Christianity, as the high-water mark of the brotherhood movement. Some of the aspects of the men's movement appeared to be echoed in the Promise Keeper's stadium crusades of the 1990s.

The YMCA. The YMCA, a parareligious Protestant organization, was imported from Britain in 1851. In the United States, it reached a peak of influence during the progressive era and carried out the philosophy of the Social Gospel movement. It was an important organizational link with many health reforms and philosophies during the second Clean Living Movement. The "Y" offered a place to hold meetings and provided speakers and tracts for various health reforms of the time.

In its early years, the YMCA offered young men, regardless of ethnic or class background, an alternative to the saloon. During the 1870s and 1880s, when social Darwinism (survival of the fittest, to be discussed in Chapter 9) and nativistic concerns began to influence its philosophy, its leaders increasingly focused on native-born middle-class Protestant youth who migrated from the rural areas to the cities, in an effort to save them from vice. The Y provided activities, such as libraries and prayer meetings, as a means to convert young men to Christianity and to exert social control over their lifestyles (Miller and Fielding 1995, 79; Putney 1991, 51–56; Calkins 1901, 143–145).

In order to attract and hold the interest of young men, the Y experimented with other activities and gradually began to incorporate sports and physical fitness into its mission. It increasingly embraced Muscular Christianity and the concept of "the whole man" (Miller and Fielding 1995, 78; Putney 1991, 49–53, 56–59). The YMCA had links to several health crusades, and it exerted a formative role in antiobscenity laws. The association sponsored the White Cross Societies of the purity movement, a crusade which promoted a single sexual standard and offered its facilities for educational programs about good health habits and the prevention of tuberculosis (Bates 1995, 255; Pivar 1973, 114). The Y was stridently antialcohol and was involved in both the temperance and the anticigarette campaigns (Tate 1995, 144–147). During the backlash era of the 1920s, decreased interest was shown in the Muscular Christian philosophy, and as a result its membership and activities began to decline, only to blossom again in the 1970s with the late twentieth-century fitness craze.

New Thought Religions and Alternative Cures

As part of the religious revival movement there was the emergence of new religious systems based upon eastern philosophies and mental healing. Gaius Glenn Atkins (1923, 283), in this era, suggested, "There was actually, between 1890 and 1930, more radical and creative religious experimentation than, very likely, since the first three Christian centuries. These experiments include between them about every imaginable and some unimaginable aspects of faith, conduct, and speculation" (Atkins 1923, 283). Religions based upon "esoteric wisdom from the east," including "Theosophy," Baha'i, and the Vedanta Society, emerged. Spiritualism, founded earlier, began to gain followers, and mysticism developed interest. Some mind-cure faiths became therapeutic movements for curing illness outside regular medical practice (Atkins 1923, 121–122; Hudson 1965, 286–287). Growth of novel religious and healing philosophies also occurred in the Jacksonian and the late twentieth-century reform era.

The inspiration for many new mental-cure systems was personified by Phineas Parkhurst Quimby (1802–1866) of Portland, Maine. After the Civil War, Quimby became intrigued by the therapeutic power of mesmerism, or hypnotism. Quimby became convinced that disease could be cured by cultivating positive thoughts instead of negative ones. He created a method to cure diseases based on his own cure by using mental imaging, and began healing others with his system (Hudson 1965, 286–287). Quimby's ideas spawned the development of several mind-cure systems under the general philosophy of "New Thought."[2] New Thought was "an attitude of mind, not a cult" (Atkins 1923, 210). The term "mental science" began to be used in about 1882 for mind cure and systems developed using this mental science. Unity was founded in Kansas City around 1887 by Charles (1854–1948) and Myrtle Fillmore (1845–1931). The Emanuel movement, a mental-healing ministry, was founded in the Boston Emanuel Episcopal Church in 1906, by Elwood Worcester (1862–1940). This movement included mind cure within an established denomination (Atkins, 1923, 112–117; Hudson 1965, 286–290).

The New-Thought movement reflected the positive feelings of the progressive era. New Thought preached that every good thing was possible through God and that negative ideas should be replaced by positive "affirmations" or thoughts (Atkins 1923, 296–297). In this era, there was also an increased interest in the "pseudosciences." "There was a widespread rebirth of faith in astrology. Men of affairs had their horoscopes read and asked permission of the stars to conduct their enterprises" (Atkins 1923, 305–306). This interest also surged in the late twentieth-century New Age movement. The most known of the New-Thought groups was Christian Science, founded by Mary Baker Eddy.

Mary Baker Eddy

Mary Baker Eddy (1821–1910) was born near Concord, New Hampshire, to a family of intensely religious Congregationalists from old-stock New Englanders.[3] Eddy was a sickly child, who as an adult was cured by the method developed by Quimby. After Quimby's death in 1866, she suffered a severe fall but healed herself and discovered the principle that underlies Christian Science, which Horatio Dresser (1919, 120–125) suggested was an adaptation of Quimby's system. She began to lecture about her experience and gathered a small group of followers in the Boston area. She married one follower, Asa Eddy, in 1877.

Christian Science can be considered an alternative health system and as such did "not draw a sharp line or distinction between mental and physical illness" (Peel 1988, 65). The First Church of Christ, Scientist, was organized in Boston in 1879 and the belief system began to grow (Atkins 1923, 289). In 1908, Eddy founded the *Christian Science Monitor*, which established a reputation as one of the country's leading daily newspapers and before she "passed on" (as the concept of death was phrased), she revised her 1875 book as *Science and Health with Key to the Scriptures*, which her followers regarded as divinely inspired. This work and the Bible formed the scriptures of this new faith.

As a religion and alternative healing system, Christian Science posed a threat to both mainstream religion and orthodox medicine. Both supporters and detractors wrote about it during the first decade of the century. Typical is a March 1907 article in *Current Literature*, titled, "Are We Standing at the Birth of a Great Religion?" Christian Science reached its peak in influence and popularity in the 1920s. It remained an active denomination throughout the twentieth century.

Evangelical Fundamentalists

The lower classes and uneducated, primarily in the southern and western states, began to fear the rapid social and theological changes taking place in the nation. Reaction to the upheavals caused by transition from a rural to an industrial society—modernism—was a factor in a rising evangelical revivalist movement during the two decades on either side of the turn of the twentieth century. This crusade had Nativist undercurrents and gave support to some health-reform movements. Members of this loosely connected movement tended to be the rural poor. Their leaders often clashed with the more staid middle-class mainstream denominations (Quebedeaux 1983, 23–24; Marsden 1983, 151–152; 1991, 42; Atkins 1923, 172). The middle class, for the most part, looked down upon these revivalists.

Three factions made up the fundamentalist revivalist movement.[4] In the last two decades of the nineteenth century, "Holiness revivals," seeking perfection in the Methodist tradition, led to the formation of a number of new Holiness denominations such as the Pilgrims Holiness church, the Salvation Army (from England), and the Nazarenes. Holiness groups tended to win converts among immigrants and the working class. During the first decade of the new century, Pentecostalism emerged. Pentecostal denominations emphasized supernatural experiences such as "speaking in tongues" and faith healing and tended to attract converts from among the very poor. The third group was "dispensational" fundamentalism, arising from a Baptist tradition. It stressed the necessity of adhering to the right doctrine, "the fundamentals," and the importance of organizing against modern and worldly trends (Anderson 1979, 49–54, 60–61, 188–191; Atkins 1923, x; Marsden 1991, 39–44; Quebedeaux 1983, 24–25).

Although these more conservative religious groups had doctrinal differences and often did not agree, they shared common traits. They all opposed modernity—what today is often called "secular humanism." They emphasized the central evangelical doctrines of the complete authority of the Bible, the necessity of a conversion experience, and the importance of a "holy life," freed particularly from "barroom vices such as drinking, dancing, card-playing, and lasciviousness" (Marsden 1983, 152). These factions coalesced as a distinct interdenominational movement after World War I to fight modernism. By the 1920s, fundamentalism had become associated with revivals, "camp meetings," mass conversions, and Bible schools (Marsden 1991, 31; Philips 1996, xv; Quebedeaux 1983, 24).

Fundamentalist and more liberal mainstream churches converged in agreement upon one issue: temperance. Fundamentalists strongly supported the Prohibition crusade (see Chapter 8). Atkins (1923, 21), for example, at the end of the era, perhaps overstated the influence of the fundamentalists when he remarked that revivalist Billy Sunday's "hatred for alcohol and the saloon . . . had much to do with making America 'dry.'" Sunday (1862–1935), the best known evangelist in the first third of the twentieth century, started his career as a baseball player. He introduced theatrics into revival meetings, including acrobatics, colored lights, and music. He was also in sympathy with Nativism (Lender 1984, 475–476).

Media attention to the movement began to wane after the renowned Scopes trial involving prosecution of a Tennessee school teacher for teaching Darwinian evolution, and after the death of William Jennings Bryan (1860–1925), the intellectual firebrand of the movement. Fundamentalism began to emerge again as a political force in the last decades of the century at the beginning of the third Clean Living Movement.

PHYSICAL CULTURE, DIET, AND NUTRITION

The more liberal religious revivalist and the Muscular Christianity movements spawned a physical-culture crusade that embraced physical fitness, sports, hygiene, and diet. This progressive hygienic movement, like Muscular Christianity, embraced the philosophy of the "whole man." The physical-culture movement was in part the child of Protestant revival enthusiasm; being physically fit became associated with being morally fit.

The Dawn of the Physical-Culture Movement

During the first Clean Living Movement (see Chapter 4), reformers championed physical fitness and exercise, but the concept was not popular. Dudley Sargent (1849–1924), a physician and gymnastic instructor, reviewed the history of the movement in the January 2, 1901 *Harper's Weekly*. He suggested that in 1848, at the waning of the first movement, a large number of Germans emigrated to the United States. They soon began to establish gymnastic—*turner*—societies in major cities and regions to which they migrated, such as the Midwest. The influx of these immigrants resulted in some interest in gymnastics. In 1856, Catherine Beecher published *A Manual of Physiology and Calisthenics for Schools and Families,* which aroused increased attention among the middle class for light exercises in homes and schools. In 1860, Dio Lewis, one of the founders of the physical-culture movement, introduced to the public the "New Gymnastics," consisting of exercises with wooden wands, dumbbells, and Indian clubs accompanied with music. This system aroused considerable enthusiasm for lighter gymnastics. In the meantime, advocates of heavier and more muscular forms of German-style gymnastics were beginning to assert themselves in colleges (Sargent 1901, 81). After the Civil War, there was a rise of interest in both gymnastics and sports. This interest dramatically increased in the 1880s, and became an integral facet of the second Clean Living Movement.

Dio Lewis

Dioclecian Lewis (1823–1888), a pioneer in physical culture and a temperance reformer, was born near Auburn, New York, to a farming family. His life and influence illustrated the link between the temperance, suffrage, and physical-culture crusades at the end of the first and the inception of the second Clean Living Movements. He practiced homeopathic medicine a short time in the late 1840s and early 1850s, but gave up treatment for prevention. In 1856, Lewis traveled to Europe to study German and Swedish gymnastics and became convinced that these activities offered Americans their best chance for health (Malone 1957, 209; Whorton 1982, 275–276).[5] During the 1850s, Lewis delivered lectures on physiology to young women. In 1861, he founded the Boston Normal Institute for Physical Education, the first physical-education teachers training institution in the nation. About a half of his students were women. In 1862, he published his most important book, *New Gymnastics,* and two years later started a school for young women in Lexington, Massachusetts, where fitness activities were mandatory (Lender 1984, 295–296; Whorton 1982, 277–280).

Similar to other health reformers, Lewis advocated "sunshine, fresh air, exercise, cleanliness, much sleep, cheerful scenery, and a wise diet" (Lewis 1871, 246). Unlike other reformers, he was not a vegetarian. Lewis championed temperance, suffrage, equal pay for equal work, and nontraditional occupations for women, such as a physician, attorney, and health educator. On his 1873 lecture tour, he sparked the women's temperance movement, discussed in Chapter 8 (Whorton 1982, 275; Blocker 1989, 1–11).

The Upswing of Physical Culture

The physical education, fitness, and personal-hygiene aspects of the second Clean Living Movement had their roots in the 1880s. By the 1920s, like most other issues of the progressive era, these concerns began to wane. Several well-known physical-education specialists of the time took note of the fitness movement. Sargent (1901) pointed out that "popular interest in bicycling, football, and golf [had] increased" during the 1890s. Luther H. Gulick (1908, 10383) contended that varying health reforms of the era were reformist manifestations of the same "physical well-being pulse." As evidence of the growing fitness movement, Gulick cited the tripled increase in YMCA attendance during the previous ten years, construction of free public gymnasiums, and the introduction of athletics into colleges and public schools. Evidence of a general health movement included national concern for sanitation and disease, passage of pure-food laws, wide interest in the "problems of diet," and "the popularity of 'health foods' and required hygiene classes in the public schools." Gulick was wise enough to know, however, that the movement and public interest in health and fitness would wane. Therefore, he recommended that changes be instituted while the movement was still at its peak. He suggested that the nation establish a national bureau of health, government-sponsored school health services, eugenics measures to ensure the rearing of healthy children, and temperance legislation.

The Physical-Education Movement:
Edward Hitchcock and Dudley Sargent

A result of the physical-culture movement was the incorporation of physical education and hygiene as a required part of school and college curricula. In 1861, Edward Hitchcock (1828–1911), a physician and son of the "Dyspepsia-forestalled" Edward Hitchock (Chapter 4), became the first hygiene and physical-education professor in the country. He held this position at Amherst College for fifty years. Hitchcock considered good health a duty to God and a prerequisite for effective

Christian service. Hitchcock was instrumental in founding the Association for the Advancement of Physical Education in 1885. This organization became the American Alliance for Health, Physical Education,
Recreation and Dance which is still the primary professional organization in this field at the beginning of the twenty-first century (Lee
and Bennett 1960, 35, 122; Whorton 1982, 283).

In 1879, Dudley Sargent became the second physical-education professor in the country, at Harvard University. In 1880, based upon several exercise systems and the philosophy of Muscular Christianity,
Sargent developed a new gymnasium, exercise equipment, and program of physical activities. It was not until the development of
Sargent's physical-education program that a concern for exercise and
physical culture became a national movement (Whorton 1982, 285; Lee
and Bennett 1960, 28–29).[6]

The concept of the whole man, which included a sound, or healthy,
mind in a sound body (*mens sana in encopore sano*), became an important concept for overall health, both in the school physical-education
and the popularized physical-culture movements. This concept was
also linked with the eugenics movement (see Chapter 9), and Sargent
was also a participant in this issue. Besides academic physical education,
Sargent (1901) reported in *Harper's Weekly* that an "era of gymnasium
building throughout the country [at] . . . Young Men's Christian Associations, city athletic clubs, sanitariums, hospitals, armories, military
posts, etc" had begun. In 1881, Sargent founded a physical-education
"normal" (teacher's training) school, still in existence today, to meet
the demand for teachers of physical education.

The Bicycle Craze

The "safety bicycle," with two wheels the same size, appeared on
the American scene in the late 1880s and became a craze by the 1890s.
These bicycles were expensive and owned mostly by the middle class.
The wheel was considered good for health inasmuch as exercise in the
open air was deemed particularly beneficial. Bike riding was also considered a cure for many diseases (Whorton 1982, 294, 307–322; Greene
1986, 228–232).

The main contribution of the bicycle, besides exercise, was to encourage women to discard the corset for more suitable clothing for
comfort and safety. Some critics branded women cyclists as "suffrag-
ettes" or immodest for wearing the Bloomer-type outfits (Whorton
1982, 319–330). Sargent, in his 1901 *Harper's Weekly* article, noted that
bicycling as an exercise was on the wane. James Whorton (1982, 330),
the fitness historian, implied that a reason for this may have been that
the bicycle provided independent speed and mobility. It uncovered a

taste for rapid private transit that eventually was supplanted by the emerging motor car.

The Popularization of Physical Culture

By the first decade of the century, physical culture included more than just exercise and gymnastics. It was a combination of proper eating, drinking, breathing, exercise, posture, rest, and cleanliness. By the end of the nineteenth century, the physical culture movement had developed two aspects. Besides athletics, sports, and exercise, supported by trained physical educators and organizations such as the YMCA, it had also become a crusade of self-appointed "health-conscious zealots outside the physical education ranks" (Whorton 1982, 295).[7] One of the most conspicuous and colorful health reformers in the popularization of physical culture was Bernarr Macfadden.

Bernarr Macfadden

Originally named Bernard A. MacFadden (1868–1955), he was born near Mill Springs, Missouri, to an alcoholic father and tubercular mother and orphaned at an early age.[8] Macfadden was an underfed and sickly child. To gain health, as a teenager, Macfadden began to work with dumbbells. He became a wrestler and coach and changed his name to Bernarr Macfadden because he thought it sounded more powerful. By the 1890s, he had embraced physical culture as a preventive health doctrine and began to teach muscle building as a self-taught physical culturist. Macfadden invented exercise equipment, opened his own gymnasium in New York City, and, in 1899, launched a popular magazine, *Physical Culture*, devoted to exercise and bodybuilding. Its motto was, "Weakness is a crime; don't be a criminal" (Ernst 1991, 1–12, 21; Maxcy and Todd 1987, 155–161; see also *New York Times*, October 13, 1955). As a health reformer, Macfadden popularized exercise and diet much in the same way as did Sylvester Graham in the first and Richard Simmons and Jane Fonda in the third Clean Living Movements. Macfadden championed diets of whole grains, raw vegetables, salads, and fruits and nuts, rejected alcohol, and denounced tobacco. By 1935, Macfadden headed a giant magazine empire aimed at the mass market of nonliterary readers (Ernst 1991, xi, 15, 21; see also *New York Times*, October 13, 1955).

Unlike Sylvester Graham, Macfadden was an advocate of sexuality and became a proponent of a healthy sexuality. Macfadden, like many other reformers of the time, supported both the birth control and eugenics movements and had concerns about the "immigrant threat." Macfadden married four times, sired a "physical culture family," and had many sexual partners throughout his lifetime. He died at the age of eighty-five from complications stemming from a round of fasting (Whorton 1982, 298–301; Greene 1986, 246–255; Maxcy and Todd 1987, 182–183).

Diet and Nutrition

An integral aspect of physical culture was concern over diet and nutrition. Increased interest in vegetarianism and diet emerged in the 1880s, reached its peak in the first decade of the twentieth century, and began to wane after 1910. Whorton (1981a, 73) contended that "the Progressive decades were in fact richer in unconventional systems of nutrition than any other period of American history." Sports and athletics were closely related to diet and it was thought that a high-meat diet was important for physical progress. Vegetarians were considered by many health enthusiasts to be poor athletes (Whorton 1981a, 61).

Vegetarianism, championed by Sylvester Graham and William Alcott during the first Clean Living Movement, reemerged in the 1890s. Vegetarian enthusiasts attempted to vindicate their diet, claiming it was better than a meat diet for athletes, based upon the results of athletic contests (Whorton 1981a, 61–64; 1981b, 81). For example, the June 10, 1893 *Spectator* reported that the first two finishers in a walking race from Berlin to Vienna were vegetarians. Many health reformers crusaded for vegetarianism with religious zeal. John Harvey Kellogg, along with Macfadden, became a leader of this "muscular vegetarianism," and Horace Fletcher developed another system of dietary reform.[9]

Diet Reform: John Harvey Kellogg and Horace Fletcher

Kellogg and Fletcher, who were friends and supported each other's nutrition and health systems, were as well known as Macfadden during their lifetimes.[10] John Harvey Kellogg (1851–1943), born in Tyrone Township, Missouri, the son of a devout Seventh-Day Adventist (see Chapter 2), was deeply involved with several health-reform crusades. He was a sickly child, threatened with an early death from tuberculosis. Kellogg's health improved after he became a vegetarian. He worked at the Adventist publishing house, taught school, attended Russell Trall's hydropathic college, and, in 1875, graduated from the Medical College of New York City. The next year he became director of the Battle Creek Hydropathic Sanitarium. His program at the "San," the pet name for the institution, banned alcoholic drinks, meat, tea, coffee, tobacco, and spices. Besides a vegetarian diet, the daily regimen included proper exercise, sensible clothing, sunshine, and rest (Whorton 1982, 203–204; Whitman 1985, 494–495).

Kellogg had unlimited energy and became involved with many activities. He developed the precooked flaked breakfast cereal "cornflakes," and a variety of meat substitutes. Both he and his brother William launched cereal manufacturing, with W. K.'s company becoming a large corporation still in existence today. Kellogg wrote countless articles and books, championed the eugenic and temperance movement, and advocated sex education and pure food and drug legislation. He attacked alcohol and "self-abuse" and was active in health advocacy until his death. He also maintained close collegial relationships with elite members of the medical profession (Whitman 1985, 494–495; Whorton 1982, 203–205; Numbers 1976, 188–189).

Horace Fletcher (1849–1919) was born in Lawrence, Massachusetts. As a youth he tried various occupations and became wealthy through various businesses. When turned down for life insurance in 1895 due to obesity, he became involved with the New-Thought religious movement. Inspired by this religious philosophy, he developed an elaborate diet system to cure his obesity. The regimen became known as "Fletcherism," a term coined by Kellogg, and advocated not eating unless one was hungry, thoroughly masticating every mouthful of food until it had lost its flavor, eating whatever appealed to the appetite, and eating only when free from anxiety and depression. It became popular among some health reformers (Whorton 1981b, 63–67; 1982, 205; Malone, 1957, 464–465).

SUMMARY

Religious ferment at the end of the nineteenth and the beginning of the twentieth century helped create interest concerning various health issues. Physical activity and diet were integrated into reform activities emanating out of religious revivalism; to be a Christian also meant to be physically fit. New religions, such as Christian Science and New-Thought denominations, rapidly grew and focused upon mental healing and positive health. Fundamentalist religions crusaded against alcohol. The religious fervor of the era became an underlying presence among reformers and the health-reform crusades of the second Clean Living Movement. Physical activity, diet, and dress reform became integrated into women's rights and physical culture became popularized among many middle-class individuals.

NOTES

1. The term "social gospel" did not come into common use until after 1900. Before then, the designation most widely used was "social Christianity." Although there were influences from Britain, "the Christian social movement in

the United States was fundamentally indigenous" (Handy 1966, 4). For more information about this movement, see Phillips (1996), Handy (1966), Hopkins (1961), and Atkins (1923).

2. The self-appointed early historian of New Thought was Horatio W. Dresser (1866–1954); see his *A History of the New Thought Movement* (1919). In this work, he discusses the similarities and differences between Mary Baker Eddy's and Quimby's philosophies. Both of Dresser's parents had been cured by Quimby and were early leaders in the New-Thought movement. They established a healing clinic and wrote articles on the philosophy. Dresser also published Quimby's manuscripts. For further information concerning New Thought, see Atkins (1923, Chapter 8).

3. The most detailed biography of Eddy is the three-volume work, *Mary Baker Eddy*, by Robert Peel (1966, 1971, 1977). For other publications which discuss her life or Christian Science, see Thomas (1994), Peel (1988), Atkins (1923), and Wilber (1913). Some of these works criticize her and others are glowingly positive.

4. The term "fundamentalism" was not used until about 1920. It refers to a series of twelve volumes concerning the fundamentals of biblical truth, published between 1909 and 1912. The work rigorously defends the infallibility of views expressed in the Bible. As this term became popular, it was often used in place of evangelicalism. Fundamentalism became associated with a rejection of the religious principles and social agenda of the more liberal churches (Phillips 1996, xv). See Marsden (1991) for more information concerning fundamentalism and evangelicalism.

5. For further information concerning Lewis, see Eastmann (1891) and Vertinsky (1979).

6. During the upward surge of the fitness movement, there were a number of competing exercise philosophies. Among physical educators of the era, this competition became known as the "battle of the systems." These systems included Swedish gymnastics, introduced into the northeast and some urban areas in the 1890s and noted for its mechanical precision; German gymnastics, popular in the Midwest and noted for strength-building activities; and the methods developed by Sargent, Lewis, and Hitchcock. A meeting held in Boston during 1889 attempted to develop a national unified concept of physical education, but it was only marginally successful. In the 1890s, several states passed legislation for school-based physical education which used one system or the other. However, it was not until just after the turn of the century that compromises began to be made. A balanced program began to evolve, which included games, sports, and other activities along with anatomy, physiology, hygiene information, and sex education (Lee and Bennett 1960, 27–29, 43).

7. During the first decade of the century, as the physical culture movement was being popularized, some saw it as a fad. Pearl (1908) suggests that a debilitating effect on the human race is "the cult of 'fads'—forever seeking health and of developing a morbid self-consciousness of the body—the water-cures, the food-cures, the fast-cures, the exercise-cures, the pathetic half-truths at which we grasp and with which we morbidly struggle, instead of going on leading normal and temperate lives."

8. For further information on the colorful life of Macfadden, see Maxcy and Todd (1987) and Ernst (1991). An entertaining biography by one of his former wives, Mary Macfadden (1956), is *Dumbbells and Carrotstrips*.

9. See Whorton (1981a, 1981b) concerning diet and vegetarianism crusades at the turn of the century.

10. For more information concerning Kellogg, see Carson (1957), Numbers (1976), and Schwartz (1970). A novel and a film based upon *The Road to Wellville* (Boyle 1993) is a fictional account of Kellogg and his sanitorium. For information concerning Fletcher, see his 1898 autobiography and Whorton (1981b).

8

Saloons, Suffrage, and Smoking

Our society . . . stands not only for total abstinence and prohibition, but for no secretarianism in religion, no sectionalism in politics, no sex in citizenship.

Frances Willard, *Glimpses of Fifty Years* (1889)

And men are temperate, not when either their food or their drink is regulated for them by law, but when they have acquired the intelligence and the power to regulate both for themselves.

Prohibition or Temperance—Which? *Outlook* (1903)

The movement is not so much against the consumption of whiskey and other alcoholic beverages as against saloons, rum-shops, bars, and the like.

Edward Lissner, *Harper's Weekly* (1907)

Public smoking has become so general that the mere suggestion of the "rights" of the non-smoker will doubtless cause some amusement to the smoker who has never taken the trouble to think of the matter.

Twyman O. Abbott, *Outlook* (1910)

The individuals involved with antialcohol and antitobacco reform and in favor of suffrage had deep religious commitments. This commitment led to campaigns to eliminate bad habits and vices, such as alcohol and tobacco use, that were perceived as enslaving the individual and leading to family dissolution, poverty, crime, and nonmarital sexual activities. The first health campaign to emerge in the second Clean Living Movement was a crusade against alcohol and the saloon.

SALOONS AND THE PROHIBITION MOVEMENT

Around the time of the Civil War, several temperance organizations, including the American Temperance Union, went out of existence and the temperance movement "stagnated" (Cherrington 1920, 163–164). Not until about a decade later did the first stirrings of a new movement emerge. The temperance movement from the 1870s until 1920 went through several eras of activity in terms of strategies or political control.[1]

From 1873 to 1893, the movement was dominated by women and church-based groups on the local and, in some cases, the state level. Although the beginnings of this era fostered moral-suasive (education and social pressure) aspects, a call for abstinence and coercive (negative sanctions) components were also evident. The coercive phase of the cycles began around 1893. From this date the Anti-Saloon League (ASL) was a major force in the movement and supported nonpartisan efforts for legislative prohibition on the local and state levels until 1913. From 1913 to 1920, the third era of strategy called for a national constitutional amendment for prohibition that culminated with the Eighteenth Amendment. The backlash phase (1920–1933) emerged with the "roaring twenties," as opposition toward prohibition from the beverage industry, urban sophisticates, the press, and other groups arose. The complacency stage, where alcohol was seen to be relatively harmless, was found in the decades of World War II until the late 1950s.

A variety of factors contributed to the national prohibition movement. These included, but are not exclusive to, health and eugenic concerns, anti-German and anti-immigrant sentiments, World War I, middle-class progressivism, and, most important, that urban crime and family disintegration was caused by alcohol and the saloon.[2]

Per Capita Consumption and the Change in Drinking Practices

Although the use of alcohol appears to have fallen precipitously in the antebellum temperance era, production and use rose again after the Civil War. It then more or less leveled off until the end of the century, when it fluctuated between one and one and a half gallons per person per year. It rose briefly for a few years in the 1870s. After 1900, per capita consumption increased for about a decade and then began to decline, because of state and local prohibition efforts, even before national prohibition was instituted. However, during the latter part of the nineteenth century, drinking preferences changed. Beer replaced whiskey as Americans' preferred alcoholic beverage. In 1865, per capita consumption of beer totaled a little over three gallons annually; by

1900, it had reached sixteen gallons, while whiskey had dropped (Blocker 1989, 65; Rorabaugh 1979, 231). Breweries began to have immense political power. As prohibition forces became more powerful, the breweries began to resist local option and statewide prohibition campaigns (Warner 1909, 32–33).

Drinking Establishments

Two types of drinking establishments became more numerous. They included the private club and the saloon for the masses.

Upper- and Middle-Class Clubs

Wealthy and middle-class Americans tended to consume alcohol at home or in private clubs or elegant saloons, a term derived from the French word *salon*. These establishments were filled with expensive furniture, woodwork, and carpets. Many of these gathering places were hotel bars that became famous, such as the Palmer House in Chicago. Smaller saloons that catered to drinkers of more moderate means were similarly decorated. Among more affluent Americans, drunkenness was unacceptable. One drank to be sociable, to relax, and to enjoy oneself. Lender and Martin (1987, 99–102), however, have suggested that temperance reformers considered middle- and upper-class drinking a poor role model for the hordes of "undomesticated" European immigrants. They considered well-to-do drinkers as much a threat to the republic as heavy-drinking westerners, immigrants, and "poverty-stricken drunkards."

The Rise of the Urban Saloon: A Workingmen's Club

The number of saloons grew quickly in the generally prosperous postwar period. Many saloons were the workingman's "social club." It was acknowledged as such in a report by the Committee of Fifty, a group (discussed later) that collected "impartial facts" concerning the "physiological, legislative, ethical, and economic aspects of the drink question" at the turn of the century (Calkins 1901, v). The committee found that "a careful study of the saloon as it exists to-day in our American cities has revealed the fact that it is performing a double office, it is satisfying a twofold thirst; it is meeting the physical craving for intoxicating liquor, but it is also meeting the thirst for fellowship, for amusement, and for recreation" (Peabody 1905, 146–147).

Saloons were important to workingmen because they provided newspapers, toilets, check cashing, recreation, fellowship, job leads, card tables, and sometimes billiards. Saloon patrons were primarily immigrants and unskilled industrial workers. Most provided a so-called "free lunch," in which "either without extra cost or for a small amount, sufficient food [was] furnished to satisfy an ordinary appetite" (Peabody 1905, 148–150). The worst of these establishments became centers of drunkenness, crime, prostitution, and political corruption. The San Francisco Barbary Coast and Chicago's Gold Coast, for example, were infamous for such activities, although they were also found in many other communities. Burnham (1993, 26) has argued that "all the problems connected directly with alcohol in American culture flourished in saloons and were symbolized for most citizens in the drunkenness and irresponsible, destructive behavior that were exactly the opposite of the careful, controlled, future-oriented conduct that connoted civilization among dominant groups at the time."

In frontier towns and mining communities, western versions of saloons were often the scene of drunken brawls. In smaller towns, where retail businesses shared space, middle-class parents could not get away from these outlets, which greatly concerned churchgoing citizens. The saloon was seen as a threat to family and middle-class values. By the turn of the century, children were warned by their parents to steer clear of bars, and young women were known to cross the street to avoid walking past tavern entrances (Blocker 1989, 68; Lender and Martin 1987, 104–106; Peabody 1905, 150). Just as "ardent spirits" in the Jacksonian era and drunk driving in the late twentieth century became initial focuses of hostility toward alcohol, so did the saloon at the turn of the century.

The Prohibition Party and the Reform Clubs

In Mansfield, Ohio, a State Prohibition Party was formed in 1868, which put forward a slate of candidates for state elections. The following year the National Prohibition Party (NPP) was formed. The group reasoned that if alcohol was eliminated so would other social problems. The National Prohibition Party contributed significantly to the antialcohol aspects of the second Clean Living Movement in that it helped clear the way for nonpartisan support of temperance political activity in later years, which finally led to the Eighteenth Amendment (Cherrington 1920, 168–169; Blocker 1989, 88, 92–93; Dillon 1944, 211).

The NPP, in alliance with the Women's Christian Temperance Union, pushed for statewide prohibition amendments and laws. Such enactments were secured in Kansas (1880), Iowa (1882), Maine (1884), and Rhode Island (1886). However, between 1887 and 1893, only two of fourteen states considering adopting state prohibitory constitutional amendments actually passed such measures, North and South Dakota. The NPP was unable to form a coalition with the Populists in 1892, a

feat which Frances Willard, the dynamic leader of the WCTU, attempted to facilitate (Cherrington 1920, 168–169, 179–180).

During this period, several religious-oriented groups were established to "reform the inebriate." Like the Washingtonians of the antebellum period, these societies were primarily aimed at men who drank
heavily. The three most prominent groups originated in Maine. These
were the Reform Club, founded in 1872 by I. K. Osgood; the Blue Ribbon Movement, launched by Francis Murphy in 1873; and the Red
Ribbon Reform Club, inaugurated in 1874 by Dr. Henry A. Reynolds.
The structure and activities of these groups was similar to the modern
Alcoholics Anonymous. They were different in that members were
required to sign an abstinence pledge. In addition, members of the
Red and Blue Ribbon Clubs often wore blue and red ribbons to signify
they were abstinent from all alcoholic beverages (Daniels 1878, 345–
387; Fehlandt 1904, 231–232).

The WCTU and Its Era of Power, 1873–1892

During the same two- to three-year period when the Reform Clubs
were founded, a women's crusade against alcohol emerged. It resulted
in the Women Christian Temperance Union, often called the WCTU or
the Union, which was the first large-scale mass movement of American women for any cause. These "white-ribbon women"—members
of the WCTU wore white ribbons and often referred to each other by
this name—cut across regional, racial, and ethnic boundaries. The
Union was the first sizable organization controlled exclusively by
women and from its inception excluded males from voting membership. Through the WCTU, women became visible leaders from coast
to coast (Gordon 1898, 161; Bordin 1981, 156–157).

The Women's Crusades against Liquor and Saloons

In 1873, Dio Lewis, a physical educator (see Chapter 7), lecturing in
Fredonia, New York, suggested that women band together and pray
at the local saloons in an attempt to close them. The next day a group
of women enacted Lewis's plan. Through newspaper accounts of the
activity and Lewis's lecture tour, this idea spread quickly. A few weeks
later, Lewis spoke at Hillsboro, Ohio. On December 24, the day after
Lewis's lecture, women marched, sang hymns, prayed, and convinced
some liquor-selling drugstores not to sell alcohol. A few days later, at
the Washington County Courthouse in Ohio, women again organized
after Lewis's lecture. Besides marching and singing, these women also
used axes to smash casks of alcoholic beverages. Thus was born the
women's crusade (Blocker 1985, 3, 10–12).[3]

The women's crusade spread throughout the country and in many communities succeeded in closing, at least temporarily, many local retail liquor outlets. At a national convention on November 18, 1874, in Cleveland, Ohio, the WCTU was officially founded. When Frances Willard became president five years later, it became the largest and most powerful women's organization ever assembled in American history. The WCTU shaped not only prohibition and woman suffrage, but also other health reforms, and shifted temperance reform to female dominance for the next two decades (Blocker 1989, 77–81; Dannenbaum 1981, 235–236).

Frances E. Willard and Health Reform

Frances Willard (1839–1898), born in Churchville, New York, of middle-class parents, was a teacher. She became a founder and president of the WCTU in Chicago and became the corresponding secretary of the national WCTU in 1877. She held the position of president from 1879 until her death (Bordin 1981, 142; Gordon 1898, 54–59, 101; Dillon 1944, 369). Willard was in many ways a symbolic link to the many health reforms of the second Clean Living Movement. As early as 1881, she campaigned for whole-wheat bread, dress reform, and exercise. As her biographer, Mary Earhart Dillon (1944, 307) suggested, "Vegetarianism was closely linked with temperance as fresh air and water seemed to be one of their tenants." Willard perennially agitated for legislation forbidding women to deform their figures by corsets and long skirts which swept the streets. She investigated phrenology and psychical research (Dillon 1944, 295; Bordin 1981, 109).

Under Willard's influence, the WCTU adopted a "Do-Everything Policy" that engaged the Union in many reform issues. Through both private charity and legislation, the WCTU attempted to address the health and social problems arising from rapid social changes. The Union formed departments devoted to "social purity," heredity, school hygiene, physical culture, antismoking, and drug education (Bordin 1981, 109). The WCTU became so powerful that it oversaw alcohol, tobacco, and hygiene education in the public schools by endorsing textbooks. This was accomplished through the leadership of Mary H. Hunt, superintendent of the WCTU's Department of Scientific Temperance Instruction. Hunt began to edit and revise textbooks that Union chapters then urged local school boards to adopt. Physiologists and other scientists, however, clashed with Mary Hunt and the WCTU over the content of public school instruction regarding the nature of alcohol and its effect upon the human system. They argued that information provided by the WCTU was not factual and only discussed the negative effects of alcohol (Paulty 1985, 366–372). The clash over factual information was similar to scholars countering the Office of Substance Abuse Prevention (OSAP) in the late 1980s. OSAP mandated that public school instruction needed to convey a "clear message" that all alcohol consumption was harmful (Engs and Fors 1988, 27).

Political Support for Local and State Prohibition, 1893–1913

During the last decade of the nineteenth century, temperance groups began to support politicians who favored prohibition, regardless of party affiliation. The Anti-Saloon League became the major pressure group for prohibition during this period. By 1906, this "non-partisan movement for prohibition had come to be generally considered as representing the most effective method of fighting the liquor traffic" (Cherrington 1920, 277). Local option had been the most popular route, but beginning in 1907 there was a push for state referenda. Between 1907 and 1917, there were thirty-eight state referenda, with a total of nineteen states passing state prohibition (Blocker 1976, 237–238; Cherrington 1920, 176–180; Kerr 1985).[4]

The Committee of Fifty

The Committee of Fifty for the Investigation of the Liquor Problem was organized in 1893. It was made up of individuals representing different trades, occupations, and opinions and was unaffiliated with temperance organizations. Its purpose was to "investigate facts" concerning the alcohol problem. The committee looked at "practical methods of temperance reform—total abstinence and moderation, legal prohibition and the licensing system" (Peabody 1905, 8). During the first decade of the twentieth century, it was one of the few voices of moderation and gave suggestions such as advising "a single glass of wine per day" for persons of middle age. It recommend that night schools, public lecture courses, free public libraries, and education classes connected with the YMCA be instituted as alternatives to the saloon (Peabody, 1905, 3–4, 9, 179; Williams 1996, 186).

Anti-Saloon League

Cherrington (1920, 249) suggested that "the year 1893 found the Prohibition movement in the United States at a low ebb. . . . Joints, camouflaged drug stores, speak-easies and numerous other institutions devised for the purpose of evading the prohibitory law, flourished in most of the Prohibition states." Only five states remained under nominal prohibition: Kansas, Iowa, North and South Dakota, and Oklahoma. During this year, the Anti-Saloon League was founded as a state society in Ohio by Dr. Howard H. Russell, a congregational minister. Its purpose was to support any candidate for local or state office who was in favor of prohibition, regardless of party affiliation. In contrast to other prohibition groups, the League was staffed by paid workers, many of whom were also clergymen. The League rapidly grew in membership and influence, and in 1895 became a national organization (Cherrington 1920, 253–259; Blocker 1989, 96, 101–105; Williams 1996, 185–187; Kerr 1985).

Up until 1900, the WCTU held the reins of power in the prohibition movement; at the turn of the century, the Anti-Saloon League became the primary force. From 1893 until 1906, the Anti-Saloon League vigorously crusaded against saloons, resulting in thousands of towns adopting state local-option measures for prohibition. In 1906, the Anti-Saloon League began to shift to a nonpartisan statewide prohibition campaign instead of local option. It also shifted from social to legislative reform and redefined the enemy as being the saloon and liquor traffic rather than the drinker (Cherrington 1920, 255–256; Williams 1996, 188).

Other Temperance Reformers

One of the most colorful figures of the second Clean Living Movement was Carry Nation (1846–1911), who became famous for wielding a hatchet to demolish barrooms, thus becoming the scourge of barkeepers and drinkers in Kansas and elsewhere. However, she received little support from the national temperance movements. Nation also opposed tobacco, foreign foods, corsets, short skirts, and barroom "nudes," and favored woman suffrage. She became a caricature of the WCTU by the mid-twentieth century. The role of other women, such as Willard, and the importance of the WCTU to health and social issues dimmed under the glare of Nation.

One of the first recruits to the Anti-Saloon League was Wayne Wheeler (1869–1927), who became superintendent and then chief executive officer of Ohio's League in 1903, a position he retained until his death. Wheeler was the force behind the League's rise to national influence. He became general counsel to the Anti-Saloon League of America. In 1905, Wheeler was elected governor of Ohio. Over the years, Wheeler personally led "assaults on alcohol in the courts" and was known for his insistence on "vigorous steps against the liquor traffic in defense of the Volstead Act." Wheeler became symbolic of the drive and political acumen of the temperance movement and pioneered the "pressure tactics" used in modern politics (Blocker 1989, 98; Lender 1984, 511–512).

Nativistic Undercurrents to the Prohibition Movement

The prohibition movement, like the Jacksonian antialcohol movement, had Nativistic undercurrents. The late nineteenth-century temperance movement, for the most part, was composed of members of the Prohibition Party, the WCTU, and the Anti-Saloon League. It drew its support from Protestant evangelical churches and native-born middle-class Americans. Prohibition crusaders noted that much of the "liquor trade" was in the hands of "low-class foreigners," such as the Irish and Germans. A steady influx of Roman Catholic immigrants from southern and eastern Europe increasingly crowded into urban areas during the two decades before and after the turn of the century. These immigrants, who continued the drinking patterns of the "old country" and resisted "Americanization," began to alarm more traditional Americans. To control drinking among immigrants, antialcohol laws were enacted in several cities aimed specifically at them (Warner 1909, 116–119, 245–246; Pittman and Snyder 1962, 112; Timberlake 1963, 15–16).

The Push for National Prohibition, 1913–1920

By 1912, the prohibition movement had claimed considerable success inasmuch as about one-half the country was "living in territory in which the liquor traffic has been forbidden by law." This had been obtained through local options and statewide prohibition (Iglehart 1911, 215; Blocker 1989, 111). Over the next seven years, many states began to adopted statewide prohibition. In 1916, temperance forces won a sufficient number of dry Congressmen to provide the necessary two-thirds vote for a Constitutional amendment. However, the prohibition issue was delayed by the United States' involvement in the European war. An amendment to the Lever Food and Fuel Control Act of August 10, 1917, a food conservation bill, banned the use of grains and foodstuffs in the production of distilled spirits for beverage purposes, which effectively shut down the distilling industry. This act also regulated beer and wine production (Blocker 1989, 114–121; Timberlake 1963, 174; Burnham 1993, 27).

At the end of 1917, Congress voted to submit to the states the National Prohibition Amendment. Lobbying by the League brought about enactment by Congress, on November 21, 1918, the War Prohibition Act. This law forbade the manufacture of beer and wine after May 1, 1919 and outlawed the sale of all intoxicating beverages after June 30, 1919. The Eighteenth Amendment achieved the ratification of the necessary two-thirds of the states by January 1919 to take effect January 16, 1920. In reality, the nation went dry under war prohibition in July

1919 rather than January 1920 (Timberlake 1963, 178–180; Blocker 1989, 114–121).

With ratification of the Eighteenth Amendment, Congress had only to enact an effective enforcement law. The Anti-Saloon League codified the prohibition laws of various states that were incorporated into a bill that Andrew J. Volstead introduced into Congress on May 19, 1919. It was passed by both houses and sent to President Woodrow Wilson who vetoed it on October 27. The next day it was promptly overridden by the House and Senate. Title II of this act forbade anyone to "manufacture, sell, barter, transport, import, export, deliver, furnish or possess any intoxicating liquor." Drinkers were allowed to make fermented cider and fruit juice for use in their own homes. It also allowed for the sale of alcoholic liquor for medicinal, sacramental, and industrial purposes (Timberlake 1963, 181–182).

Heady with the triumph of national prohibition, the Anti-Saloon League now raised its sights even higher and embarked on a campaign to extend the benefits of prohibition to the entire world. It was not successful, as the "American Experiment" was bewildering to many European nations where drinking was an essential part of the culture (Timberlake 1963, 180).[5]

The Backlash Phase: The Roaring Twenties and Repeal

As with many other health-reform issues discussed in this work, the antialcohol movement began to lose its force as the movement went into the backlash stage. Backlash phases of health-reform cycles have been precipitated by segments of the population that are opposed to the reform. These have included individuals, industries, the media, and others who for personal, economic, political, or social reasons are against the measure. The backlash phase against national prohibition encompassed a number of factors, including sensationalized press reports, sophisticated urban writers opposed to what they perceived as "puritanical" rural values, efforts on the part of the alcohol beverage industry to change perceptions of drinking, hostility against government intervention, and increased crime and lawlessness due to black market alcohol.

Opposition to the Eighteenth Amendment

Burnham (1993, 28) has argued that "Contrary to myth, prohibition was substantially successful. The saloon, the disreputable public drinking place, disappeared—the obvious goal of the Anti-Saloon League. Moreover, despite the many legal sources of intoxicating beverages, the per capita consumption of alcohol declined by the 1920s . . . medical conditions associated with alcohol consumption declined . . . and social conditions also showed definite changes."[6] However, not all historians or sociologists agree with this point of view. Many have considered the great experiment of prohibition a failure that led to increased social problems. For example, Zimmer and Morgan (1992) point out that the decrease in alcohol-related problems actually began before the enactment of widespread prohibition laws and began to increase again in the late 1920s before repeal. Not only did prohibition fail to prevent the consumption of alcohol, it led to the extensive production of unregulated and untaxed alcohol, the development of organized crime empires, increased violence, massive political corruption, and contempt for the law. It also spawned underground drinking establishments. These included "speakeasies" and sophisticated dinner clubs and cabarets in urban areas frequented by the upper middle class and other urban sophisticates.[7] This type of illegal drinking, where intoxication was often the rule, was echoed in the late twentieth-century movement. A high proportion of university students under the age of twenty-one began to drink in "underground" situations when it became illegal to purchase alcohol in 1987. This resulted in an increase in alcohol-related problems among this group (Engs and Hanson, 2000).

Decline of the Movement

After 1920, a decline in support for prohibition among women had developed and local leadership in the WCTU changed in social composition. The percentage of women from upper-middle-class backgrounds waned, while the percentage from lower-middle-class and lower-class backgrounds waxed upward. Upper-middle-class women began to gravitate toward associations that opposed the prohibition amendment (Bordin 1981, 163). The WCTU gradually become a caricature of its former self. By the 1960s, Carrie Nation had become stereotyped as the essence of the WCTU. Forgotten were the accomplishments achieved under Willard's charismatic leadership and the organization's advocacy of a variety of health and social reforms. By the last decades of the twentieth century, the WCTU continued to publish educational materials on alcohol, drugs, tobacco, and other health issues.

SUFFRAGE AND ITS LINKS TO THE TEMPERANCE MOVEMENT

Emergence of women's antialcohol groups and women's rights were intimately intertwined. Both movements questioned the nature of democracy and the means of social control within the American culture.

During the peak of prohibition and suffrage agitation, one suffrage leader commented that "many consider the temperance and woman suffrage movements as practically identical" (Stewart 1914, 143). From 1874 until about 1900, as noted previously, the WCTU was both the leading temperance and the leading women's organization in the United States. After 1900, the National American Woman Suffrage Association became the main force for suffrage and the Anti-Saloon League was its counterpart for prohibition. Symbolic of the union of several reform movements among women was an International Council of Women conference in 1888, at which there were representatives from the "purity," temperance, and suffrage causes (Paulson 1973, 118–120; Bordin 1981, xviii; Brown 1916, 93).

Suffrage was first granted to women in Wyoming soon after the Civil War to encourage women to migrate west. However, forty years of struggle ensued before passage of the Nineteenth Amendment, which gave women the same voting right as men. Numerous works have chronicled the woman suffrage movement. Therefore, it will be discussed only briefly as it relates to prohibition and other health reforms of the era.[8]

The WCTU and Its Influence on Woman Suffrage

The WCTU was the major vehicle through which American women developed a changing role for themselves in society. Before 1873, most northern women had worked only in their churches. Through the Union, women learned of their legal and social disabilities, gained confidence in their strengths and talents, and became certain of their political power as a group and as individuals. The organization provided the underpinnings for the surge of interest in woman suffrage after 1900 and made the Nineteenth Amendment possible. Leaders of the WCTU realized that suffrage for women was necessary as a "weapon for home protection," and the Union began to actively campaign for suffrage (Bordin 1981, 157).

Susan B. Anthony

Susan B. Anthony (1820–1906), a prominent temperance and suffrage leader, was born of Quaker parents in Adams, Massachusetts. Anthony began her first public crusade on behalf of temperance. However, discouraged by the limited role ascribed to women in the established temperance movement, she, along with Elisabeth Cady Stanton, formed the National Woman Suffrage Association in 1869. That same year, the American Suffrage Association was founded by Lucy Stone. In 1872, Anthony demanded that women be given the same civil and political rights that had been extended to black males under the Fourteenth and Fifteenth Amendments. She was arrested several times when she went to the polls and attempted to vote. From then on, she campaigned endlessly for a federal woman suffrage amendment until her death (Barry 1988).

The Fight for Woman Suffrage on the National Level

Emergence of the Peoples Party (Populists) in the early 1890s raised the hopes of both suffragists and prohibitionists. Willard tried to unite the Prohibition and Populist Parties, while Susan B. Anthony and other leaders attempted to secure endorsement for woman suffrage from the Populists. Both failed in their attempts (Paulson 1973, 136). There had been continuous appeals to the national political conventions to recognize the enfranchisement of women as part of their party platforms. However, only two parties, the Prohibition Party, organized in 1872, and the Socialist Party, which emerged in 1901, declared for woman suffrage. Constitutional amendments for suffrage were defeated in 1887, 1914, and 1915. Suffrage suffered setbacks and defeat between 1896 and 1910, a period known among suffragists as "the doldrums." Suffrage by constitutional amendment was only adopted in seven states over this era (Harper 1922, vi, 702; Catt 1940, 161–162; Blocker 1976, 237–238).

The woman suffrage movement began to gain momentum at the end of the first decade of this century. The movement increasingly became more militant, as women held parades, organized outdoor meetings, and barnstormed their states in automobiles. In 1913, two suffrage leaders organized the Militant Congressional Union and announced intentions of conducting a vigorous campaign for a federal woman suffrage amendment. These more militant activities began to pay off. Between 1910 and 1914, eight states enfranchised women (Beeton 1995, 115; Flexner 1975, 259, 263–265).

The Great War began in Europe in 1914. Concerns with the war and increased nationalism began to strengthen the call for more democratic suffrage. In January 1917, women picketed the White House, asking, "How long must women wait for liberty?" Throughout the war years they were sometimes attacked and jailed for suffrage activities. In April 1917, the United States entered the war against Germany. As men went to the European trenches, women began to fill traditional male occupations, such as working on farms, in munitions plants, and as clerks (Harper 1922, 728–730, Flexner 1975, 298–299).

Following the signing of the armistice on November 11, 1918, both political parties were concerned about the women's vote in the 1920 election. Thirty states now had woman suffrage by constitutional amendment or legislative act. Congress met in a special session in 1919 and passed the Nineteenth Amendment. Ratification of the amendment by two-thirds of the states occurred on August 18, 1920, at which point women in the United States were enfranchised on an equal basis with men (Flexner 1975, 294–297, 314–324; Catt 1940, 161–164, 172). Prohibition and suffrage, interlinked from the beginning of the second Clean Living Movement, had both become the law of the land.

SMOKING THE "DEVIL'S STICKS"

Cropping up concurrently with the prohibition and woman suffrage crusade was an anticigarette campaign. In many cases, opponents of the "evil weed" and "little white slaver" were the same diligent individuals and groups as the antisaloon and liquor agitators.[9] Temperance workers' overriding concern with liquor prevented them from pressing the anticigarette campaign with full vigor to the national level. Difficulties in enforcing newly enacted state anticigarette laws resulted in their being ignored or repealed within a few years. These and other factors, including the popularity of "smokes for soldiers" during World War I, prevented cigarette bans from attaining the national notoriety of liquor prohibition during the backlash era of the roaring twenties. In spite of this, between 1896 and 1921, nineteen states had passed laws prohibiting cigarettes. The last of these laws was repealed in 1927. As has been repeatedly found, most prohibition legislation against "vices" such as alcohol and tobacco are difficult to impose on segments of the population that do not want them. By the 1940s, prohibition of cigarettes had disappeared like fading smoke.

The Growth of Cigarette Smoking

Until about 1884, cigarettes were hand rolled by skilled European workers in New York and other urban tobacco shops. These cigarettes were composed of expensive imported "Turkish" tobaccos and were smoked primarily by upper-class and bohemian urban dwellers. In 1885, following the invention of a practical cigarette-rolling machine and a shift to domestic tobaccos, cigarette production increased. To promote these new cigarettes, advertising took a new turn. Cigarette boxes were fitted with "photo-art" pictures of actresses and sports figures, which were popular among boys. In addition, they contained redeemable coupons for mantlepiece clocks and other items. Advertisement was also accomplished through newspapers, billboards, and sporting events. These new forms of advertising spurred cigarette sales (Robert 1949, 141–146; Dillow 1981, 96, 101).

Chewing tobacco declined after 1890, when laws were introduced to forbid spitting in an effort to prevent tuberculosis (Teller 1988, 21). The cigar, after reaching a peak in 1907, began a long decline and then reached a plateau (Heimann 1960, 216–217, 244). Cigar sales only began to rise again in the 1990s as an upper-middle-class backlash against the antismoking crusade of the late twentieth-century Clean Living Movement.[10]

During World War I, the use of cigarettes by servicemen was sanctioned by both official edict and public consensus as necessary for the war effort. Congress included cigarettes in the rations issued to solders overseas. Even the Salvation Army and YMCA, which had previously opposed the use of cigarettes, cheerfully dispensed them during the war. The impetus for this may have come from manufacturers. By 1921, cigarettes became, and still are, the leading form of tobacco consumption (Tate 1995, Chapter 4; Burnham 1993, 95; Heimann 1960, 216–217, 244).

The Antitobacco Crusade

Despite the dramatic increase in cigarette smoking, they quickly developed a negative reputation. A crusade emerged not only against tobacco but also for nonsmokers' rights to a smoke-free environment. Similar to the last two decades of the twentieth century, reformers advocated laws to require restaurants to have accommodations for nonsmokers, "where they will not be subjected to the inconvenience and discomfort of inhaling tobacco" and to prohibit smoking in public places (Abbott 1910, 766). Throughout this era there were concerns that cigarette smoking led to beer drinking, alcoholism, wife beating, and crime ("Some Cigaret Figures" 1914).

A late twentieth-century myth suggested that the antismoking movement at the turn of the twentieth century was primarily morally and not scientifically based. However, antismoking activists during the second Clean Living Movement articulated virtually every health issue that was debated in the late twentieth-century movement. For example, an article entitled the "Anti-Cigarette Crusade" (1901) considered smoking "more hurtful than cigar-smoking because cigarette smokers so often inhale the smoke into the lungs." Data from insurance companies suggested that regular tobacco use reduced life span (Tate 1995, 6, 149–150; Dillow 1981, 101).

Moral Suasion: Education against Tobacco

The WCTU developed a Department for the Overthrow of the Tobacco Habit in 1884. It cited the health hazards of smoking and suggested the best opportunity to make headway against this practice was with the young. It introduced antismoking education in the schools. In 1895, the WCTU argued the merits of fresh air and advocated that smoking be permitted only if it did not interfere "with the rights and freedoms of any other individual." Various WCTU affiliates then deluged Congress with petitions demanding a federal ban on cigarettes on grounds they were causing insanity and death in thousands of American youth. In 1914, Thomas Edison and Henry Ford, who refused to employ smokers, wrote tracts expounding the health dangers of smoking (Bordin 1981, 109; Wiley 1916, 91–92; Tate 1995, 75).

Lucy Page Gaston and the Antismoking Crusade

The noisiest warrior in the anticigarette campaign during the second Clean Living Movement was Lucy Page Gaston (1860–1924). Born in Delaware, Illinois, of staunch abolitionist and prohibition parents who were friends of Willard, she attended the Illinois State Normal School, where she led raids on saloons, gambling dens, and tobacco shops as an active member of the WCTU. As part of her campaign in the 1890s, in imitation of the "cold-water armies" of a previous generation, she and other reformers urged children to sing antitobacco songs, wear pins, join parades, and take the "Clean Life Pledge" (Warfield 1930, 244; Robert 1949, 169; Tate 1995, 119–122).

In 1899, a group of businessmen helped Gaston create the Chicago Anti-Cigarette League, which became the National Anti-Cigarette League in 1901 and the Anti-Cigarette League of America in 1910. This organization strove to secure laws to prohibit the manufacture and consumption of cigarettes and to prosecute violators of the law (Warfield 1930, 245; Dillow 1981, 102–106; Tate 1995, 119–140, 170–177).

Coercion: Legislation and Other Sanctions against Cigarettes

Many antitobacco groups formed during this era. Constant anticigarette agitation by all these advocacy groups quickly led to the coercion phase of the antitobacco cycle, which coexisted with moral suasion throughout this period. Laws against tobacco use were aimed mostly at the "little white slaver" and not pipes or cigars. The August 12, 1905 *Harper's Weekly* implied this was because cigarettes were new, inexpensive, and tended to be smoked by boys and poor immigrants. In 1888, parents and antitobacco crusaders registered outrage against advertisements and enticements that encouraged boys to smoke. Cigarette manufacturers were pressured to eliminate these tactics, similar to efforts during the last decades of the twentieth century (Tate 1995, 159; Dillow 1981, 101).

By 1900, most states had banned cigarette and tobacco sales to minors. In 1901, the March *Outlook* reported that "only two states, Wyoming and Louisiana, have not given some attention to cigarette-smoking." Approximately nineteen states at some point during the first two decades of the century passed bans (or prohibitive taxes) against cigarettes.[11] When anticigarette laws were found to be unenforceable, states began to repeal them. By 1915, only nine states still prohibited cigarettes, and, by 1930, cigarettes were again legal in every state. Most states, however, still prohibited cigarette sales to minors (Dillow 1981, 107; Robert 1949, 249–250; Sullum 1998, 30; Troyer and Markle 1983, 41).

The Backlash Phase

Despite the reformers' antitobacco campaigns, tobacco consumption continued to increase. During the reform movement, the Tobacco Trust began fierce lobbying to prevent total prohibition of tobacco and cigarettes. A change in attitude occurred. In 1900, it was considered vulgar for a woman to smoke. However, fifteen years later many women began to smoke as a symbol of suffrage and emancipation. The cigarette became part of the flapper costume in the 1920s (Kluger 1996, 40; Martin 1900, 631; Robert 1949, 253).

SUMMARY

During the second Clean Living Movement, agitation arose against alcohol and tobacco and for woman suffrage. After many years of polemics and politicking, alcohol was prohibited on the national level, women were granted the right to vote, and cigarettes were prohibited in about nineteen states. However, a backlash to the legal curtailment of alcohol and tobacco occurred, often called the Roaring Twenties.

NOTES

1. Different time periods for eras of control or strategies, or even separate reform cycles for this antialcohol movement, have been suggested. Cherrington (1920) suggests a continuous reform movement with five phases: Partisan movement against liquor traffic, 1869–1893; Nonpartisan cooperation for local prohibition, 1893–1906; Nonpartisan state prohibition movement, 1906–1913; Nonpartisan movement for national constitution prohibition, 1913–1919; and movement for national prohibition, 1919–1920. Historian Jack Blocker (1989) suggests a temperance cycle dominated by women and the WCTU (1860–1892) was followed by a cycle dominated by the Anti-Saloon League (1892–1933).

2. Hundreds of works have chronicled the prohibition movement, along with various interpretations as to the factors that led to the passage of the Eighteenth Amendment and its repeal. A few contemporary secondary references include Aaron and Musto (1981), Blocker (1976, 1985, 1989), Burnham (1993), Clark (1965), Gusfield (1986), Hamm (1995), Kerr (1985), Rorabaugh (1979), Rumbarger (1989), Timberlake (1963), and Tyrrell (1979). Earlier sources include Cherrington (1920) and various works by the Committee of Fifty.

3. The Hillsboro march is generally the symbolic beginning of the women's crusade. After Ohio, the next leading crusade states were Indiana, Illinois, Michigan, and New York, while most cities experienced crusades they were generally weaker than in small towns (Blocker 1989, 78).

4. The only states that "stood firm until national prohibition went into effect in 1920" during this whole era were Maine, Kansas, and North Dakota (Cherrington 1920, 181). Many other states passed and then immediately repealed or declared the state prohibition laws unconstitutional.

5. Sweden, Iceland, and Finland adopted some prohibition legislative measures after being evangelized by American missionaries. For information concerning efforts in Europe, see Engs (2000), Eriksen (1990), Kerr (1985), and Levine (1992). See Engs (1995) for the history of the origins of drinking cultures in Western Europe.

6. Some other authors, including Aaron and Musto (1981) and Moore and Gerstein (1981), have also come to this same conclusion. See Burnham (1993, Chapter 2) for details concerning the influence of the alcohol beverage industry, the press, and others who organized for repeal.

7. For information concerning the backlash era and the failure of prohibition, see Allsop (1961), Engleman (1979), Kobler (1973, Chapters 10–13), Hanson (1995, Chapter 3), and Sinclair (1962, Chapters 9–15).

8. Hundreds of works have been written about woman suffrage and the women involved with the movement. Some contemporary works include Buhle and Buhle (1978), DuBois (1997), Flexner (1975), Graham (1996), and Wheeler (1995). For older publications by suffrage crusaders, see the six-volume *History of Woman Suffrage* (Stanton et al. 1969), published between 1881 and 1922, and Catt (1940). Paulson (1973) and Bordin (1981) have examined the relationship between suffrage and prohibition.

9. One of the best sources for information concerning the anticigarette movement and its relationship with other health issues is found in a dissertation by Tate (1995). Other sources that discuss the anticigarette movement during the second Clean Living Movement include those by Dillow (1981), Robert (1949), Kluger (1996), Kiger and Gaston (1997), and Sullum (1998).

10. See the article by Randi Epstein in the *Washington Post*, January 7, 1997. This feature article discusses the increase in cigar smoking, "cigar bars," and martini drinking as a backlash to the late twentieth-century health-reform movement.

11. A typical law of the era was that of New Hampshire: "No person, firm, or corporation shall make, sell, or keep for sale 'any form of cigarette.' The gift of a cigarette to minors is made a misdemeanor quite as much as the sale to adults" (anticigarette crusade 1901). Authors differ, both during the early twentieth century and in contemporary times, as to which states passed prohibitory laws against cigarettes. This may be due to the fact that some authors include states that immediately repealed their laws, states that passed prohibitory taxes, or states in which cities passed local laws. The total count ranges from fifteen to nineteen states, based upon the contemporary sources of Sullum (1998), Tate (1995), Troyer and Markle (1983), and Dillow (1981).

9

Eugenics, Purity, and Birth Control

Man is an organism—an animal; and the laws of improvement of corn and of race horses hold true for him also. Unless people accept this simple truth and let it influence marriage selection human progress will decrease.

Charles Benedict Davenport, *Heredity in Relation to Eugenics* (1911)

Our knowledge is now so accurate that it is possible to predict almost exactly the kind of children that will be born to parents whose heredity and mental habits are known.

Norman Barnesby, *Forum* (1913)

We ask your attention to our white cross pledge of equal chastity for man and women; of pure language and a pure life.

Frances Willard, *Glimpses of Fifty Years* (1889)

We want children to be conceived in love, born of parents' conscious desire, and born into the world with healthy and sound bodies and sound minds.

Margaret Sanger, *My Fight for Birth Control* (1931)

EUGENIC AND HEREDITARIAN CONCERNS

Eugenics, as stated by Charles B. Davenport, a prime mover of the eugenics movement, is the "science of the improvement of the human race by better breeding" (Davenport 1911, 1). Eugenic attitudes evolved from Darwinian evolutionary theory and were imported from Britain. Francis Galton, a British scientist and cousin of Darwin, after studying the pedigrees of eminent men, concluded that "nature was more important than nurture."[1] He postulated that genius is hereditary, which he reported in his first important work, *Hereditary Genius* (1869). Here, he argued that the theory of evolution implies that "it would be quite practical to produce a highly gifted race of men by judicious marriages during several consecutive generations" (p. 1). These thoughts quickly traveled to the academic community in the New World.

In the United States, the ideology became an underlying influence for several health campaigns of the second Clean Living Movement.[2] Mark Haller (1963, 5) points out that "eugenics at first was closely related to the other reform movements of the Progressive era and drew its early supporters from many of the same persons. It began as a scientific reform in an age of reform."[3] Unlike other health crusades of this era, such as prohibition and tuberculosis, the eugenics movement never became popular among the masses. Eugenics largely remained a movement of the upper middle class. It was a kind of secular religion for academics, social workers, and criminologists, who dreamed of a society in which each child might be born endowed with vigorous health and an agile mind. Opponents considered eugenics "a religious cult" or a "panacea for all human ills." Some religious organizations, in particular the Roman Catholic Church, were against eugenic reforms (Bruehl 1928, 52–53, 183; Haller 1963, 3–5, 177; Hague 1914, xxix–xxx; Pickens 1968, 4, 36).

The movement can be divided into three stages. During the first, from about 1870 to 1905, hereditarian attitudes took root among a variety of professionals. The second phase, the years of the movement's greatest impact, ranged from about 1905 through the late 1920s, when both moral suasive and coercive measures were implemented. After 1930, based upon new knowledge from genetics and psychology, the scientific basis upon which much of the movement rested was found to be invalid and the movement waned. The chilling use of negative eugenics to foster a superior race in Hitler's Germany discredited eugenics throughout the rest of the century (Haller 1963, 6–7; Pickens 1968, 4–5).[4] However, eugenic practices began to emerge again during the third Clean Living Movement in the 1980s.

The Roots of the Movement

The scientific community in the late nineteenth century included both environmentalists and hereditarians. The environmentalists stressed education and varying opportunities for personal success, while the hereditarians emphasized innate character, differential fecundity among social classes, and genetic determinism. By 1870, natural selection and inheritance of acquired characteristics had become the explanation of human heredity for both schools of thought (Pickens 1968, 39). Charles Rosenberg (1976, 35), a public-health historian, argues that the period of most enthusiastic hereditarianism, from 1885 to 1920, coincided with unbridled enthusiasm and acceptance of the germ theory of disease. A conclusion drawn from the germ theory suggested that since constitutional maladies such as cancer, insanity, heart disease, and feeblemindedness were not bacterial, they therefore must have hereditary origins. It followed that since these conditions were hereditary, selective breeding or "sanitary marriages" should be encouraged to promote the most desirable traits and eliminate the negative ones.

Race Degeneracy

"Race degeneracy" was a phrase first introduced as an offshoot of social Darwinism in the 1880s. Based upon earlier precepts, Robert Rentoul (1906, 1), a British physician, defined someone who could transmit mental or physical disease to an offspring as a "degenerate." This view implied that if the unfit propagated, the downfall of the human race would result. Based upon these beliefs, eugenicists categorized individuals and their resulting offspring as to two types. These included the "aristogenic," who were genetically fit and produced long lines of renowned men (outstanding women were rarely mentioned), and the "cacogenic," the unfit, who produced many generations of both male and female degenerates (Davenport 1914, 4–5).

At the turn of the twentieth century, reports on several families suggested that hundreds of the feeble-minded, insane, criminal, or poor could be descended from one defecting ancestor. These works included *The Jukes: A Study in Crime, Pauperism, Disease, and Heredity* (1910) by Richard Dougdale (1841–1883), in 1877, and *The Kallikak Family* (1912) by Henry Goddard (1866–1957), a popular book. These families were mentioned in many eugenics publications as support for the theory of inherited degeneracy and to promote eugenics legislation. However, the accuracy of these studies is questionable today.

Grave concerns about the degeneracy of the population spawned three factions in the nascent eugenics movement. Haller (1963, 5–6) has suggested that these included social-welfare professionals and institutional caregivers concerned about the prevention of crime, disease, and poverty; Nativists alarmed by the massive influx of poor immigrants from southern and eastern Europe; and academics interested in genetics. All were concerned about "race suicide."

Race Suicide

At the turn of the century, increased concerns emerged over the decline of the birth rate in western civilizations and uncontrolled population growth among "less advanced and unfit civilizations." Edward A.

Ross (1866–1951), a sociologist from University of Nebraska, called the declining birthrate among northern-European-derived people and the middle class "race suicide" (Ross 1901, 88). American nativists feared that the Anglo-Saxon lineage would die out because southern European immigrants and the unfit were producing more children than the more capable old stock. Many works during the first two decades of the century addressed race suicide. *The Passing of the Great Race* (1970), a 1918 book by Madison Grant (1865–1937), a New York attorney, which glorified the culture of blond and blue-eyed Nordics, epitomized this attitude.

However, not everyone agreed with Anglo-Saxon superiority and the "great white race." Franz Boas (1858–1942), an anthropologist (1894, 301–303), criticized what he called negative attitudes toward other races when he suggested that the standards of white culture were naïvely posited as a norm, and every deviation from that norm was automatically considered characteristic of a lower type. Boas attributed European cultural superiority to the circumstance of their historical development rather than to inherent capabilities.

Coalescence of the Movement

The problems of heredity and the prevention of inherited diseases and conditions dominated the meetings of many reform groups in the first few years of the twentieth century. In 1903, the first organization of the eugenics movement, the American Breeders' Association, was formed by agricultural breeders and university biologists. At the second meeting of this association in 1906, a committee on eugenics was established, with Charles Davenport as its secretary. This eugenics committee brought together institutional caregivers, Nativists, and academics, and was the first group in the United States to have the term "eugenics" in its title (Haller 1963, 62–65, 173; Fink 1938, 204–205).

Charles Benedict Davenport

Charles Benedict Davenport (1866–1944) was the driving force of the eugenics movement. Davenport was born and raised in Stamford, Connecticut, the son of a proud and stern Puritan family who could trace its ancestry back to the Norman conquest of England. He graduated from Harvard University with a Ph.D. in biology in 1889, and in 1904 helped establish and became director of the Carnegie Institute of Washington's Station for Experimental Evolution at Cold Spring Harbor on Long Island. In 1910, this became the Eugenics Record Office and a center of eugenics publications. Throughout his life, Davenport crusaded for caution in the selection of marriage partners, a ban on racial mixing, and exclusion of undesirable immigrants from the United States (Fink 1938, 204–205; Haller 1963, 63–66; Gillispie 1971, 589–590; Pickens 1968, 51).

Maturity of the Movement

In 1909, two events symbolized the burgeoning maturity of the movement. The American Academy of Political and Social Scientists (AAPSS) published a series of conference papers called *Race Improvement in the United States*. This publication brought together many professionals and progressive reformers concerned about social issues. During 1909, the American Breeders' Association's eugenics committee was upgraded to a section. In 1913, this section had gained enough influence to have the name of the organization changed to the American Genetic Association and its journal renamed the *Journal of Heredity* (Haller 1963, 173–174; Hofstadter 1959b, 162).

Positive and Negative Eugenics:
Moral Suasion and Coercion Aspects of the Movement

The eugenics movement, like other health-reform movements, had both moral suasive and coercive aspects; they were termed "positive" and "negative" eugenics. In 1914, Harvey Ernest Jordan (1878–1941), an embryologist from Johns Hopkins University, suggested, "Positive eugenics seeks to improve the race by encouraging greater reproductivity among the racially fitter, the civically more worthy, stocks. Negative eugenics aims to prevent contamination and degeneration by prohibition of parenthood to the obviously and grossly unfit. The peculiar means employed by positive eugenics are mainly educational, by negative eugenics legislative" (p. 110).

Positive Eugenics. Articles promoting positive eugenics began to become common in middle-class publications at the end of the first decade of the century. There was "encouragement of parenthood on the part of the worthy" (Saleeby 1911, 19). Popular books, tracts, and magazine bylines implied it was the duty of healthy and clean parents (free of sexually transmitted diseases) to reproduce in order to prevent degeneracy of the population. Advice was given for appropriate mate selection, parenting, child rearing, and actions individuals could take to produce better and healthier babies (Hague 1914, xxi; Baker 1912, 113–114; Saleeby 1911, 24–41). Positive eugenics also included the avoidance of "racial poisons," a term coined by Saleeby in 1906. Racial poisons included lead, alcohol, tobacco, the diseases syphilis and gonorrhea, and even war. These substances and conditions were thought to injure the "germ-plasm"—reproductive cells—and to prevent "healthy, effective and intelligent offspring" (Saleeby 1911, 58–60; Ellwood 1914, 221–222; Pernick 1996, 42–43).

The "campaign for better babies" was at the heart of positive eugenics. Eugenics groups and other organizations came together to promote this concept. They were most concerned about preventing syphilis from being transmitted to babies, which caused profound physical and mental deformities. Various organizations pushed for laws to require the "marriage certificate, a health certificate as a clean bill of health for those about to marry" (Daggett 1912, 230). Many states required premarital blood tests for syphilis and examinations during this era before a marriage license was granted.[5]

Negative Eugenics. Negative eugenics laws were also passed. Most eugenicists rejected negative measures such as euthanasia, infanticide, and abortion, but were in favor of sterilization and segregation of the unfit.[6] However, most states allowed for sterilization of institutionalized "confirmed criminals, idiots, imbeciles, and rapists" if the institution's board agreed. The laws varied from state to state, but in general a combination of lax enforcement and court decrees left them relatively innocuous. Many were tested and found unconstitutional (Laughlin 1922, 1–6; Hart 1912, 3–4).

The eugenics movement began to wane in the 1930s. Heredity emphasis was giving way to a form of "environmental naturalism," and social scientists explored the implications of culture on human ability. Lack of scientific evidence, the depression, and the sterilization and killing of millions under the Third Reich contributed to the death knell of the eugenics crusade by the mid-1940s.

THE ANTISEXUALITY SOCIAL PURITY MOVEMENT

The antisexuality movement included the "vice-society," antiobscenity, and "purity" or "social purity" movement. It had its roots in the 1870s. This broad movement had ties with the temperance, suffrage, and eugenics movements. The movement peaked in influence in the decades on either side of 1900. Three main factions characterized the crusade, and during the course of the movement their leaders and philosophies overlapped or merged in some cases. These factions included the antiobscenity and vice-societies campaigns on the part of Anthony Comstock and others, the fight against regulated prostitution and agitation for a single standard of sexual conduct for both men and women, and the social-hygiene movement sponsored by professionals who advocated educating Americans, including students, about eugenics, birth control, and venereal disease. The antiobscenity and prostitution crusades, for the most part, used coercive techniques, while the social-hygiene education programs relied upon moral suasion, except for marriage laws.

The Antiobscenity and Censorship Crusade

The antiobscenity and vice-society aspects of the purity movement spawned coercive activities to prohibit materials that leaders considered immoral. In 1866, the New York City Young Men's Christian Association surveyed young working men and became concerned about their weakness for pornographic books, saloons, and prostitutes. To fight at least the "licentious books" and other printed matter, YMCA officials launched a campaign for stricter state obscenity laws.

Anthony Comstock

Anthony Comstock (1844–1915) was the prime mover of the antiobscenity movement. His life, other than his last years, spans the Victorian era, when prostitution flourished and nice women were not expected to like "that sort of thing." Comstock was born in New Cannon, Connecticut, of a devout Congregationalist family (Trumbull 1913, 39–40).[7] After serving in the Civil War, Comstock went to New York City to work as a dry goods clerk and, in 1868, after one of his friends had been "led astray," launched a crusade to entrap pornography dealers and illegal saloons. He married in 1871, and the following year was paid by the YMCA to continue his antismut campaign. From 1873 until his death, he served as a special agent on vice for the U.S. Post Office Department and was authorized to crack down on so-called acts of depravity and given the power to arrest (Dennett 1926, 30–32; Trumbull 1913, 50–56; Broun and Leech 1927, 148–154).

Much like some antialcohol and antidrug crusaders of the third Clean Living Movement, who considered the concept of teaching responsible drinking as giving permission for wholesale drunkenness among youth, Comstock vehemently argued that "if you open the door to anything, the filth will all pour in and the degradation of youth will follow" (Hopkins 1915, 489). He took this position even if it involved only dispensing contraceptive information for physicians and their patients. Over his career, he persecuted and arrested numerous individuals for breaking vice and obscenity laws. Many were poor European immigrants struggling to make some kind of living. Comstock often bragged about the number of individuals he had arrested who committed suicide or died early (Broun and Leech 1927, 148–154).

The Antiprostitution and Moral Education Movement

Both antiprostitution and moral education groups emerged in the 1870s and coalesced to become the social-purity movement in the early 1880s. This movement developed a broad range of interests, including sex and moral education, child rearing, age-of-consent reforms, elimination of the "double standard," temperance, and, later, social hygiene, in addition to the abolition of prostitution (Pivar 1973, 6–7, 11; Grittner 1990, 43).

Neoabolitionists and Vigilance Societies

Neoabolitionists and vigilance societies became the coercive elements of the purity movement. Many early purity crusaders were former abolitionists with strong religious convictions who considered prostitution another form of slavery. In the early 1870s, some reformers attempted to regulate prostitution in several states. Susan B. Anthony and still other reformers began opposing these bills, as their goal was to completely eliminate "white slavery." These new abolitionists launched a mass campaign against regulation, and this crusade, under the WCTU and Frances Willard, evolved into a moral crusade for social purification. The victory of home and church values over those of the saloon and brothel became, for purity and temperance reformers, a struggle between the forces of light and darkness. By the late 1880s, regulation was no longer considered a respectable reform measure (Pivar 1973, 51–52, 85, 274–275).

Reformers became increasingly concerned about young girls being recruited into prostitution. Many states had fixed the age of sexual consent at ten, while Delaware had set it at seven years of age. Reformers recognized that low-age laws were a persistent threat to family purity inasmuch as they allowed the recruitment of preadolescent girls into brothels. In 1885, the WCTU began agitating for raising the age of consent. By 1895, the age of consent had been raised in many states (Pivar 1973, 104–105, 140–144).

Similar to other reform movements, the antiprostitution crusade had nativistic and eugenic undertones. Grittner (1990, 4) reported, for example, that "between 1909 and 1914, novels, silent films and religious tracts warned young, native-born white women of foreign panderers lurking in the urban shadows" to entice them into brothels. In reality, the chief victims of prostitution were immigrant women. He further suggested that the myth of white women being victimized by Catholic, Jewish, and Chinese immigrants in addition to eugenic concerns, alarm over alcohol and drug use, and diseases among immigrants helped develop sentiments that led to restrictive immigrant laws (Grittner 1990, 129–130).

Moral and Child-Rearing Education

Reformers began to realize that adolescent girls went into prostitution because of few, or low-paying, job opportunities. Organizations sprang up in eastern cities to educate working girls about urban dangers, including moral education. A major thrust of moral education was chastity until marriage. As part of the general purity movement, the White Cross Society of the British Anglicans, whose primary goal was a single standard of sexual morality for both men and women, was adopted. The WCTU added White Cross and White Shield, the female equivalent of the society, as adjuncts to its other purity activities. Frances Willard gave public lectures and published pamphlets to publicized these groups. Other organizations, such as churches and the YMCA, included purity reform as a component of their work. The White Cross Society became a mass movement and augmented the women's movement (Pivar 1973, 107–114, 177–179; Willard 1889, 428).

Besides a campaign for purity, in 1886 the WCTU initiated a massive campaign to educate women in new child-rearing techniques that served to popularize the purity movement. It included child development from conception to maturity. Groups of mothers met at "mothers' meetings" to discuss child rearing and other topics. They introduced moral education into the high school curricula. This mothers' crusade evolved into the National Parents Teachers Association (Pivar 1973, 174–175, 228–229).

Social Hygiene: Sex Education and the Venereal Disease Education Movement

Purity reform as a social movement evolved into a social-hygiene movement about the turn of the century. This new movement, supported by health professionals concerned over sexually transmitted diseases, advocated sex education. During the mid-1890s, journal articles reflected concerns of a few physicians concerning adequate sex education for the prevention of venereal diseases. Women physicians and women's clubs crusaded for sex education in the schools. By 1912, "sex hygiene [was] taught in 138 schools and colleges throughout the country" (Daggett 1912, 230). It was suggested that sex education should be the sum product of the three great forces in society, "the school, the home, and the church" (Pacific Coast Social Hygiene Conference 1914). However, as was found in the late twentieth-century Clean Living Movement, bitter school board clashes regarding sex education also arose.

Venereal disease education was important to social-hygiene reformers. Social purists, similar to the American Tuberculosis Association discussed in Chapter 11, turned from volunteerism to reliance on professional expertise and administration. Physicians became more involved with the movement (Pivar 1973, 243). In 1906, the National Vigilant Committee, a convergence of social hygiene and social medicine, was formed and led by Prince Morrow, a physician. By 1910, this group had gained national status. Another independent institution, the Bureau of Social Hygiene, was funded by John D. Rockefeller Jr. This bureau collected data on social purity questions and funneled the information to numerous vice commissions. Both of these associations combined into the American Social Hygiene Association (ASHA) in 1913 with "the purpose of promoting public health and morality" (Eliot 1914, 1; Pivar 1973, 243–244; Grittner 1990, 74).

The ASHA brought together many persons dedicated to the growing belief that sex education, rather than prudery and secrecy, could best prepare young persons for life. If individuals were satisfied in marriage, prostitution and the double standard would not be necessary. Many academics joined this association. Education concerning venereal disease, sexual hygiene, and eugenic implications for choosing a mate and planning a family were advocated. It promoted "activity and the common use of the recognized safeguards against sexual perversions—such as bodily exercise, moderation in eating, abstinence in youth from alcohol, tobacco, hot spices, and all other drugs which impair self-control, even momentarily" (Eliot 1914, 3). Under the influence of the ASHA, red-light districts adjoining armed-forces training camps were closed in 1917 when the United States entered the war (Grittner 1990, 75). This group, along with the eugenics movement, pushed for the prevention of the spread of venereal disease to wives and the unborn. By 1922, thirteen states had laws promoting restrictive marriages because of venereal diseases (Laughlin 1922, 345–346). The ASHA is still active today and focuses upon sexually transmitted diseases and sex education.

THE BIRTH-CONTROL MOVEMENT

The birth-control movement emerged at the crest of the second Clean Living Movement, The idea of birth control—coined by Margaret Sanger in 1914—ran counter to romantic love and fidelity to conjugal ties in the nineteenth century. There was a belief that birth control led to moral irresponsibility and "free love." It was not considered respectable. Contraception was associated with libertine practices, such as those of Humphrey Noyes of the Oneida Community and nonmarital sexuality (Pickens 1968, 70–71). In reality, birth control was being used by the educated middle class. Information about methods were quietly passed among networks of women and between wives and husbands. Small families became increasingly fashionable among the middle class by the turn of the century, leading eugenicists to be concerned about racial suicide (Chesler 1992, 71–72).

The birth-control movement emerged from several currents of the progressive era. It was an extension of the campaign for women's rights, it emerged from a rebellion against the laws which forbid even physicians from discussing or disseminating contraceptive information, and it became a eugenic technique. Contrary to some of the other health reforms during the second Clean Living Movement, where restrictive laws were passed against drinking and smoking, birth-control supporters, like the woman suffrage movement, agitated for more personal freedoms, especially for women.[8]

The birth-control movement, like the suffrage and temperance movements and certain aspects of the purity movement, was primarily supported by white upper-middle-class or wealthy women. In the decades before World War I (see Chapter 8), women agitated for change. Increased job and educational opportunities allowed women to challenge the historic attitude that assumed that they were naturally inferior and needed to depend upon men for economic support. The birth-control movement, as perceived by Margaret Sanger, its primary leader, offered freedom from mandatory childbirth, expressed a drive for equality in marriage, and was intimately linked to the suffrage movement (Pickens 1968, 58, 72–73, 79; Chesler 1992, 66).

Margaret Sanger

Margaret Higgins (1879–1966) was born to Irish-immigrant parents in Corning, New York.[9] Somewhat sickly with tuberculosis as an adolescent, Higgins nevertheless completed two years of practical nursing training and in 1902 married William Sanger, an artist and architect. Working as a nurse in the New York City tenements, Sanger found many poor women did not want the burden of more pregnancies but did not know how to prevent them. Literature concerning birth control, because it was perceived both as pornographic and threatening the integrity of the institution of marriage, was difficult to obtain. In 1914, Sanger began distributing a pamphlet called *Family Limitations,* which discussed contraceptive methods and challenged existing laws against birth control. She also published a militant journal, *Women Rebel*, that urged legalization of birth control (Kennedy 1970, 22–26).

In August 1914, Sanger was indicted by the Department of Justice on grounds she violated postal regulations regarding distribution of her journal, and faced a possible prison sentence of forty-two years. Sanger fled to Canada, and then to England. She remained in Europe for about a year, visiting clinics and learning techniques on fitting diaphragms (Kennedy 1970, 26–34). In 1916, the government dropped its charges against her and, during that same year, in defiance of the law, Margaret and her sister opened the first birth-control clinic for contraceptive instruction in the nation. However, the police soon closed it and Margaret was arrested and convicted. In an appeal, the judge Frederick Crane ruled that physicians could give birth-control information to married women for the cure and prevention of venereal disease. Sanger was jailed for a month, giving more visibility to the movement, just as it had for the woman suffrage crusade during this same era (Reed 1978, 106–107).

In 1923, the Birth Control Clinical Research Bureau, a contraceptive clinic, was formed. During its first year, over a thousand women visited the clinic. Diaphragms were provided, which had been smuggled into the country. A follow-up study of more than 1,000 patients at the clinic concluded that diaphragms were safe and effective. By the late 1920s, they were being manufactured in the United States and sold to physicians (Reed 1978, 113–115). In 1921, Sanger established the American Birth Control League. In 1929, she formed the National Committee on Federal Legislation for Birth Control in a continuing effort to get a "doctors-only" bill passed. This bill, first submitted in 1923, proposed allowing physicians to dispense contraception information and devices rather than repealing the federal law (Dennett 1926, 200–202; Kennedy 1970, 224–225).

By the early 1930s, several hundred physician had learned about contraceptives at the Clinical Research Bureau and, by 1938, 300 birth-control clinics had emerged in the United States. In 1936, the *United States v. One Package* court case eliminated contraceptive methods from the obscenity law and allowed contraceptive materials to be sent through the mail to physicians. The right of individual citizens to bring such devices into the country for personal use was not established, however, until 1971 (Reed 1978, 117–121; Grant 1988, 365).[10]

At the beginning of the movement, Mary Ware Dennett launched her own crusade while Sanger traveled in Europe. In 1915, several feminists, under the leadership of Dennett, formed the National Birth Control League, which instituted an education and lobbying campaign to change laws rather than defy them (Sanger 1931, 124–124). Congressional resistance to changing the laws on contraception encouraged Dennet (1926, iii–iv) to publish *Birth Control Laws* to educate the public on "just what the present laws provide . . . how they happened to be the way they are . . . various proposition that have been made for changing the laws . . . and the basis on which to differentiate between sound and spurious legislation." Although these anticontraceptive laws were more or less nullified by a series of court decisions in the 1930s, the Comstock clauses on contraception were not repealed until 1971, almost a hundred years after their enactment.

Proponents and Opponents of the Birth-Control Movement

For the most part, leaders of the eugenics movement supported birth control because, like sterilization, it constituted a method of achieving the goals of ensuring healthy and genetically fit babies. Many health reformers argued that educating the unfit and alien classes on contraceptive methods could decrease their birth rate. Some eugenicists, however, did not agree with birth control on the grounds it contributed to racial suicide (Pickens 1968, 73–74; Haller 1963, 92). However,

Sanger herself noted in 1931 that "over time many Protestant leaders, physicians [and] scientists rallied to the movement" (Sanger 1931, 349–351). Some critics argued that birth control would lead to immorality and free love. Primary resistance to the birth-control movement came from the Roman Catholic and Mormon Churches. Catholic writers, with the blessings of the Church, produced tracts and books condemning birth control as immoral. The Mormon Church considered birth control an "evil practice" on the grounds it ran counter to the biblical command to "be fruitful and multiply" (Bush 1992, 18–22; Haller 1963, 90).

By the late 1930s, the crusade era of the movement had waned and Sanger went into semiretirement. In 1939, the Birth Control Clinical Research Bureau and the ongoing Birth Control League merged. This new organization became known as the Planned Parenthood Federation in 1942. It is still active at the turn of the twenty-first century and provides women's health care, including routine examinations and cancer screening, assessment and treatment of sexually transmitted diseases, contraceptive information and devices, and, in some communities, pregnancy terminations.

SUMMARY

The eugenics movement became intertwined with many other movements of the progressive era. It was an underlying factor in temperance, antismoking and antidrug campaigns, physical culture, Nativism, and the public health crusades of the second Clean Living Movement. The antisexuality campaigns evolved into a movement in which sexuality and sexually transmitted disease education was considered important. The birth-control movement emerged as a rebellion against strict Victorian morality and laws.

NOTES

1. Francis Galton (1822–1911), coined the term "eugenics" in his *Inquiries into Human Faculty and Its Development* (1883, 24): "Eugenes, namely, good in stock, hereditarily endowed with noble qualities. . . . The word *eugenic* would sufficiently express the idea." Besides eugenics, other terms, including "race-improvement," "race-regeneration," "racial-hygiene," and "sanitary marriages," were common. Opposite to eugenic was "dysgenic," or racial degeneracy due to the breeding among the unfit. Terms such as "degeneracy," "unfit," "defective," "insane," and "feeble-minded" were commonly used by professionals and nonprofessionals alike during the progressive era. They were considered the correct technical terms during this time, although today they are likely to be considered offensive.

2. Several works discuss the eugenics movement as an aspect of the progressive era. See, in particular, Haller (1963), Pernick (1996, 1997), Paul (1995), Pickens (1968), and Larson (1995). Many eugenicists were concerned that

through charity and medicine the unfit were being kept alive to breed more unfit, which resulted in some clashes between the eugenics and public-health movements.

3. An example of the interlinking of eugenics with other health-reform movements is illustrated by the 1909 lectures published from the Thirteenth Annual Meeting of the American Academy of Political and Social Science, entitled *Race Improvements in the United States* (1909). Most of the health reforms of the day were discussed, including public health and disease prevention, purity, physical culture, birth control, sex education, prohibition, social gospel, pure food and drugs, woman suffrage, and venereal disease education, among others.

4. There is a tendency today for the eugenics movement to be completely discounted as a "racist crusade" or to have its influence on various progressive reforms minimized. Donald Pickens (1968, 55) reminds us that "during the first thirty years of the twentieth century, reputable men of science in the United States formulated the eugenic creed." He further argues that "the American eugenicists from 1859 to 1930 were both creatures and creators of their intellectual history. It would be of little profit to use present-mindedness against the eugenicists; rather, [it is important] to understand the eugenicists with their naturalistic Darwinian and sociological presupposition as part of [the] problem of man's nature." Many states still have eugenics laws on their books which were passed during the progressive era. The most common is the premarital exam and/or blood test for certain diseases before a marriage license can be granted.

5. Some states began to forbid the contracting of marriage if either party were "insane, an idiot, feeble-minded, epileptic or had not been cured of syphilis or gonorrhea." In some states, indigence, being a "habitual drunkard," or applying for a license while intoxicated were grounds for denial of a license (Rentoul 1906, 133–143).

6. Martin Pernick (1996, 81–82, 143) discusses a film entitled the *Black Stork*, which was "the most explicit depiction of negative eugenics to reach the silent screen." It was shown beginning in 1916 for almost thirty years in different editions. The film depicts defectives as a repulsive, dangerous, and costly menace to society and argued for eugenic measures.

7. Several works concerning Comstock have been written over the years by both supporters and detractors. See Bates (1995), Bennett (1971), Beisel (1997), Broun and Leech (1927), Trumbull (1913), and, in particular, Fisher-LaMay (1989), which examines Comstock's career in terms of the Victorian precepts that governed public thinking on sexual behavior, and a dissertation by Johnson (1973).

8. Mary A. Hopkins (1915) wrote a series of six articles concerning all sides of the birth-control debate for *Harper's Weekly* in 1915. This series is symbolic of the burgeoning public interest in birth control and the rise of the movement.

9. Information about Sanger can be found in her autobiography (1931), and in works by Chesler (1992), Reed (1978), and Kennedy (1970).

10. My maternal grandmother stated in the late 1960s that when she immigrated from Canada to the United States in 1915, after spending a decade in Germany, she smuggled in cervical caps, as she knew she could not easily obtain them in North America.

10

Pure Food and Drugs and the Elimination of "Dope"

It is clearly the duty of the State to close opium dens and restrict the sale of poisons, and in regard to the sale of patent and proprietary medicines containing poisonous drugs the contents should be expressed on the label and the word poison added.

George M. Kober, *Science* (1897)

The prevalence of the drug habit, the magnitude of which is now startling the whole civilized and uncivilized world, can be checked only in one way—by controlling the distribution of habit-forming drugs. With the Government as the first distributor and a physician as the last, drug-taking merely as a habit would cease to be.

Charles B. Towns, *Century* (1912)

The evils of drug addiction are found among all classes, ages and conditions of society—persons of the high and low walks of life, children of tender years and very aged persons, the latter have in many instances been habitues for over half a century.

"A Year of the Harrison Narcotic Law," *The Survey* (1916)

Interwoven with each other, and with other progressive health campaigns during the second Clean Living Movement, was a pure-food and an antidrug movement. The moral suasive aspect of these two movements were generated in the 1890s by public-health professionals concerned about adulterated foods and patent medicines containing addicting drugs. In the last decade of the nineteenth century, the dangers of addiction began to be realized. After 1900, the popular press began to discuss these topics and campaigns for uncontaminated food and the accurate labeling of patent medicines began. This resulted in the passage of the Pure Food and Drug Act of 1906.

A perceived increase in narcotic addiction, resulting from loopholes in the Food and Drug Law, led to escalated coercive measures that cumulated in passage of the Harrison Narcotic Act in 1914 and other laws in the early 1920s.[1] The Harrison Act stemmed, in part, from supposed opium and cocaine use among the so-called "dangerous" social classes. These strata included Chinese opium smokers, black cocaine users, and the criminal underworld. The attitude of the middle class toward drug users shifted. Over the course of the first two decades of the century, drug users began to be seen as criminals rather than being sick. During the backlash phase, a lucrative black market arose to supply drugs that had previously been legal and repressive measures were taken against users. As a result, both drugs and the user were demonized. Although the main thrust of the antidrug movement had waned by the mid- to late 1920s, during the 1930s some other legislation passed stricter food, drugs, and cosmetics laws. The nadir of illicit drug use was from the late 1930s through the 1940s. It was not until the last three decades of the twentieth century that the fervor of the early twentieth-century movement emerged again in campaigns for food labeling and the war against drugs.

THE PURE-FOOD CAMPAIGN

The pure-food movement began on the state level in 1879. By 1881, New Jersey, New York, and Michigan had passed laws to prevent the adulteration of food and drugs. Twenty years later, almost every state had passed legislation regulating some aspects of food, but few of these laws were actually enforced. Bills submitted to Congress through the 1890s and early 1900s were not passed because of a lack of public support and because of lobbying on the part of food and proprietary drug groups (Kober 1897, 797–798; Mason 1900, 405; Temin 1980, 27–28).

Popular Support for Pure Food

Popular magazines in 1900 began to warn the public about food adulteration and urged "an honest label" in terms of ingredients. Particular concern arose regarding "oleo-margarine, filled cheese and mixed flour" (Crampton 1900, 308). To determine the extent of harm of some of the adulterants, a "poison squad" was organized by Harvey Wiley in 1902. A dozen volunteers restricted themselves to diets adulterated with common food additives which had been linked to ill health (Lender 1984, 515).

The story of this "poison squad" was printed by the "muckraker"—journalists who sensationalized the news during the first decade of the century. These "yellow journalists" fanned the flames of the movement with a series of publications in 1905 and 1906 which attacked poisons in food. Growing public support for stricter legislation regarding pure foods resulted in President Theodore Roosevelt's advocation of pure-food legislation in his annual message to Congress in December 1905 (Young 1992b, 309–310; Temin 1980, 28).

The two most prominent crusaders concerned with food adulteration and contamination were Harvey Wiley, the "father of the food and drug laws," and George M. Kober, a sanitarian and public-health crusader.

Harvey Washington Wiley

The chief architect of the Pure Food and Drug Act was Harvey W. Wiley (1844–1930). Wiley, "one of the most prominent figures of the Progressive Era," provided a symbolic link between the "Temperance Movement and the broader reform impulse of the period" (Lender 1984, 515). Born in Indiana, Wiley was very religious as a boy. Harvey Young (1992b, 309), a historian of the food and drug movement, considered the movement a secular outlet for Wiley's religious convictions. Trained in chemistry and medicine, Wiley became chief chemist of the federal Department of Agriculture in 1883. Over his almost thirty years in the post, he transformed the Bureau of Chemistry into one of the most effective agencies of the federal government. Besides being involved with food and drug reforms, Wiley also was an advocate of other public-health campaigns including prohibition and eugenics (Lender 1984, 515; Pernick 1997, 1770; Temin 1980, 32; Young 1992b, 308–319).

George M. Kober

George M. Kober (1850–1931), born and reared in Hessen-Darmstadt, Germany, emigrated to the United States in 1867. He received his medical training while serving with the United States Army at several schools and hospitals. In addition to his involvement with the campaign to establish a national public-health department and sanitation to prevent disease, Kober became president of the National Tuberculosis Association and pushed for pure food and drug laws and the elimination of narcotics. He produced numerous articles on the need for these various public-health reforms (Knopf 1922, 360–363).

The Pure Food and Drug Act of 1906

Early in 1906, Upton Sinclair (1878–1968) published a pivotal work, *The Jungle*. The book constituted a conscious attempt to convert readers to socialism by presenting the grim lot of packingtown workers.

Rather than promote socialism, the book fermented a national outrage against the meat industry; sales of meat products fell dramatically. The book proved to be a prime force in promoting the passage of pure food laws (Young 1992b, 314). In June 1906, Congress passed the Pure Food and Drug Act. Another bill that passed the same day gave the Department of Agriculture direct authority to inspect animals in meat-packing plants (Young 1989, 262; Temin 1980, 27–29).

THE PATENT-MEDICINE CRUSADE

Modern patent-medicine regulation in the United States has its roots in the progressive era, when a movement to properly label ingredients and eliminate "poisons" from patent medicines flowered. Two classes of drugs were distinguished at this time. The first were formulary drugs, whose compositions were listed in official publications. The second were patent or proprietary medicines manufactured by "secret processes" from unknown ingredients and sold under trademark names. Because these patent medicines presumably relieved the symptoms of common aches and pains at a time when physicians offered few cures, they proved to be very popular. Health reformers became increasingly alarmed about the lack of labels that pinpointed the poisonous and addicting substances found in these nostrums ("The 'Patent Medicine' Crusade" 1905; Temin 1980, 24–25; Kober 1897, 799).

A Call for Honest Labeling

Popular magazines, such as the *Ladies Home Journal* and *Collier's Weekly*, began publishing articles about the dangers of patent medicines after the turn of the century. An article by Maud Banfield (1903) in the *Ladies Home Journal*, for example, pointed out that "the reason why patent medicines are so dangerous is because they often contain large quantities of alcohol, opium, or cocaine, and thus induce or encourage dangerous habits, which often times they specifically profess to cure."

Antialcohol and other health reformers exerted increased public pressure on Congress to legislate restrictions on the proprietary medicine business, which led to the coercive phase of the pure-food and drug movement. These pressures coalesced with the passage of the Pure Food and Drug Act, despite the strenuous opposition of the Proprietary Medicine Association and the National Wholesale Liquor Dealers Association. The law stipulated the identification of dangerous drugs, including alcohol, on the packages of various preparations (Timberlake 1963, 159; Young 1989, 265–268).

As a component of the new law, labels that manufacturers placed on their medicines were required to be truthful. "Before the passage of the Food and Drug Act, it was the general custom of manufacturers to put upon the labels some reassuring legend such as 'contains nothing injurious to the youngest babe,'" even if these "soothing syrups" contained opiates, chloroform, and cocaine, as described by Hall (1910) in *Good Housekeeping*. After passage, if certain substances were listed as not being present, they, in fact, could not be in the nostrum. Adulterated or misbranded articles were subject to government seizure and prosecution.

Not satisfied with loopholes in the 1906 Act, reformers began to push for legislation regarding a "standard of purity for drugs." After continued pressure from reformers and the public, the Sherley Amendment was enacted in 1912. This amendment added the requirement that labels not contain any false or fraudulent statement regarding curative or therapeutic effects. The Net Weight Act of 1913 required that all packages shipped in interstate commerce "be plainly and conspicuous marked to show the quantity of the contents," as reported in an article entitled, "Extensions of the Food and Drug Act" (1914). The next step in the campaign against dangerous drugs was for their complete eradication from society.

A WAR AGAINST DRUGS AND "DOPE FIENDS"

The Food and Drug Law of 1906 led to a reduction of the narcotic contents of patent medicines and a decrease in their sales. However, this new labeling, combined with popular education concerning the dangers of drugs, did not reduce overall drug addiction. To the contrary, an increase in the nonmedical use of opiates and cocaine emerged (Courtwright 1982a, 114). Concerns about patent medicines merged into a generalized antidrug movement during this time as the social class of users shifted and addicts began to be seen as criminals rather than sick.

The typical addict in the late nineteenth century was a white upper-middle-class matron who was addicted through the medical use of proprietary or prescription medication. These women were generally regarded sympathetically and considered innocent victims. Opiate addiction peaked among this group in the mid-1890s, and then began to decline as fewer physicians prescribed them. Opiates and other drugs were also used by literary figures who were considered eccentric (Booth 1996, 191–193; Schieffelin 1909, 208; Courtwright 1982a, 1–2, 100–102; Zentner 1974, 49; Kober 1897, 798). During the early twentieth century, these high-socioeconomic-class addicts were supplanted by "fast men and women" and lower-class males living in urban areas. As the addict population changed, drug use began to be regarded as corrupt and its users as loathsome criminals. Addiction shifted from a medical to a criminal problem. By the 1920s "dope fiends" were considered self-indulgent, irresponsible, lower-class members on society's periphery, such as prostitutes, criminals, and jazz musicians (Booth 1996, 191–193; Courtwright 1982a, 1–2, 100–102; Zentner 1974, 49–50; Kober 1897, 798). These attitudes are still found today.

Moral Suasion: Education and Treatment

The moral-suasion phase of the antidrug movement is illustrated in titles of articles from popular magazines aimed at women. Examples include "The 'Patent-Medicine' Curse," "Why Headache Remedies Are Dangerous," and "Drugging the Baby" during the first decade of the twentieth century. Such articles and publications strove to convince consumers to avoid using the drugs found in patent medicines. At the beginning of the second decade, the movement began to enter the coercive phase. Scare articles appeared, such as "The Peril of the Drug Habit" and "The Drug-Endangered Nation" in an effort to convince the public that stricter laws were needed against drugs.[2]

Treatment of "Inebriates" and "Dope Fiends"

In the early part of the antidrug movement, treatment was advocated for innocent victims of drug addiction. During the last decade of the nineteenth century, both alcoholism and drug addiction were considered diseases that could be cured. Alcoholism was viewed as a disease found primarily among those who "dwelled in the land of cold winters." Treatment, however, could cure this disease.[3]

A popular "scientific" treatment for alcohol and drug addiction was the Keeley cure. This treatment, developed by Leslie E. Keeley, a physician, consisted of a "reconstructive Nerve Tonic having the Double Chloride of Gold and Sodium for its basis, which will in every case, without exception, *forever* relieve the nervous system of the acquired necessity for Alcohol, Opium, Morphine, or any other stimulant or narcotic." Both opium- and alcohol-addicted individuals went to Keeley treatment centers, which had been established across the country. Keeley claimed about 95-percent effectiveness. However, because little research is available as to this method's efficacy, it probably had a short-term placebo effect. Other forms of treatment for drug and alcohol addiction included asylums, sanitarium, and water-cure establishments.[4]

Nonmedical Drug Use and Fear of Minorities

Opium smoking became associated with western Chinese immigrants and cocaine sniffing with Southern black laborers and the urban underworld over the course of the second Clean Living Movement. The underlying fear and hostility toward these "dangerous classes" on the part of the dominant middle class played a role in agitation for more stringent laws against opiates and cocaine as the moral-suasion phase merged into the coercive phase of the movement. As had been found with alcohol and tobacco in both the mid-nineteenth-century and late twentieth-century Clean Living Movements, cocaine, opium, and its derivative heroin became demonized.

Opium and Chinese "Coolies"

In the 1860s and 1870s, Chinese "coolies," or laborers, began to arrived on the West Coast, bringing with them their opium habit and the institutionalized opium den. The den, similar in function to the saloon for European immigrants, offered, in addition to opium, gambling, prostitution, loan sharking, and companionship. Most of these laborers were indentured servants under the control of merchant creditors and secret criminal societies or "tongs." Once the laborers had worked off their debt, they were theoretically free; however, many of them became deeper in debt due to opium addiction (Booth 1996, 193; Zentner 1974, 45–47; Courtwright 1982a, 67–68).

Because most of these Chinese immigrants did not plan to stay in the country, there was little incentive to abandon old ways and adapt to the new culture. Instead, they remained isolated. Ambivalence or hostility toward them and a growing fear of cheap coolie labor, which threatened American workers' sense of security, fueled virulent anti-Chinese campaigns culminating in the 1882 Exclusion Act to limit immigration. Laws were also passed in many states restricting the occupational mobility of these immigrants. This led to Chinese-operated businesses, such as restaurants and laundries, often associated with opium dens and gambling casinos (Weir 1909, 330; Musto 1987, 282; Booth 1996, 193; Zentner 1974, 45–47; Courtwright 1982a, 70).

As the Chinese migrated eastward, they introduced opium to other areas of the country. Opium-smoking whites began to frequent the Chinese opium dens and the habit spread through contacts with individuals who were already users. Unlike the medical addict who was regarded with sympathy, these smokers were blamed for their dependence (Zentner 1974, 47; Courtwright 1982a, 70–71; Kober 1897, 798; Booth 1996, 194).

Opium use was more or less tolerated as long as it was confined to the Chinese. When it began to spread among whites in the mid-1870s, there were alarming reports in the popular press that the "idle rich" were beginning to frequent the dens. Although opium smoking was not as widespread as morphine injecting, the public viewed it with horror after stories of young white girls being forced into prostitution were published (Booth 1996, 195–196; Courtwright 1982b, 28).

The fear of miscegenation and the "yellow peril" translated into restrictive legislation against opium in cities with large Chinese populations. However, the laws, even when passed, were rarely enforced. Crackdowns generally occurred only when whites and Chinese smoked together in common establishments. As a result, whites began to smoke in their own dens and obtained their opium from Chinese dealers (Courtwright 1982b, 28; Booth 1996, 195–196).

Cocaine, Blacks, and the Underworld

Cocaine was first identified in the mid-nineteenth century. However, the medical properties of the drug were not realized until 1878, when W. H. Bentley in the United States used it to cure morphine addiction. Based upon reports it was a cure, such practitioners as Sigmund Freud (1856–1939) used cocaine to treat patients with depression, morphine addiction, alcoholism, and other problems. It soon found its way into proprietary medicine and was considered a "wonder drug" (Ashley 1976, 33, 219; Gold 1993, 14–16; Courtwright 1982a, 96–97).

During the 1880s, cocaine was widely sold in patent medicines and tonics, particularly those to cure chronic cough, sinusitis, and hay fever. Cocaine was also used in soft drinks. In 1886, John Pemberton of Atlanta, Georgia, introduced a syrup containing cocaine and caffeine, from the kola nut, called "Coca-Cola." It was advertised as a temperance beverage and a therapeutic agent for many ailments. Cocaine was removed from the drink in 1903 as a result of public pressure, as the dark side of cocaine use, including dependence, was soon apparent. After passage of the Pure Food and Drug Act, a decline in use occurred in many nostrums. However, nonmedical use of cocaine increased (Ashley 1976, 66, 86; Courtwright 1982a, 114; Musto 1989b, 4–5; Schieffelin 1909, 208).

The press portrayed cocaine use as a particular problem of the black community. Articles aroused fear by reporting supposed violent rampages among African-Americans who allegedly were under its influence. Charles B. Towns (1912), head of a New York City drug-treatment hospital, claimed that southern overseers "deliberately put cocaine into the rations of his Negro laborers in order to get more work out of them to meet a sudden emergency." These laborers were then supposed to have spread the habit throughout the South to cotton plantations, railroad work camps, and levee construction sites (Foster 1996, 547–564; Musto 1987, 7–8; Courtwright 1982a, 97–98; Grinspoon and Bakalar 1985, 39).

White middle-class fear of increasing nonmedicinal use of cocaine throughout black and also poor white communities resulted in repressive measures.[5] Several authors over the past twenty years, including Courtwright (1982a, 197–198), Musto (1987, 7), and Ashley (1976, 67–92), however, have suggested that most of the material published at the turn of the century concerning the violent behavior of black cocaine users was probably anecdotal tales.[6]

Cocaine use also permeated the criminal class of society. Between 1895 and 1900, nonmedical use of the drug became common in the white underworld in both northern and southern cities, where it was generally sniffed in powdered form called "snow" (Courtwright 1982a, 97–98). In the early part of the second decade of the century, cocaine began to be portrayed in the media as more evil than opiates. Towns (1912) considered cocaine "the most harmful of all habit-forming drugs." He suggested it "quickly deteriorates its victim" and was a "shortcut to the insane asylum." When its recreational use was perceived as spilling out of the black community and the underworld into the middle class, reformers called for further restrictions. Reports in the popular press concerning the use of cocaine among children were also described. One author suggested "several cases have been reported where groups of school-children have been taught to use the drug" (Schieffelin 1909, 209). When cocaine and other drugs were seen as infiltrating the rest of society, reformers called for more restrictive measures against these evils.

Coercion: Negative Sanctions and Legislation against Drugs

Some state or local ordinances were passed in the last decade of the nineteenth century to curb the abuse of cocaine and opiates. By the second decade of the new century, these drugs became increasingly demonized. In addition, drug use began to take on a criminal and deviant identity (Burnham 1993, 116–117). Anticocaine laws had been passed in forty-seven states by 1914 and twenty-seven states by 1915 had passed antiopium smoking legislation. Most of the laws against opium were aimed at closing the public dens, rather than forbidding the practice outright. Laws against cocaine attempted to restrict the use of cocaine to dentists and physicians for use in their practices and not for resale. In general, the penalties for cocaine were more severe, reflecting the anticocaine hysteria generated by the news media. In New York state, under the Boylan Act of 1914, for example, the illegal sale of heroin was considered a misdemeanor and a violation of the state public-health law, while the illegal sale of cocaine was a felony violation under the penal code (Kennedy 1985, 96–98; Booth 1996, 196; Courtwright 1982a, 98; Schieffelin 1909, 210–211).

The greatest impact on American opium smokers and cocaine users resulted from federal import and tax laws. Federal control over narcotic use would have been considered unconstitutional at the turn of the century. However, by the end of the first decade, near the peak of the progressive era, federal laws and taxes began to be imposed on a variety of health-related issues, paving the way for more restrictive antidrug measures. These included taxes on foods (such as colored oleomargarine), labeling of patent medicines, and prohibition of transporting prostitutes or alcohol across state lines (Courtwright 1982b, 29; Schieffelin 1909, 210–211; Musto 1987, 9–10).

Some International Pressure

As a result of international politics and concern over increased opium use in Far Eastern territories under the control of European countries and the United States, an international movement to regulate the drug emerged. Attempts to check the use of habit-forming drugs on the international level forced federal measures in the United States. American missionaries pressed Theodore Roosevelt to support an international conference planned for the winter of 1909 in Shanghai. However, the American delegation realized that a complete lack of domestic antinarcotic legislation would limit their leadership in the call for suppression of the Far East opium traffic. To save face, a bill was quickly drafted to prohibit the importation and use of opium for other than medical purposes in the United States. It was signed into law in 1909, a week after the conference convened in Shanghai (Courtwright 1982a, 81–82; Low 1913; Booth 1996, 196–197).

This Smoking Opium Exclusion Act of 1909 banned all imports of the drug other than by registered pharmaceutical firms, and imposed stiff penalties on traffickers. At The Hague in The Netherlands, an international agreement "to prevent the manufacture, exportation, importation, or use of opium for smoking purposes" was signed in January 1912. Restrictions from these acts, however, resulted in a black market to supply drugs (Booth 1996, 197; Courtwright 1982a, 84–85; 1982b, 29).

The Harrison Narcotic Law of 1914

The U.S. Congress ratified The Hague Convention in 1913. However, Europe was soon plunged into war and, as a result, "the narcotic problem—if they thought of it at all—seemed the least of their troubles" (Gavit 1927, 16). Opiate and cocaine use increased in the United States, but the Great War interrupted the antinarcotic movement on an international level. Because both cocaine and heroin use were perceived as increasing among the criminal element and minorities, and spilling over into more affluent social classes, a push for new laws to curb these evils emerged.

In 1914, President Woodrow Wilson signed the Harrison Act. Historian David Courtwright (1982a, 106) remarked that "in many respects the Harrison Act was a classic piece of progressive legislation: reform effort (restricting the sale of narcotics) met business self-interests (rationalizing the narcotic market) to produce a compromise measure." Framers of the law considered it the domestic implementation of the Hague Opium Treaty. Over the next decade, legislation to tighten up the Harrison Act became a priority as a result of increasing perceptions that addicts were criminals rather than sick. In 1919, an amendment to the act further restricted opiates and cocaine as the coercion phase of the antidrug movement peaked. This amendment made it more difficult to export bulk morphine for reimportation into the United States and made it illegal to sell, purchase, or dispense cocaine except in its original government-stamped package. During this same year, the Supreme Court ruled it illegal to prescribe narcotics for known addicts unless they were being treated in federally licenced clinics. However, just three years after the first clinic was opened the Supreme Court ruled that it was illegal to prescribe drugs in maintenance clinics after all (Kennedy 1985, 100; Musto 1987, 128–140).

This change in the law forced drug users further into the criminal underworld. In 1922, importation of cocaine and coca leaves was prohibited other than as a small amount for medical use under the Narcotic Drug Import and Export Act. This act also established the Federal Narcotics Control Board. Congress outlawed all domestic use and production of heroin in 1924. However, heroin use and smuggling continued (Courtwright 1982a, 206; Booth 1996, 201–202). These additional laws and increased hostility toward control were factors in a backlash against the antidrug, prohibition, and other restrictive crusades of the era.

The Backlash Era: The 1920s and the Jazz Age

Joseph Kennedy (1985, 102), in a controversial essay about cocaine, suggested that during the decade after World War I, "a pleasure-seeking constituent in the nation went to war against the reactionary establishment to regain the freedom of personal consumption" of drugs. This was similar to the "me generation" of the 1970s, when young people and others stressed creature comforts and the importance of having a good time, including drug experimentation. The Roaring Twenties backlash era was characterized by open revolt against the moral strictures of any prohibitive legislation that might prevent pleasure, including alcohol, drugs, and tobacco. In reaction to flaunting of the laws, reformers tightened enforcement and in the process turned ordinary citizens into criminals. These included social drinkers, occasional drug users, and, in some states, tobacco smokers, as discussed in Chapter 8. By 1928, about one-third of federal prisoners were violators of the Harrison Narcotics Act. During the 1920s and 1930s, the goals of American government policy were to stop the supply and to force addicts to seek treatment (Kennedy 1985, 103; Musto 1987, 184, 193; Booth 1996, 202; Burnham 1993, 118).

Cocaine use began to decline in popularity in the 1930s and was replaced by amphetamines around 1932. The decline of use in cocaine was due to its extreme negative effect on users, including paranoia and severe psychological dependency. Kennedy (1985, 111) has argued that "the pursuit and misuse of cocaine in the previous decade created a sordid atmosphere around the drug that made it unattractive, if not repulsive." By the 1940s, cocaine had become a rare and esoteric vice and was no longer considered a topic of much attention. It played an insignificant part in American culture in the 1950s and early 1960s and was rarely seen even in groups that had been associated with the drug, such as jazz musicians (Kennedy 1985, 114–116). Burnham (1993, 118) has suggested that for all drugs "throughout the interwar period, almost the whole of the public believed that all users were either deviant or criminal or both."

SUMMARY

An important aspect of the second Clean Living Movement was a crusade to regulate the purity of foods and drugs. A campaign for the proper labeling of patent medicines over a period of about twenty years evolved into an war against cocaine and opiates when they became associated with undesirable elements of society. This antidrug crusade tended to criminalize the behavior, along with substances that during the previous generation were legal. Rebellion against restrictive drug laws on the part of some, often considered deviant individuals, was a factor in the so-called Roaring Twenties backlash era.

NOTES

1. The term "addiction" was not commonly used during the early part of this era. Popular terms were "vice," "habit," or "opium eaters" when referring to morphine or opium use. "Addiction" in this book refers to both physiological and psychological dependence on any substance (see Courtwright 1982a, Chapter 2, for further information). "Narcotic" was the general classification for any addicting drug, including opiates, cocaine, and cannabis. Pharmacologically, narcotics are depressants derived from opiates, or synthetic opiates. Alcohol is a depressant, while cannabis and cocaine are stimulants in terms of their physiological effects.

2. *The Ladies Home Journal, Good Housekeeping, Literary Digest,* and *Century Magazine,* in particular, had many articles concerning the peril of drugs and drug users from about 1909 until 1915.

3. The "disease concept" of alcoholism is not a product of current thought. An attorney, John Flavel Mines (1891) chronicles his treatment at a Keeley clinic where he considers his alcoholism a disease. He stated, "For twenty years I had been a victim of the disease of drink," and "My own diagnosis told me that my trouble was a disease." Engs (1991b, 1995) has described the development of the southern European, northern European, and blended patterns of alcohol use and the reasons why northerners are more likely to be problem drinkers. These include the lack of Romanization (urbanization and cultural change of indigenous populations), and other factors such as latitude, climate, weather, political–economic system, and agricultural practices. The observation that alcoholism is more likely to be found among northern Europeans can be traced to antiquity and is documented in both classical Roman and Greek literature.

4. See the works by White (1998) concerning the Keeley treatment and Jonnes (1996) concerning other aspects of the drug use and treatment at the turn of the century.

5. Foster (1996, 559) hypothesizes that open recreational use on the part of blacks violated the white upper-middle-class norm of private medicinal drug use in the "sanctity of the home." Unlike opiates, cocaine was used openly and became the natural target of the dominant culture.

6. Courtwright (1982a) offered a plausible explanation of why so many contemporaries were convinced of the link between cocaine use and crime among blacks. These include excuses for repression of blacks, more powerful firearms for police, and a sense that cocaine use indirectly contributed to crimes against property. I would also add other hypotheses, including white middle-class fear of a rapidly changing society; eugenic fears of race degeneration; and a belief that through the elimination of cocaine, alcohol, and other drugs a golden age free from crime, disease, family disintegration, and other social problems would be more likely to emerge.

11

Tuberculosis, Public Health, and Influenza

Epidemic diseases, like empires, rise, peak, and decline.
Old Saying

Quite recently ... there seems to be a growing interest in sanitary matters in our cities, and people are asking whether the death-rates are higher than they ought to be ... and to what extent it is worth while to expend money to secure pure water, clean streets, odorless sewers, etc.
John Billings, *Forum* (1893)

[There is] a worldwide movement to put an end to the most deadly and most needless scourge with which humanity is afflicted.
Charity Organization Society,
A Handbook on the Prevention of Tuberculosis (1903)

If [immunization's] promise is borne out in general practice, [it] will work a revolution in the health, happiness, and length of life of the human race.
Leonard Keene Hirshberg, *World's Work* (1913)

Interwoven with the temperance, physical-culture, and the pure food and drug crusades was a sanitation and disease-prevention movement. Koch's confirmation in 1882 that microorganisms caused disease led to this movement, which focused specifically on tuberculosis and included the expansion of public health, preventive medicine measures, and the formation of voluntary organizations such as the National Tuberculosis Association. However, in spite of improved sanitation, newly discovered immunization and other preventive measures, along with strong optimism that disease finally had been conquered, nature had a surprise. The fatal Spanish Flu epidemic raged at the end of World War I as the second Clean Living Movement began to wane.

THE ANTITUBERCULOSIS MOVEMENT

Over the course of the second Clean Living Movement, the leading cause of death shifted from infectious to chronic disease. At the turn of the century, pneumonia and tuberculosis were the two leading causes of death. By 1920, heart disease had become the major killer. Decreased death rates for these respiratory and other infectious diseases in the early twentieth century were largely brought about by improved living conditions, including better nutrition, housing, and working environments. In addition, reform campaigns for environmental sanitation, specific immunization, and therapy were also important for the elimination of communicable diseases. To address tuberculosis in particular, a health-reform crusade arose to eliminate this ancient scourge.[1] The TB movement pioneered many contemporary methods of public health. These included the voluntary association focused against a specific disease, a model for close cooperation among health professionals, lay members, and public and private agencies, and campaigns of mass public education (Teller 1988, 1).

The Nature of the Tuberculosis Epidemic

Evidence of tuberculosis has been found in Egyptian mummies and documents from other ancient civilizations. Over the centuries, tuberculosis, like most infectious diseases, has waxed and waned in terms of severity.[2] For generations it had been noted that TB tended to "run in families." In the nineteenth century, tuberculosis was thought to be inherited. At the dawn of the "bacteria age," at the turn of the twentieth century, TB's familial occurrence was equated with a common source of infection in the household (Dubos and Dubos 1952, 188). By the end of the twentieth century, inherited genetic traits were again considered a factor, at least in terms of lack of susceptibility to the disease.[3]

In the United States, the first statistics concerning tuberculosis date to around 1850. It was noticed that states that were newly settled, such as the Rocky Mountain areas and the Southwest, were free from the disease and even acquired a reputation as health resorts for patients. As they became urbanized, TB morbidity increased. The more crowded the cities, the higher the death rate from consumption. Richard Shryock (1957, 32), a medical historian, has observed that "tuberculosis was a major menace to the evolving urban civilization of the last two centuries." The death rate from TB in major cities, including New York,

Boston, and Philadelphia, rose after 1850 and remained high until after 1880, when it began to decline (Shryock 1957, 31–32). Many observers of TB now attribute the decline chiefly to socioeconomic improvements, including less crowding, better nutrition, better ventilation, natural selection, and shortening of the work week (Bates 1992, 321–325).

Immigrants, Poverty, and Tuberculosis

New York City at the turn of the twentieth century was not only a center for the tuberculosis epidemic but also for the TB movement. Poor peasants from Ireland and southern and eastern Europe packed into already crowded slums. These immigrants contributed to the epidemic just as immigrants had contributed to the cholera epidemic during the Jacksonian era. Irish immigrants had a TB rate almost three times that of native-born whites and about twice that of other European-born immigrants. The "colored" component (African and Chinese descent) had a TB rate nearly five times that of native-born whites in New York City. This was attributed to their so-called "dirty" living habits. Italians, Russians, Hungarians, and Poles were considered much less likely to die from TB, even though they also lived in the tenements of New York and other large cities. This was because they were considered to have more moderate drinking habits (Charity Organization Society 1903, 52–57).

The Beginning of the Tuberculosis Movement

The campaign against tuberculosis, called the tuberculosis movement, began in the last decade of the nineteenth century and reached maturity in 1917, when the last state agency was formed (Teller 1988, 1). The crusade consisted of four stages: the *sanitorium, public-health, voluntary,* and *health-education* phases. Each period grew out of the preceding one and generally overlapped subsequent stages. Similar to other movements in the reforming surge, the movement had phases of moral suasion and coercion. Although it reached a complacency phase after World War II, it did not go through a backlash, as most citizens agreed with and adopted the hygiene measures fostered by the movement.

Like many other health crusades during the three Clean Living Movements addressed in this book, the campaign against TB did not intensify until after the problem was already on the wane. The germ theory was not accepted in medical circles until about 1880, the tubercle bacillus was only seen for the first time in 1882, and the movement for treatment and segregation of patients in sanitoria did not gain momentum until the 1890s. However, the mortality from tuberculosis began to fall after 1880. By 1900, the annual mortality from this disease had already "fallen to 200 per 100,000, half the figure reached a few decades earlier." But even at this lower level, tuberculosis remained the leading cause of death. Therefore, it was not surprising that "many physicians and public health officers remained for a time unaware of the downward trend that had begun spontaneously" (Dubos and Dubos 1952, 186). Over the course of the twentieth century, the prevalence of TB continued its downward trend until the mid-1980s, when it rose for a few years.

Stage One: The Sanitorium Movement

The initial focus of the tuberculosis movement was on the isolation and treatment of "open"—active—cases of TB in sanitoria. This movement had its beginnings in 1885, with Edward Trudeau's founding of the Adirondack Cottage Sanitorium at Saranac Lake, New York. Following the success of this center, sanitorium construction began to grow in the late 1890s.[4] This stage of the movement peaked during the second decade of the twentieth century.

Edward Livingston Trudeau

Edward Trudeau (1847–1915), a New York City physician, contracted consumption. Thinking he was dying, he retreated to the Adirondack region of upstate New York to die in the open air and wilderness. Instead, he found he recovered from the disease. He moved his family to the mountains and treated others with the condition at his sanitorium. This small facility grew to become an influential center for both research and treatment of TB. Because of the successful personal experiences on the part of Trudeau and some other physicians, the sanitorium was advocated as the primary treatment modality. Treatment was considered to be more effective in special institutions than at home, because it prevented the spread of the disease to the rest of the family and the community (Shryock 1957, 28, 113–114; Dubos and Dubos 1952, 177–180; Knopf 1922, 12, 313–317).

As part of the sanitorium movement, in conjunction with the public-health aspects of the TB crusade, a number of alternative-treatment institutions emerged for poorer patients in the first decade of the twentieth century. They included "school camps," "open-air classes," and "preventoriums" for children who were considered at risk for the disease. At all these facilities, rest and good nutrition was provided. Health education, including personal hygiene, bathing, and tooth-brushing, was also taught (Teller 1988, 113–116).

Stage Two: The Public-Health Movement against Tuberculosis

During the mid-1890s, an "official" public-health movement against the white plague emerged. Programs to make the environment more sanitary and to identify cases ensued. The first official public-health activity against tuberculosis occurred in 1894.[5] The Department of Health of New York City, after a period of preliminary study and observation, adopted a series of resolutions designed to suppress the disease (Jacobs 1908, vi–vii). Hermann M. Biggs (1854–1923), medical director of the Board of Health, secured adoption of a resolution providing for reporting cases, free examination of sputum, and home visitation of consumptives as part of the sanitary code. By 1897, this code was amended to make the notification of pulmonary tuberculosis compulsory for all patients, including those under the care of private medical practitioners (Drotlet and Lowell 1952, xxii; Teller 1988, 20–21).

In 1901, the New York Board of Health adopted a "regulation to permit the compulsory segregation of recalcitrant cases of tuberculosis," which represented the beginnings of the coercive phase of this campaign. The effectiveness of this measure was limited by the lack of special wards or buildings where patients could be isolated for treatment. Officials also came to believe that moral-suasive and educational methods were more effective in encouraging patients to go to institutions for treatment than were police measures (Drotlet and Lowell 1952, xxii).

Public-health measures rapidly increased in other areas during the first decade of the new century. Between 1905 and 1914, nearly every state legislature in session was considering tuberculosis laws or appropriations. By 1908, all but fifteen states and most of the large cities had adopted public-health measures. These included antispitting, case-reporting, and registration laws, the disinfection of houses, and educational programs to prevent the spread of the disease. In many areas of the Untied States, several more years would pass before anti-TB measures were fully enacted as part of the sanitation movement to prevent many diseases (Shryock 1957, 118; Jacobs 1908, 347–414).

Stage Three: The Voluntary Health and Prevention Campaign

Development of voluntary agencies began the third stage of the movement. These agencies focused upon measures to educate the public in methods of preventing the spread of the disease. Today we tend to take for granted the idea of national voluntary societies focused upon a single health issue. However, these organizations date from the turn of the twentieth century (Shryock 1957, i). In 1892, the Pennsylvania Society for the Prevention of Tuberculosis was founded by

Lawrence F. Flick (1856–1938) for the purpose of "educational and preventive work in the tuberculosis field." Flick was one of the first physicians to accept the contagiousness of TB and labeled the fight against TB a "crusade." This organization, which launched an educational and prevention campaign throughout the state, was unique in that it was founded on a principle of medical, public-health, social-work, and lay-member cooperation. This structure became a model for many other voluntary health associations formed during the progressive era (Jacobs 1908, vii; Shryock 1957, 52; Teller 1988, 27–28).

During the first decade of the twentieth century, numerous antituberculosis associations organized in most states for the purpose of case finding and preventing the spread of infection. These organizations also supported the facilitation of public-health measures and the construction of treatment centers (Drolet and Lowell 1952, xxvii).

The Committee on Prevention of Tuberculosis of the Charity Organization Society

The Committee on Prevention of Tuberculosis of the Charity Organization Society of the City of New York, a social-work group, was formed in 1902. It eventually grew into the New York Tuberculosis and Health Association. The Committee highly recommended and fostered coordinated action among various groups, agencies, and medical services, and became a model for other groups. The prevention campaign of the committee included educational pamphlets, exhibitions, and lectures to educate the public about the communicability of consumption through "sputum, dried and powdered and floating in the air as dust" (Charity Organization Society 1903, 252). These programs encouraged keeping the body strong so as to prevent the disease by drinking plenty of pure water, sleeping eight hours a day, and eating "plain good food" (pp. 263–264). As a part of the second Clean Living Movement, its educational philosophy interwove with temperance, dietary reform, and personal hygiene.

National Association for the Study and Prevention of Tuberculosis

Many organizations or committees from other reform or health groups came onto the scene in the fight against TB in the first few years of the century. However, these groups often became rivals and did not cooperate with each other. This lack of coordination concerned leading tuberculosis physicians. In 1904, a number of leaders, including Trudeau, Biggs, and Flick, founded the National Association for the Study and Prevention of Tuberculosis, which was renamed the National Tuberculosis Association (NTA) in 1918 and the American

Lung Association (ALA) in 1973. This group allowed nonphysician members and accepted the concept that TB was a preventable curable disease (Shryock 1957, 75; Knopf 1922, 23–32; Teller 1988, 31). This prototype health organization developed an innovative approach to obtain funding; namely, the sale of "Christmas seals." These popular stamps were used for decades. The idea took root at Christmas 1904 in Denmark, where stamps were sold to collect funds to aid sick and especially tuberculosis children (Shryock 1957, 128–129).

In 1907, an article was published in a popular American magazine about these Christmas stamps. Emily P. Bissell and Dr. John Black, struggling to maintain a "tuberculosis shack" outdoor camp near Wilmington, Delaware, after reading about this fund raising effort, decided selling stamps might be a good method for securing their own funds. In December of that year, the first "seal" was sold, sponsored by the Delaware Red Cross (Leonard 1908). The sale was a financial success. More important, the sale educated the public about the disease. The average person at this time still considered TB to be "incurable, non-contagious, and hereditary." They had never thought about either curing or preventing it. The next two years a successful national sale was conducted under the direction of Red Cross chapters and women's clubs (Knopf 1922, 55–56).

After seeing the success of the Red Cross drive, the NTA leaders, in 1910, negotiated to form a liaison with the Red Cross in the Christmas seals. Sales were held each year, with the exception of 1918, during the midst of the influenza epidemic and World War I. In 1920, the Red Cross withdrew from this campaign and gave exclusive rights to the NTA. With the success of the Christmas seal, the tuberculosis movement had involved a large segment of the population in the crusade against the disease (Teller 1988, 33–34; Knopf 1922, 57–63; Shryock 1957, 131).

Stage Four: Education and the Modern Health Campaign

The fourth stage of the tuberculosis movement emerged in the second decade of the century. It included health-education campaigns for both adults and children. The education programs promoted personal responsibility for maintaining good health so as to build up resistance to the disease through personal hygiene, nutrition, exercise and rest. These programs were carried out by public-health groups, voluntary groups, and schools. The best example of this educational campaign was the "Modern Health Crusade" sponsored by the NTA.

In 1917, the NTA inaugurated a movement for teaching health practices among school children. This Modern Health Crusade was not an organization, but rather a "system of health education." It was aimed at correcting nutritional defects and habits, fostering chaste practices, and promoting correct posture, proper exercise, rest, general physique, and the building of resistance against disease. S. Adolphus Knopf (1857–1940), a physician, professor, and historian of the early NTA, in 1922 proclaimed, "It is hoped that eventually the crusade will become as much a part of a child's required schooling as the 'Three R's'" (Knopf 1922, 43–44).

The movement brought together the cooperation of the government, voluntary associations, and education and treatment organizations. It became a model for other chronic-disease health campaigns. Unlike many other health-reform issues during the first two Clean Living Movements, concern about tuberculosis did not disappear at the end of the era. As TB declined over the course of the century, the National Tuberculosis Association broadened its interest to encompass all pulmonary diseases. It became a leader in the antismoking campaign at the beginning of the third Clean Living Movement.

THE PUBLIC-HEALTH
(PREVENTIVE-MEDICINE) MOVEMENT

The progressive era's public-health and preventive-medicine movement dramatically lowered the mortality rate, especially among young children and infants.[6] Advances in standards of living coupled with general sanitation improvements resulted in dramatic strides in overall health, beginning in the last decade of the nineteenth century. In addition to food and water sanitation, other new practices included immunization against certain communicable disease, more specific treatments, and personal-hygiene education. These techniques resulted in the greatest increase in human health compared to any other period in history. Antibiotics and advanced surgical and technical methods in the last half of the twentieth century have primarily kept more people alive in their later years.

Not everyone supported the public-health movement. Some religious groups believed such developments were "against God's will." Some individuals in the eugenics movement (see Chapter 9) attacked medicine and public-health efforts for preserving lives they considered hereditarily unfit. Eugenic and public-health advocates battled over whether heredity played a significant role in infectious disease (Pernick 1997, 1767; Rockafellar 1986, 111).

A nativistic element also surfaced in the public-health movement. The Quarantine Act of 1893 gave broader powers to the Board of New York to prevent individuals from entering the city if suspected of carrying infectious diseases. Between 1892 and 1893, eastern European Jews were impounded on "quarantine islands" in New York harbor to prevent a typhus and cholera epidemic from entering New York City.

When Bubonic Plague was found for the first time in the United States in San Francisco's Chinatown during 1900, the Chinese were quarantined in their section of the city. Discriminatory public-health efforts were also based upon social class (Markel 1997, 174–175, 194–198).

The Campaign to Develop a National Health Department

By 1872, most urban areas had full-time local health departments. The first state health department was formed in Massachusetts in 1878. By the end of the nineteenth century, most states had established health boards, but the majority of these boards proved to be powerless and ineffective. The creation of a national health organization was a difficult, protracted matter, fraught with politics, that became a national campaign spanning the second Clean Living Movement (Duffy 1992, 152–153; Marcus 1979, 202).

In 1878, a devastating yellow fever epidemic swept up the Mississippi Valley. Because the disease was known to have entered the country through the port of New Orleans, authorities were charged with laxity. As a result, the American Public Health Association, formed in 1872, along with the Marine Hospital Service, established in 1798 to meet the medical needs of sailors, sponsored legislation for a national health department. After much political wrangling, the National Health Board was established, which wielded quarantine powers. However, further political maneuvering on the part of local Louisiana politicians, suspicious of federal interference, and of Surgeon General John Hamilton, who wanted to retain power, prevented the board from being reinstated. After four years, the organization returned to the Marine Hospital Service, whose primary job was to examine and quarantine immigrants for contagious diseases and keep mortality statistics (Duffy 1992, 162–172; Kober 1897, 796; Markel 1997, 173–176).

As part of other progressive legislation during the first decade of the twentieth century, momentum for coordination of public health on a national level increased. Pressure by many groups spurred Congress in 1912 to create the United States Public Health Service (USPHS) for nationwide disease prevention. It incorporated the Marine Hospital Service. The new monitoring agency was headed by a surgeon general and was chartered to study and investigate the "full range of diseases and conditions influencing the propagation and spread thereof," including sanitation sewage and both direct and indirect pollution of navigable streams and lakes through the country. This service institutionalized the late nineteenth-century notion of effective disease prevention based on the interdependence of all health agencies (Marcus 1979, 202–203).

The Optimism of Preventive Medicine

Preventive medicine, as opposed to treatment, was a concept that began to gain scientific credibility around 1890. The movement first fostered sanitation efforts, then specific immunizations to prevent disease. By 1909, preventive medicine was generally held to have "done far more to alleviate suffering and to prolong life than the average man is aware" (Torrey 1909, 536). A decrease in annual mortality was attributed primarily to the elimination of infectious diseases during the first five years of life. Vaccination against smallpox, immunization against diphtheria and tetanus, quarantine of the sick, extermination of the mosquito which caused yellow fever—all these were examples of the successful battle against disease (Henson 1909, 1044–1047).

The Sanitation Movement

The sanitation movement to provide clean water and dispose of sewage and garbage evolved in the late 1880s from the earlier movement now rationalized by the germ theory of disease. By the mid-1890s, sanitation was considered to be the most important factor for preventing enteric illnesses, and in particular the general water supply. Typhoid fever in a community was looked upon as a measure of the pollution level of drinking water. In the late 1890s, concerns were raised over the spread of disease from one locality to another. Articles in popular magazines began advocating more stringent sanitation measures to eliminate disease. This push for increased sanitation resulted in the inspection of milk and meat in sixty-two cities by 1904 (Shryock 1957, 67). By 1909, epidemics of typhoid, cholera, or dysentery were beginning to be considered inexcusable. Such epidemics occurred because of carelessness in maintaining the purity of the public water system or milk supply, or in preventing foods from coming in contact with polluted water (Torrey 1909, 537).

Elimination of insect pests was part of the sanitation movement. During the first decade of the new century, the housefly was seen as a frequent source of infection because it alighted "on infected human excreta, later settling on food and carrying the infection to our tables" (Henson 1909, 1046). Magazines published advice to the public on methods for controlling flies, including such measures as using screens on windows and covering excreta in "open closets" with dirt. Extermination of mosquitoes that carried malaria and yellow fever had begun in the first couple of years of the century. Swamps were drained and standing ponds were coated with petroleum to kill mosquito larvae. Because it was impossible to drain all swampy areas, it was suggested that "verandas should be screened if used after sundown, and all beds should be covered with mosquito canopies." To prevent malaria in infested areas, taking quinine several times a week was advised (Henson 1909, 1044–1047).

Personal-Hygiene Campaign

Personal cleanliness and responsibility began to be advocated to eliminate some diseases. Billings (1893) suggested that public bathing and washing facilities be built for poor people as a measure to eliminate disease. It was noted that in clean environments, where bathing and clothes washing was frequent, there was less likely to be typhus. It was considered a civic duty to comply with quarantine laws that isolated children with measles, whooping cough, or scarlet fever in their homes so as to prevent the spread of these childhood diseases (Henson 1909, 1046).

At the turn of the twentieth century, personal-hygiene education, both for the public and school children, began to be advocated (Fall 1897, 275). "Anti-spitting" education and the use of disposable "Japanese paper napkins, which may be destroyed by fire" were suggested to prevent the spread of tuberculosis and other respiratory diseases (Charity Organization Society 1903, 252).

The Immunization and Specific-Therapy Campaign

For centuries it had been known that contracting of certain infections, such as smallpox and measles, conferred lifetime immunity. After the discovery of microorganisms in 1882, experimental investigations with animals using different bacteria began. They attempted to determine if immunity could be induced. In France, Louis Pasteur found that repeated injections into animals with certain attenuated or weakened microorganisms caused immunity and prevented illness (Torrey 1909, 537).

The age of vaccination, immunization, and antitoxins began in the late 1890s. By 1909, there was a "growing realization of the truth that it is better to prevent diseases than to cure" (Torrey 1909, 544). Within a decade of the discovery of several causative organisms, vaccination against disease was attempted. In 1896, crude preparations of killed typhoid bacillus were used to immunize British soldiers against typhoid fever (Hirshberg 1913, 685). After more research on the vaccine, all American military personnel were immunized in 1911, which all but eliminated the disease among troops encamped along the Mexican border (Hirshberg 1913, 686; Torrey 1909, 539).

The cholera bacillus was identified in 1883, and in 1902 a vaccine to immunize against the disease was developed in Japan. The plague bacillus was identified in 1894, but it took until 1906 to discover the rat–flea connection. In 1907 immunization against the plague in India reduced the attack rate to less than one-third of the noninoculated. For the infected, there was also a faster recovery rate. Based upon this information, immunization, quarantine, and the elimination of rats were used to control a 1907 plague in San Francisco (Torrey 1909, 539–540; Smith 1941, 318–325).

Cities along the Mississippi River had frequent typhoid fever epidemics due to contamination of water supplies from river flooding. In 1912, a sudden outbreak of the disease occurred in Memphis. The local health department took measures to stop the pollution of the water supply and citizens were immunized against the disease. These actions halted the epidemic. "Very few of the persons who were vaccinated contracted the disease," and if they did, the "violence of the attack was minimized. . . . Thus, the people witnessed an impressive exhibition of the value of preventive measures when unimpeded by politics or quackery" (Hirshberg 1913, 686). By the second decade of the century, public-health departments found vaccination and other preventive measures to be cheaper than treatment.

The "Spanish Lady" and Public Health

By 1913, various reform activities against disease and social problems, as part of the glowing optimism of the progressive era, came to be seen as the salvation of the future. On the eve of the Great War, "sanitary reform was considered to have done more for real happiness of mankind and has the potential to eliminate poverty and misery, remedying industrial disputes and contributing to the cause of international peace." Many statesmen were "now coming to discern in preventive medicine the pillar of fire lighting the way" (Huber 1913). This heady optimism and smugness, however, was short lived.

In 1918 and 1919, the Spanish influenza pandemic erupted, serving as a sneer against the health crusades of the previous two decades. The epidemic, in three waves, raged for about a year and killed ten times more people than World War I. It took about a half million lives in the United States and over 22 million worldwide. Richard Collier (1974, 303), in his popularized history of the pandemic, calls it the "most appalling epidemic since the Middle ages." Since it overlapped with the end of the war it did not receive heavy press coverage and for several years afterward the full extent of the pandemic was not known. Curiously, it became a forgotten plague by the mid-twentieth century. Only in the last few decades of the century was its history resurrected (Collier 1974, 304; Beveridge 1977, 30–33).[7]

The public-health agencies on all levels lacked organization, but they did attempt to implement anti-influenza measures. At the end of September, the USPHS appointed a director for influenza in each state. The service recruited volunteer doctors and nurses to care for the ill. However, sufficient numbers of medical personnel were unavailable, since many were already involved in the war effort. The epidemic undermined people's faith in the application of public health. During the postwar period, a more cynical public resisted regulative measures on the part of health officials. The 1918 disaster, however, pointed out the lack of coordination among various agencies. It persuaded many people to call for extensive research on influenza and led to a centralized national department of health with powers far greater than before. School nurses examining children for illness during the epidemic pointed out other health problems and a need for continuous health education in the schools and a greater coordination in all health services (Rockafeller 1986, 111–113; Crosby 1976, 50–51, 312–313; Walters 1981, 143–144).

The overall public-health movement had been so successful that, by 1920, despite the war and influenza, a decrease in all infectious diseases resulted. Heart disease was now the leading cause of death. Pneumonia had become the second leading disease and tuberculosis number three (Drotlet and Lowell 1952, xvi). The peak of the public-health movement came about in 1914. The Great War halted its progress, not only in the United States, but particularly in Europe. After that year, a temporary increase in tuberculosis, malaria, typhoid, yellow fever, typhus, and diphtheria occurred, especially in Europe.

SUMMARY

This chapter discussed the tuberculosis movement and the rise of public health and the elimination of many infectious diseases by immunization and various preventive measures. The tuberculosis movement became a model for the modern voluntary organization and the Spanish influenza epidemic increased awareness of how much still needed to be done in terms of public health and preventive medicine.

NOTES

1. Several publications during the twentieth century have focused upon the antituberculosis movement. Selected sources include Bates (1992), Drotlet and Lowell (1952), Dubos and Dubos (1952), Jacobs (1908), Teller (1988), Knopf (1922), and Shryock (1957).

2. As part of an "epidemic cycle," most diseases, including TB, first appear as a few sporadic cases. This early phase is followed by one of great prevalence, virulence, and severity. Then new cases become progressively fewer and the incidence of the disease declines. The beginning of a new cycle is signaled by an increase in cases (Dubos and Dubos 1952, 187). The yearly influenza cycle is a typical example of this "epidemic–endemic" curve. From

limited evidence, the TB epidemic cycle is thought to be about 200 years. Based upon the theory of epidemic waves, Dubos and Dubos (1952, 187), in the mid-twentieth century predicted that the incidence of TB would start to increase again at the end of the twentieth century. This has proven to be the case, with a rise of more than 18 percent between 1985 and 1991. This increase has been attributed to a decrease in funding for TB prevention and treatment programs and to the AIDS epidemic which began in the early 1980s. Between 1992 and 1996, TB began to decrease or level off in most of the country, except for impoverished urban areas (Bryant 1992, 29–31; Center for Disease Control 1997, 695–700). It remains to be seen if this decline is temporary or if the incidence will begin to rise again, indicative of a 200-year cycle.

3. It has been observed for decades that Ashkenazim (eastern European) Jews appear to have a resistance to TB (Charity Organization Society 1903, 55). It is now hypothesized that carriers for the recessive genetic condition Tay-Sachs syndrome, found among eastern European Jews, are less likely to become infected or die from TB.

4. In 1904, there were 96 sanitoria or special hospitals for treating TB in the United States. By 1914, there were 550 sanitoria and 400 dispensaries (local clinics). In 1920, construction of sanitoria and dispensaries grew more slowly. From 1904 to 1919, the mortality rate from TB declined 33 percent (Jacobs 1908, vi; Knopf 1922, 12, 53, 407; Shryock 1957, 116). However, as pointed out by Bates (1992, 321), "Many observers now attribute the decline of tuberculosis chiefly to socioeconomic changes." As treatment facilities began to be built, the standard treatment for tuberculosis included rest, fresh air, food such as "milk and raw eggs," and cod-liver oil. Many urban victims of the disease were impoverished, often working ten to twelve hours a day. They were undernourished and lived in substandard housing, and the clean and restful environment of the sanitorium improved many aspects of their health (Charity Organization Society 1903, 337–339; Dubos and Dubos 1952, 139–140).

5. In 1893, the Michigan Board of Health required notification of TB. However, the regulation was not well observed. Various municipal boards of health, such as that in Boston in 1896, adopted antispitting regulations, but, again, they generally were not enforced (Jacobs 1908, 375, 369).

6. "Public health" and "preventive medicine" are different terms for the same movement. Physicians were, and are, more likely to use the term "preventive medicine." In this book, these terms are used interchangeably.

7. In 1998, the Armed Forces Institute of Pathology identified the influenza virus from the frozen remains of a native Alaskan buried for nearly eighty years. It was also isolated from autopsy samples from two soldiers who had died during the fall of 1918. To prevent such a pandemic from returning, the virus is being studied for a possible immunization should this strain again become active (Taubenberger et al. 1997). For more historical and sociological works that discuss the epidemic, see Crosby (1989, 1976), Beveridge (1977), and Collier (1974).

PART III

The Third Clean Living Movement, 1970–2005

> Statements of principles issued by popular health reform movements of the mid-nineteenth and early twentieth centuries all sound as though they were somehow copied from holistic-health handbooks, or a lecture on high-level wellness, or the promotional literature for a Well-Being Workshop of the eighties.
>
> James C. Whorton, *Other Healers: Orthodox Medicine in America*
> (1988)

> We are in the midst of a "new clean living" movement. . . . A delicate balance must be maintained between social legislation and personal choice as trends sometimes get out of control, resulting in harm to the individual and society.
>
> Ruth C. Engs, *Journal of School Health* (1991a)

> The [health] movement has drawn its adherents disproportionately from the middle and upper-middle classes, who have more disposable income, time, and energy to invest.
>
> Michael S. Goldstein, *The Health Movement:*
> *Promoting Fitness in America* (1992)

> The United States is currently in its Fourth Great Awakening, which began about 1960. . . . It is a rebellion against preoccupation with material acquisition and sexual debauchery; against indulgence in alcohol, tobacco, gambling, and drugs; against gluttony; against financial greed; and against all other forms of self-indulgence that titillate the senses and destroy the soul.
>
> Robert W. Fogel, *Brigham Young University Studies* (1995)

There were profound social, cultural, economic, and technological changes in the post–World War II era. In reaction to this rapid change, a religious awakening emerged.[1] In its wake, the millennial Clean Living Movement surfaced over the last decades of the twentieth century. Beginning with the civil rights movement in the 1960s, many social and health reform movements began to stir. Hugh Heclo (1996, 42), a public-policy historian, has suggested "in many ways, [the civil rights movement] was the exemplary model for other movements. Activists for a variety of causes were not only inspired by its righteous confrontation . . . but also were educated by its grassroots mobilizing strategy and effective use of the media to dramatize its case. . . . Although each of the sixties movements had its own history, they were also interconnected, sometimes by overlapping memberships, but most especially by activists' mutual inspiration and critical motifs."

These social movements were initiated among members of the postwar "baby-boom" generation, which demanded women's rights, free speech, the ending of the Vietnam War, and other social changes. Many baby-boomers also experimented with drugs, extramarital sex, and alternative lifestyles. From the early 1960s until the mid-1970s, social unrest and violence tore at the fabric of the American society. President John F. Kennedy, his brother Robert, and the civil rights leader Martin Luther King Jr. were assassinated. Antiwar demonstrators were killed and thousands of young men fled the country to avoid military service.

By the mid-1970s, more conservative Christians and older Americans began to react against what they perceived as immoral and unpatriotic behaviors. Their anger coalesced into political action. The resulting agitation included campaigns against the use of drugs, alcohol, and other activities of the 1960s and 1970s. In addition, a more secular health-reform movement, that to some became a "religion," surged out of the youthful generation. Fitness and exercise, diet, alternative religions and medicine, consumers rights, smoke-free environments, and other health reforms became prime concerns of the day. Amid these health-reform initiatives, as had been the case during the previous two movements, a widely popularized deadly new disease— AIDS—cast a dreadful pallor onto the scene.

In the late twentieth-century health-reform movement, reformers were often well-financed, large, grassroots, not-for-profit, and even government organizations founded, or led, by activists. By the end of the twentieth century, some scholars suggested that American culture had become increasingly secular. For example, Hugh Heclo (1996, 46) argued, "With 'sin' passe, self-blame was out and system-blame was in." Some reformers began to blame the system rather than encouraging individuals to take personal responsibility for their behaviors. This attitude led to reform crusades that included litigation against tobacco manufacturers, alcoholic-beverage distributors, and pharmaceutical and other corporations. It also led to advocacy against fast-food and ethnic restaurants that favored high-fat items. However, other reformers still advocated personal responsibility.[2]

With elimination of most infectious diseases during the postwar era, the public-health community began to focus on chronic problems. Behaviors once thought to be "sins" or "bad habits" had now become "diseases." Reformers, rather than condemning sinful behaviors, now used moral suasion to argue against unhealthy behaviors that led to illness. This *Diseasing of America* (Peele 1989) became integral to health reform during the last two decades of the century. For example, Jacob Sullum (1996), a critic of government health policies, suggested that health legislation was instituted to "control illness and injury by controlling behavior thought to be associated with them. . . . Less drinking means less cirrhosis of the liver, less smoking means less lung cancer, less gun ownership means less suicide." When moral suasion was perceived as ineffective, coercion was enacted for many reform efforts.

The third Clean Living Movement was characterized by many crusades and countercrusades. Activities that surged in the earlier years of the era were often met with countermovements about ten years later. For example, women's liberation was countered by a pro-family movement; the use of marijuana and other drugs was followed by a war on drugs; lowering of the drinking age was followed by a raising of the drinking age; nonmarital sexual activity was challenged by a new purity movement; and legal rights to obtaining abortions were met with agitation against abortion.

The third Clean Living Movement began in the 1960s with a religious revitalization, women's rights, and antismoking campaigns. During the early 1970s, concern about fitness and improved diet emerged, followed by agitation against drunken driving in the late 1970s. Alternative religions and medicine also became more popular during this decade. During the 1980s, an antidrug campaign intensified. At the peak of the movement, during the 1990s, a new eugenics movement smoldered and gained momentum as the old millennium closed.

NOTES

1. For more information on this religious revitalization, the fourth Great Awakening, and its etiology, see McLoughlin (1978, 179–216), Fogel (1995, 31–43), and Wilson (1980, 29–30).

2. Some authors have implied that health-reform crusades were, in fact, still against sinful behaviors, as they were largely against intemperance, fornication, abortion, homosexuality, gluttony, and other self-indulgences. See, for example, works by Burnham (1993), Fogel (1995), and Tate (1995).

12

Religious Awakening, New Age Religions, and Wellness

> When we look at the religious New Right in America today we cannot say whether it marks the dawn of a new spiritual era, a phase in recurrent cycles of social and spiritual anxiety, or the last gasp of an old order. All we can agree on, perhaps, is that theories of secularization that predicated correlations of scientific-technological advance and spiritual decline are in deep trouble.
>
> George M. Marsden, "Preachers of Paradox" (1983)

> The past decade and a half has been characterized mostly by change and uncertainty in the religious realm—including new religious movements, a resurgence of evangelical and fundamentalist involvement in politics, declining membership in mainline Protestant and Catholic churches, and much experimentation with new forms of spirituality.
>
> Robert Wuthnow, *The Crisis in the Churches* (1997)

> During the late 1960s and 1970s, there emerged on the American scene a large number of "new religious movements" or "cults," as their critics termed them.
>
> Richard Quebedeaux, *The New Charismatics* (1983)

> In most societies throughout most of history, magic, religion, and medicine have been intertwined, practiced together, and seen as having a common origin. . . . Far from being simply the absence of disease, health is a dynamic and harmonious equilibrium of all the elements and forces making up and surrounding a human being.
>
> Andrew Weil, *Health and Healing* (1983)

Beginning in the late 1950s and early 1960s, a wave of religious enthusiasm and spirituality, or the fourth Great Awakening, emerged in the United States. The first stages of this revival manifested themselves in increased religious expression, both outside and within the Christian tradition. In the late 1970s, the religious fervor from more conservative Christian groups, concerned about profound social changes, coalesced into political action. This new movement, often termed the Christian Right, advocated against nonmarital sexuality, drugs, and other behaviors perceived as immoral that were exhibited by "liberal" youth of the 1960s and 1970s (McLoughlin 1978, 196–200; Wilson 1980, 29–30; Fogel 1995, 32–38; Lewis and Melton 1992, ix–x).

In the middle stages of religious Great Awakenings, McLoughlin (1978, 14–20) has implied that alternative sects evolve and advance new religious and social norms. Beginning in the 1970s, a large-scale, decentralized religious subculture drawn from the occult, paganism, metaphysics, and eastern mystical traditions began surfacing. Many participants in this movement were part of the postwar "counterculture" generation. By the 1980s, this surge had become an integral part of American culture and was termed the "New Age" or "New Religious" movement. Interwoven with New Age beliefs were concerns about diet, meditation, alternative healing, and holistic health (Lewis and Melton 1992, ix–xii; Lucas 1992, 190–195).

Similar to the revivalist spirit in the Jacksonian and progressive eras, as discussed in Parts I and II, leaders emerged who sought to either bring America back to a Golden Age or create a new society of peace and prosperity.[1] This fervor, in turn, generated a number of health-reform crusades. The religious zeal of the fourth Great Awakening, as of the turn of this new century, is still producing effects on American society and precipitated the current Clean Living Movement.

THE CHRISTIAN RIGHT

At the beginning of the late twentieth-century awakening, church membership swelled across all denominations; however, the most dramatic growth was found in the more "enthusiastic," evangelical, and ceremonial churches. Economist Robert Fogel (1995, 32) suggested there was a "sharp shift of membership away from mainline Protestant churches, which were identified with a rationalistic approach to religion, to the more mystical churches, which appeal to emotions as much as to the mind—to a religion of passion and sensation." These churches stressed personal conversion and personal salvation through faith. They called on their adherents to strive for a mystical experience that would cleanse them of their earlier sins and lead to their spiritual rebirth. As had been found in previous religious awakenings, movements that embraced this revival enthusiasm also blamed social changes on a collective failure to adhere to the established beliefs, mores, and values of the culture. They advocated a return to a more moral and traditional lifestyle. By 1976, a prayer-revival movement had cut deeply into regular membership of mainline churches and drew many "unchurched" persons into their fold. Over the last decades of the century, membership in the mainstream Protestant and Roman Catholic churches declined, while membership in the more conservative and enthusiastic churches nearly doubled (McLoughlin 1978, 14, 196–200; Wuthnow 1997, 5; Lucas 1992, 190–191). Many reformers who established grassroots organizations or advocated various health and moral reform causes were associated with these religious faiths.

The Rise of the Christian Right

Similar to the fervor to change society found in America's other great awakenings, a commitment arose to eliminate perceived social problems in the late 1970s and early 1980s. A loose collection of the more "rightist" Christians began to form around moral and ethical issues. These individuals became alarmed by the increase in divorce, crime, sexual promiscuity, out-of-wedlock births, drunken driving, pornography, sex education in the schools, and advocacy for abortion and homosexual and women's rights. Political strategists reasoned that there was an untapped political base and constituency that could be mobilized around these issues. This new political coalition, the "New Right" or "Christian Right," comprised a mix of fundamentalists, evangelicals, and neo-Pentecostals. Members of this movement for the most part lived in the southern or southwestern regions of the country and could be identified by common views that considered the role of women should be the traditional one within the family (Fogel 1995, 34, 38–39; Lienesch 1993, 2, 15–16; Wilcox 1992, 212).

This interweaving of politics and religion was also found in the previous reform eras. Marsden (1991, 85) observed that "for better or for worse, mixes of religion and politics have always been one part of the American political heritage." As in the past, this link resulted in attempts to create social pressures and sanctions against certain activities. Lienesch (1993, 8) has contended that in mobilizing the late twentieth-century movement, leaders consciously chose to build a mass movement based upon moral concerns. Since their inception, the religious–political organizations focused upon highly controversial issues such as abortion, homosexual rights, and sex education in the school. This rightist religious and political enthusiasm found expression in the Moral Majority in the late 1970s and the Christian Coalition in the late 1980s. It also took the form of Christian grassroots groups, such as Concerned Women for America and the Family Research Council (Lienesch 1993, 3, 8–12; Wilcox 1992, 212; Snowball 1991, 13–15).[2]

Pat Robertson

Marion Gordon "Pat" Robertson (b. 1930), born in Lexington, Virginia, was one of the most powerful leaders of the Christian Right in the late twentieth century. The son of a United States senator, he enjoyed a privileged youth and pursued a law degree. In 1956, Robertson became a born-again Christian and entered a Biblical seminary. While working as an associate minister, he underwent a Pentecostal experience and subsequently helped spread this message to traditional churches (Melton et al. 1997, 288–291).[3]

During the last three decades of the twentieth century, Robertson built an empire. He founded and headed a gigantic multimedia and entertainment enterprise, founded and became chancellor of Regent University for graduate students, and founded and became president of the American Center for Law and Justice, the Christian Coalition, and a charitable organization, Operation Blessing. He also campaigned for president in 1988. Robertson, like previous reformers, crusaded against behaviors he considered immoral. These included abortion, homosexuality, sex education in schools, and pornography, among other issues (Boston 1996, 158; Foege 1996, 111–112, 195–196; Melton et al. 1997, 288–291). This political advocacy against a variety of health-related and "personal behavior" issues was reminiscent of moral reformers during the progressive era, who also pressed their agenda into the courts and political system.

Robertson was considered a controversial figure in the 1990s. For example, a detractor, Alex Boston (1996, 240), a commentator for Americans United for Separation of Church and State, argued that Robertson was "a dangerous menace whose political power must be checked. The influence and power of his Christian Coalition must be challenged by the facts confronted with its own unreason."

The Moral Majority and Christian Coalition

The Moral Majority was founded by Jerry Falwell in 1978 as a vehicle through which believers could unite on a national program of political restructuring.[4] Some of the stated missions of the organization could be summed up as pro-life, pro–traditional family, antipornography, anti–illegal drug trade, and anti–ERA (Equal Rights Amendment). In attempting to form coalitions and promote candidates, leaders echoed the emotional rhetoric of the Prohibition and Purity movements during the early twentieth century (see Chapters 8 and 9) and often demonized politicians who did not agree with them. The pro-family movement strove to bring disparate religious groups, including the Roman Catholics, into this political coalition.[5] However, in order to attract such diverse constituents, organizers were forced to expand their platform to include nonfamily political positions. Support for this political coalition began to wane near the end of the Reagan administration, and the Moral Majority was disbanded by Falwell in 1989 (Bruce 1988, vii, 81–82; Lienesch 1993, 11–12, 247; Snowball 1991, 16–17, 111–118; Fogel 1995, 38–39).

The collapse of Robertson's presidential campaign and revelation of various sexual and monetary indiscretions among some televangelists contributed to the decline of the Christian Right in the late 1980s (Lienesch 1993, 15–17; Fogel 1995, 38–39). However, out of this demise a new organization, the Christian Coalition, was founded by Robertson and Ralph Reed, a young history doctoral candidate, in 1989 as a political lobbying group for right-wing causes. This rightist activist group was established to further the causes of evangelicals and Roman Catholics and to exert influences at local and regional levels on school boards and with state legislators. Like other components of the Christian Right movement since the late 1970s, it supported a return to traditional "family values," opposed abortion, and the like (Foege 1996, 126–133, 196–198; Melton et al. 1997, 288; Fogel 1995, 39; Bruce 1988, 81–82).[6]

In the mid-1990s, leaders from more liberal religions, such as the Universalist Unitarian Church, viewed infusion of moral issues into the Religious Right's political campaigns as a general threat to personal and religious rights. For example, Reich (1996), in a review of Alex Boston's 1996 book suggested that the Christian Coalition and Pat Robertson's multibillion-dollar empire would "probably endure for a long time to come, continuing to threaten civil rights and religious freedom."[7]

A Neo-Men's Movement and the Promise Keepers

Similar to the men's movement and Muscular Christianity during the turn-of-the-century reform era, a rightist Christian men's movement began to evolve in the 1980s. Jerry Falwell in the early 1980s decried the lack of male leadership in families, churches, and the nation and suggested to men that "Jesus was not a sissy." There began to be a growth in a "manliness syndrome" in the colleges supported by the evangelical right, taking the form of short haircuts, cold showers, and winning at rigorous contact sports (Wacker 1984, 305–306).

In 1991, the Promise Keepers was founded by Bill McCartney (b. 1940), a football coach at the University of Colorado. Reminiscent of Billy Sunday (the early twentieth-century baseball-player revivalist discussed in Chapter 7), stadium revivals of men featuring born-again athletes were held over the course of the 1990s. The movement embraced seven promises based on strict interpretations of the bible to help men to become better fathers, husbands, friends, and churchmen. Critics suspected that the Promise Keeper's mission had political undertones that favored subjugation of women, curtailment of personal lifestyles, and promotion of a right-wing political agenda. For example, Close (1997), in an issue of *Newsweek*, reported that the Promise Keepers contended that "homosexuality is a sin, along with extramarital sex and pornography." Men were urged to "reclaim leadership from their wives." Since there is no historical perspective on this movement as of the turn of this century, it is too early to tell what effect it might have on society in terms of health-related issues.

In some respects, the Christian Right movement echoed the perfection crusades of the previous Great Awakenings and Clean Living Movements. The movement fostered campaigns to save society's soul, to redeem it from the forces of secularity, and in the process, demonized and waged war against those who disagreed with them. Lienesch (1993, 19) has noted that the movement "defined their enemies as feminists, homosexuals, liberals, and radicals of all kinds, including Christian and even evangelical ones—as the forces of evil." They also demonized the newly forming alternative religious practices and "cults."[8]

"MAY THE FORCE BE WITH YOU": THE RISE OF THE NEW RELIGIOUS MOVEMENT

In the early 1970s, another spiritual awakening grew out of the counterculture. It was "a large-scale, decentralized religious subculture that drew its principal inspiration from sources outside of the Judeo-Christian tradition" (Lewis and Melton 1992, ix). In contrast to the fervor from the Christian right to bring America back to nineteenth-century values, the alternative religious movement strove to create a new society, a new Golden Age. Emergence of this new spiritual vigor outside America's traditional religious systems has been referred to as the New Age or the New Religious movement. Religious scholars James Lewis and J. Gordon Melton (1992, x–xii) suggest that many adherents within this broad spiritual movement do not accept the label "New Age" because media coverage has often focused on more unusual groups and "outlandish aspects of the New Age." Michael D'Antonio (1992) suggested that adherents often use "new consciousness" or a "spiritual renewal."[9]

During the 1970s, groups proliferated based upon eastern religions and practices such as transcendental meditation (TM) and other meditation techniques designed to tap into the "universal energy." A symbol of the emergence of this new religious movement into public consciousness was the late 1970s movie *Star Wars*, in which "the Force," a universal spiritual power, constituted an integral part of the plot. The film series could be seen as an allegory on finding one's spirituality through the guidance of a teacher and fighting against the powers of evil. Margot Adler's (b. 1946) *Drawing Down the Moon* (1979) gave popular awareness to Wiccan and Neo-Pagan beliefs and was a factor in the increased interest in nature and "Goddess"-based religions. Kelly (1992, 136) contended that the "Neo-Pagan Witchcraft movement in America was a new religion, that, like almost all new religions, claims to be an old religion."

In the 1980s, occult and Spiritualist techniques such as "channeling"—being in touch with a spiritual entity—and other psychic phenomena came into the public eye (Lewis and Melton 1992, xii). Lewis and Melton (1992, ix–x) suggested that *Out on a Limb,* a late 1980s TV miniseries concerning the spiritual journey of movie actress Shirley MacLaine (b. 1934), spurred the mass media to begin seriously investigating the new religious movement. Up until that time, the media had primarily focused upon high-profile groups such as the Moonies, Hare Krishna, Scientology, and other cults and had presented the New Age phenomenon as a passing fad. By the early 1990s, Lewis and Melton (1992, x) argued that the new spiritual movement was now a persistent part of the American culture. This alternative spiritual awakening, like previous awakenings that spawned new religions, also influenced social and health-related issues. Holistic health, including fitness and diet, stress-reduction techniques, healing meditation, concern for the environment and pure water, and rejection of tobacco and drugs, were concerns and practices of many of these new religions.

The New Religious movement was divided into three submovements in terms of practices or beliefs. These included the eastern mysticism human-potential systems, metaphysical-occult-psychic traditions, and Wiccan, Neo-Pagan, nature-based groups (York 1995, 99). However, in some cases an overlapping of practices or beliefs could be found among these three broad systems. As an example, a woman who considered herself a Neo-Pagan Wiccan might also practice eastern meditation, and read tarot cards.

Eastern Mysticism and the Human-Potential Movement

In 1965, the U.S. Congress rescinded the Asian Exclusion Act, which had kept Asians out of the country. This allowed millions of new Asian immigrants, including a number of religious leaders to enter the country. These Indian gurus, Zen masters, and Sufi sheikhs came as teachers to spread their faith among "western materialists." Conversely, some Americans went east to find a teacher or guru. Harvard psychologist Richard Alpert (b. 1931), for example, went to India, where his life was transformed. He returned to the United States a new person with a new name, Baba Ram Dass, and in 1971 published *Be Here*

Now. Melton (1992, 20–21, 291) has suggested that publication of this work was a useful benchmark in dating the beginning of the New Age movement.

Transcendental meditation, also from India, became popular in the mid-1970s and was undertaken by many middle-class individuals. Various practices among the eastern traditions, including meditation, yoga, and a vegetarian diet, became increasingly popular. Beliefs such as reincarnation, karma, and the energy flow through chakras emerged from Hindu tradition into mainstream America (Diem and Lewis 1992, 48; Melton 1992, 20).

The human-potential movement, a blend of Eastern religion and humanistic psychology, began to spread from the Big Sur area of California, and in particular at Esalen Institute, a personal growth center, in the late 1960s. Although differences existed among various arms of this belief system, some common beliefs included the concept of a mystical or "peak experience" and advocation of a "life-force" which could be found within everything. Various breathing, imaging, and other meditative techniques are employed to tap into this "flow of energy" to enhance spiritual enlightenment. Focusing on the present, "the here and now," rather than looking to the past became a key component of the human-potential system. These ideas spread into the contemporary culture and into mental-health and social-psychology practices (Alexander 1992, 36–37, 42–43).

The Occult and the Metaphysical Sciences

The occult and metaphysical movement of the New Religious spirituality was based upon a synthesis of many different preexisting movements, including theosophy and spiritualism. Practices included astrology, tarot-card reading, channeling, crystal healing, and other types of psychic readings. However, the New Age aspects of these belief systems could be distinguished from the older traditions in that the current movements emphasized transformation or change. For example, the use of tarot cards and astrology in the older traditions were used to predict or give the most auspicious time to carry out an event. In contrast, New Age practitioners focused on how individuals could use the information derived from these tools for self-understanding so as to change behaviors, avoid pitfalls, and lead healthier lives. To facilitate this personal transformation, diverse activities, such as massage, spiritual meditations, natural diets, and renewed human relationships, were fostered (Lewis and Melton 1992, xi; Melton 1992, 18–19).

A leader in this diverse movement was David Spangler (b. 1945). Spangler, a theosophist/channeler, traveled to England and lived at Findhorn, a spiritual community, in northern Scotland. In 1971, he wrote about his experiences and spiritual journey at this community in *Revelation: The Birth of a New Age*. This and other later works provided a theoretical basis for the metaphysical aspect of the New Age movement (Melton 1992, 21).

Neo-Paganism and Wicca

One of the fastest growing religious movements in the last two decades of the century was the Neo-Pagan and Wiccan movement. The May 1, 1998 *Chicago Tribune* suggested that there were upward of a half-million practicing Pagans in the United States. It noted that "paganism encompasses all manner of practitioners from Wiccans and Druids to feminist Goddess worshipers and a variety of polytheistic religions, some inspired by Celtic, Greek and Norse mythology, shamanism or even the visions of science-fiction writers. . . . [It] is a religion without a middleman, although there are priests and priestesses, everyone in a group is involved in creating and carrying out the rituals." This movement also included Native American and other nature-based religious practices. These groups generally accepted both the male and female spiritual principle and the forces of nature. In some, the focus was on the Goddess, or the female principle of the universal spirit or power. Concern for Mother Earth, nature, and the environment were often of interest to these groups.

Margot Adler (1996), a Pagan Universalist Unitarian (UU), remarked that Neo-Pagans, contrary to most other religions, did not have a written scripture nor a well-formed creed. Neo-Paganism was a religion based upon practice and experience in opposition to belief.[10] In addition, Adler implied that the Wiccan movement evolved out of the women's rights movement. Many of these groups became an extension of the women's movement (see Chapter 14).

Hostility toward Alternative Religions

Many of these alternative religions were not acceptable to more traditional Americans. Members were physically attacked and or even killed for their beliefs. As discussed in Chapter 2, this also happened to the Mormons in the mid-nineteenth-century awakening. Melton (1986, 245–247) described hostility against several new religious groups in the late twentieth century. For example, a Hare Krishna compound in Virginia in 1978 was attacked by "local gunmen." In the 1970s and 1980s, members of several alternative religions, particularly the Unification Church (Moonies), were kidnaped by "deprogrammers" who attempted to coerce them out of their religious beliefs (Galanter 1989, 166–172). One of the most tragic and violent incidences against an alternative religion occurred in 1993. About eighty members of the Branch Davidians, an offshoot of the Seventh-Day Adventists, were burned to death in their Texas compound after altercations with federal agents.

Adherents of the new religions tended to embrace holistic health and alternative healing practices, such as vegetarian diets, exercise, and mental healing. They also had concerns about the environment and "healing the earth." The influence of the New Age could be seen in health and medicine. D'Antonio (1992, 398) suggests that "during the roughly twenty-year lifetime of the New Age, mainstream medicine has moved from an outright rejection of the body–mind connection to a cautious acceptance. A substantial amount of research had been done to support the notion that people in the best state of mental health suffer few illnesses and recover from disease more quickly."

ALTERNATIVE MEDICINE AND THE HOLISTIC-HEALTH MOVEMENT

During of the last two decades of the twentieth century, New Age also came to imply alternative healing and treatment approaches. As the New Religious movement began to surge, so did nonorthodox treatment techniques. These methods were often dismissed by the regular medical establishment. One critic of the alternative medicine movement, James Harvey Young, considered it "pseudomedicine." Young (1992a, 87), a medical-quackery scholar, suggested, "Astrology, tarot cards, palmistry, numerology flourish, along with a host of new religions, many of them mighty weird. In such an atmosphere, quackery will certainly abound." This mixing of quackery, or alternative medicine, with new religions could be found in many popular publications, beginning in the late 1980s. One example was *Body, Mind and Spirit* (Campbell and Brennan 1994). This book listed and defined alternative medicine procedures along with religious and spiritual practices that had become common.

A vast difference was evident between the way conventional—orthodox, allopathic, and biomedicine—and alternative medicine was practiced. Over the course of the century, mainstream physicians increasingly became authoritative experts and patients receptive participants. Physicians tended to give their patients standardized treatments, such as drugs or surgery, and advice based upon standardized symptoms. In contrast, alternative health practitioners more likely prescribed individualized treatment and tended to be client centered. Emphasis was placed on the patient's responsibility in healing. Most of the alternative treatments, however, had been relegated to the fringe by the third decade of the century. Practices such as chiropractic manipulations, folk medicine, or diet and exercise regimens, such as those fostered by Sylvester Graham and Bernarr Macfadden (see Chapters 4 and 7), were dismissed as quackery by the established biomedical community (Dossey and Sawyers 1994, xxxviii–xxxxix; Gevitz 1988, 2).[11]

After World War II, conventional medicine became highly technical and expensive and underwent changes in how it was delivered. Dramatic cures of bacterial infections, lifesaving surgery, and technological advances were developed, which led patients to expect a magical cure for all illnesses. However, many diseases, especially chronic conditions, could not be cured. The majority of physicians began to specialize and the number of primary-care physicians, who had been more likely to consider all aspects of the patient's life, decreased. Physicians became increasingly isolated from public-health interests and issues that influenced health. In turn, the rights and needs of patients as whole persons were often ignored. Trust in the conventional system began to falter as consumers increasingly insisted on some control over their medical treatment. To meet these needs, many Americans began to seek alternative treatments outside conventional medicine (Knowles 1977, 1–4; Dossey and Sawyers 1994, xxxvii).

During the 1970s, unorthodox healing practices grew increasingly popular and concepts of holistic health and wellness developed. These ideas made up the alternative health, or holistic health movement.[12] The movement was grounded upon prevention and advocated health as a balance between spiritual, mental, and physical dimensions. An article discussed this new movement in the September 2, 1980 *Washington Post*. It reported that the movement grew out of the alternative health services of the 1960s, including "free clinics, drop-in centers, and crisis centers that gave care, shelter and counseling to the disaffected young of that decade." The article described the growing wellness movement as embracing self-care, patient education, prevention, fitness, and exercise. Adherents used alternative treatments ranging from meditation to acupuncture and eastern herbal medicines. By 1980, there were about one hundred holistic and wellness centers in the United States.

The growth in the holistic health movement in the 1980s mirrored consumers' growing disillusionment with orthodox medicine. With new strains of antibiotic-resistant diseases, an incurable HIV/AIDS epidemic, and an increasing lack of cures for chronic conditions in an aging population, confidence in regular medicine further eroded. A number of newsletters and health advisories emerged regarding alternative treatments, nutrition, diet, and self-care. By 1992, approximately one-third of all Americans were using some type of alternative healthcare, often without the knowledge of their "regular" physicians. Alternative therapies represented a significant part of Americans' healthcare expenditures, primarily for chronic illness (Eisenberg et al. 1993, 246–252).

Certain older practices, which had long been considered quackery, gained acceptance, including chiropractic, meditation, and acupuncture. The role of fruits and vegetables, vegetarian diets, and supplemental nutrients in preventing or inhibiting serious diseases became increasingly considered. Throughout the 1980s and 1990s, numerous books on alternative or natural healing methods were published by alternative practitioners and some regular physicians. In addition, some corporations had launched wellness programs. Lawrence (1990), for example, reported that to control runaway healthcare costs many employers were investing time and money to ensure healthy workers. Exercise and stop-smoking programs were becoming standard.

Acceptance of Alternative Medicine among Some Orthodox Physicians

In the mid-1970s, a few physicians, much to the chagrin of other regular medical practitioners, began to consider alternative techniques in a positive light. One of the first to suggest a link between mind and body was Herbert Benson (b. 1935), who studied meditation, which he called "the relaxation response" the title of a book he published in 1975. A March 31, 1997 interview in *USA Today* remarked that Benson "was ridiculed twenty-five years ago" when he suggested a body–mind connection, even though his studies showed "mental-relaxation training could lower blood pressure and improve other bodily functions."

In the early 1980s, Dean Ornish (b. 1953) researched a successful treatment regimen for seriously ill cardiac patients, consisting of a lifestyle change including a low-fat vegetarian diet, exercise, yoga, and mediation as opposed to surgery. During the 1990s, some insurance companies began to accept this regimen. In 1991, Julian Whitaker (b. 1943) launched *Health and Healing: Tomorrow's Medicine Today*, a monthly newsletter that "utilizes treatments that enhance the body's ability to heal itself." This publication recommended vitamin supplements along with exercise and other alternative methods. It also discussed research studies to support these recommendations.

Andrew Weil

In the early 1980s, one of the most influential physicians to advocate holistic health and alternative medicine was Andrew Weil (b. 1942). Born and reared in Philadelphia, Weil was the only child of owners of a millinery-supply store.[13] He was a precocious child, who graduated from Harvard University and medical school. In 1968, Weil helped conduct the first double-blind study on the effects of smoking marijuana on humans. After a short stint with the National Institute of Mental Health, he spent thirteen years as a research associate in ethnopharmacology at the Harvard Botanical Museum. In this capacity he studied native medicines, psychoactive plants, and altered states of consciousness. Weil also studied other means of consciousness changing, such as mediation and yoga. In 1972, he published *The Natural Mind* concerning the basic need to change conscious awareness, and argued that legislating against drugs was useless. Many considered him controversial during the growing antidrug movement of this era.

Around 1980, Weil began studying nontraditional health methods, such as homeopathy, chiropractic, acupuncture, herbal medicine, and psychic healing. He first began to discuss the use of alternative medical techniques in his 1983 work, *Health and Healing: Understanding Conventional and Alternative Medicine*, in which he argued that future healthcare should incorporate alternative methods and emphasize prevention. Weil became one of a few physicians to promote holistic health as being complementary to regular medicine. In 1993, he founded the Center for Integrative Medicine in Tucson, Arizona, dedicated to the integration of ideas and practices of both conventional and alternative medicine. Weil summarized the essence of alternative medicine and holistic health in a *Good Housekeeping* (Rubin 1997) article, contending, "You cannot look after the needs of your body without addressing the needs of the mind and spirit."

Some Federal Interest in Alternative Practices

By the early 1990s, interest in alternative medical practices finally caught the attention of Federal health authorities. Berman and Larson (1994, x) suggested that the Public Health Service (PHS) "recognized the need to completely revamp the current approach to health and illness when it released *Healthy People 2000.*" This report enumerated challenges and goals for improving the nation's collective health by the turn of the century and to improve disease prevention and health promotion. As part of this mandate, alternative healthcare options were deemed worthy of investigation. In 1992, Congress established the Office of Alternative Medicine (OAM) within the National Institute of Health (NIH) to more adequately explore "unconventional" medical practices (Berman and Larson 1994, xii).[14] The OAM subdivided alternative medicine into six categories. The first category consisted of *mind–body interventions*, which included the placebo effect produced by good doctor–patient relationships as well as meditation, support groups, imagery, hypnosis, biofeedback, yoga, prayer, and mental healing. *Bioelectromagnetic* applications encompassed the use of magnets and nonionizing radiation therapy, such as laser and radio-frequency hyperthermia. *Alternative systems of medical practice* consisted of many practices common to other cultures, including acupuncture and traditional oriental medicine, and homeopathic, naturalpathic, and community-based healings. *Manual healing methods* embraced chiropractic science, the laying on of hands (biofield therapeutics), and massage therapy. *Pharmacological and biological treatments* included the use of a wide range of alternative drugs and vaccines. *Herbal medicine* incorporated natural herbs and vitamins. *Diet and nutrition medicine* included the use of various high doses of vitamins or food supplements—sometimes called "orthomolecular medicine"—to prevent and reverse certain chronic conditions (Berman and Larson 1994, xii–xxii).

The OAM and its mission to objectively research unconventional medical practices for possible benefits, however, were not readily accepted by the mainstream NIH organization, which had the authority to select and support research projects. Daniel Greenberg (1997), editor of a Washington science newsletter, suggested that the OAM "from the start operated in a hostile environment." During the 1990s, a decrease in funding resulted for research concerning alternative remedies inasmuch as most were considered unscientific to mainstream medicine and many advocates refused to test treatments using standard tests of validity.

The Anti–Alternative Medicine Movement

Even though many Americans began adopting alternative medical and holistic health practices in the early 1980s, many mainstream physicians considered these practices quackery or were concerned about potential harm to patients. Individuals who promoted these alternative treatments were at first considered con artists, and the holistic movement was discounted. An article in the September 2, 1980 *Washington Post* on the burgeoning holistic movement stated, "Dr. Samuel Bessman of the University of Southern California is a . . . severe critic of the new movement. He attacked the moneymaking 'high priests' of new, unscientific 'cults' who discourage patients from seeing doctors when sick."

By the early 1990s, even though some traditional physicians had begun to accept certain alternative techniques or had integrated the concept of wellness into their practices, many critics of these procedures abounded. For example, James Harvey Young (1992b, 177), a critic of alternative medicine, attacked nutritional approaches. He stated, "As life-style changes assumed an ever larger role in pseudo-scientific preventive and curative regimens, nutritional eccentricities retained their status at the apex of the nation's health delusions." In the late 1990s, a book by Hebert Benson (1997), which suggested spiritual belief could cure many illnesses, was condemned by William Jarvis, president of the National Council Against Health Fraud. The March 31, 1997 *USA Today* quoted Jarvis as insisting, "Religion and science are two different realms, and anyone who thinks the twain meet 'is delusional.'" However, the following year, at least one study demonstrated that those who had a strong religious belief recovered from serious illnesses with fewer complications.

As the holistic movement began to take form, federal and state legislative bodies attempted to curtail certain practices or punished those practicing certain healing techniques, especially if it involved children. Practitioners of mental healing, for example, were subject to legal sanctions. Robert Peel (1988, 110–111), in his history of Christian Science medicine, reported that in 1967 a Christian Science mother in Massachusetts was convicted of involuntary manslaughter for the death of her five-year-old daughter as a result of Christian Science treatment. A few years later, the Massachusetts legislature, however, amended the welfare statute to recognize conscientious spiritual healing. In 1986, the state of California prosecuted some parents and charged them with manslaughter for turning to spiritual healing instead of seeking medical aid for a child who died (Peel 1988, 114).

The Food and Drug Administration (FDA), founded during the second Clean Living Movement (see Chapter 10), prohibited or confiscated alternative substances and unproven cures and sometimes prevented individuals from engaging in experimental treatment procedures. Desperate consumers often went to Mexico and other countries to obtain these treatments. This was particularly true for cancer and HIV/AIDS patients. However, in the late 1980s, due to pressure on the part of HIV/AIDS patients, the FDA adopted speedier clinical trials for drugs used to treat this disease (Young 1992a, 88, 270–275). During the last three decades of the century, the FDA, on several occasions, urged passage of laws to restrict the sale of vitamins and nutritional supplements. As of the turn of this century, conflict still exists between the FDA and American citizens on access to varying strengths and types of vitamins, nutritional supplements, and herbs.

By the end of the twentieth century, numerous orthodox physicians still did not accept unconventional practices and continued to consider them quackery. However, use of alternative methods, including nutritional supplements such as high doses of vitamins to prevent various illness, became increasingly popular with many Americans on the eve of the new millennium.

SUMMARY

A religious revival, the fourth Great Awakening, arose in the 1960s. This movement consisted of a growth in Christian enthusiastic religions and the development of new religious faiths. The more conservative Christians embraced traditional moral values concerning sexuality, the place of women in society, and a desire to bring society back to a Golden Age. In contrast, adherents of new religious groups often sought to create a whole new perfect society. In order to reach these objectives, the Christian Right advocated social and legislative sanctions to eliminate abortion, sex education in the schools, alcohol, drugs, and women's and gay rights. The New Religious movement fostered agendas in favor of choice concerning abortion, women's rights, gay rights, and alternative healthcare. Intertwined with the New Religious movement was a resurgence of nontraditional medical practices, such as meditation, exercise, nutrition, and other approaches that had been rejected by orthodox medicine.

NOTES

1. Michael D'Antonio (1992, 395), who has chronicled selected New Age communities, has noted that "the New Age and Christian America are also connected by their fascination with apocalyptic prophecy. . . . New Agers told me that a cataclysm would soon destroy nearly all of the Earth. It would be followed by the 'New Age' of idyllic peace and prosperity. . . . These beliefs mimic the Biblically based apocalyptic scenario predicted by countless conservative Christian preachers and subscribed by millions of their followers."

2. An article, "The Rise of Born Again Politics" (1980) in a *Newsweek* report illustrates the linking of religion and politics that included health-related issues in the Christian Right. The article stated that Jerry Falwell's "agenda for the 1980s—of the Moral Majority's" born-again politics was "a pro-family, pro-life, pro-morality platform. . . . The Moral Majority—and its evangelical allies—are against abortion, ERA, gay rights, sex education, drugs, pornography."

3. For more details concerning the life and political activities of Robertson from various perspectives, see, in particular, Foege (1996), Boston (1996), and Robertson's 1986 autobiography, *America's Date with Destiny*.

4. For details concerning the rise and fall of the Moral Majority, see, in particular, Bruce (1988), Jorstad (1987), Lienesch (1993), and Snowball (1991). See, in particular, Wilcox (1992) for statistical analysis of demographic information and issues supported by the Christian Right.

5. Alex Foege (1996, 231), a contemporary communication specialist, suggests that "family values" actually means "born-again" Christian values.

6. The stated objectives of the Christian Coalition from their home page (http://www.cc.org/about.html, last visited August 30, 1998), were strengthening the family, protecting innocent human life, returning education to local and parental control, easing the tax burden on families, punishing criminals and defending victims' rights, protecting young people and our communities from the pollution of pornography, defending the institution of marriage, and protecting religious freedom.

7. There were differing opinions among contemporary writers as to the status of the Christian Right as a movement in the 1990s. Some authors at the end of the 1980s, such as Bruce (1988), in *The Rise and Fall of the New Christian*

Right (as per the title), saw the movement's demise after the defeat of Pat Robertson. Lienesch (1993) suggested that after that date the movement was on the wane but still a persistent force in the culture. Other authors, including Boston (1996) in his *The Most Dangerous Man in America?* and Foege (1996) in *The Empire That God Built,* claim that the Christian Right is a very powerful and even dangerous force that will continue to exert considerable influence on various social and moral agendas into the twenty-first century.

8. Quebedeaux (1983, 233) implies that those who are opposed to a spiritual or religious belief system which differs from their own often label these groups as "cults." However, most mainstream denominations today originally began as small cults—including Christianity. In the United States, this has included the Mormons and Seventh-Day Adventists in the mid-nineteenth century, and Unity, Christian Science, and other New Thought groups in the early twentieth century (see Chapters 2 and 7). Today, the term "cult" is generally used as a pejorative. Pat Robertson, cited by Boston (1996, 151–154), has even labeled established religions as cults, including the ancient Hindu religion along with Mormons, Unitarians, and Christian Scientists. Since we are still in the wake of the late twentieth-century spiritual awakening, it is too early to tell what new religious traditions, which at present may be considered cults by some, may also become part of mainstream religious practice in the United States in the future.

9. There have been numerous popular publications and a few scholarly works about the various new religions. For scholarly publications, see, in particular, Barrett (1996), Hanegraaff (1996), Heelas (1996), Lewis and Melton (1992), York (1995), Galanter (1989), Bromley and Hammond (1987), and Melton (1986). Selected more general popular works include a dictionary of terms and ideas common to this movement by Campbell and Brennan (1994), and a description of selected new religious communities by D'Antonio (1992).

10. In 1985, within the Unitarian Universalist Church, the Covenant of Unitarian Universalist Pagans (CUUPS) was founded. By 1990, there were sixty chapters in the United States of this Neo-Pagan group. By the late 1990s, this had increased to seventy official chapters within the UU Church (Kelly 1992, 143; see http://www.cuups.org, last visited September 9, 1998).

11. See Gevitz (1988) for details about the history of several alternative treatment systems. See Starr (1982) for the transformation of American medical practice and its influence in eliminating alternative systems.

12. The term "wellness" was first defined in a book by Herbert L. Dunn, *High-Level Wellness,* in 1961. Dunn defines it "as an integrative method of functioning which is oriented toward maximizing the potential of which the individual is capable. It requires that the individual maintain a continuum of balance and purposeful direction within the environment where he is functioning" (pp. 4–5).

13. Biographical information for Andrew Weil is taken from the *Current Biography Yearbook 1996* (pp. 620–624).

14. A description of various alternative medicine approaches, along with a detailed biography of research exploring these methods, was found in *Alternative Medicine: Expanding Medical Horizons,* edited by Berman and Larson (1994). This federal government publication examines various alternative treatment methods in an objective manner, rather than as quackery.

13

Drunk Driving, Smoke-Free Environments, and the "War against Drugs"

As we look at the ways in which the U.S. has addressed issues related to alcohol, we might ask whether prohibition is the inevitable—if brief—culmination of temperance movements. Is our Puritan tradition of uncompromising moral stances still supplying righteous energy to the battle against alcohol?

David F. Musto, *Scientific American* (1996)

Just say no to drugs.

Nancy Reagan, *Washington Post* (1983)

Americans have reason enough to be critical about "wars" declared from Washington, especially those against crime and drugs. Administration after administration unfurls its martial banners, proclaims war on criminals and drug dealers and vows to keep fighting until total victory is achieved. Brave slogans are employed: "zero tolerance" and "unconditional surrender."

Haynes Johnson, *Washington Post* (1989)

For many adolescents, the first pack of cigarettes leads not only to a lifelong addiction to nicotine but also to other drug use, including heroin and cocaine. Recognizing the link between tobacco and hard drug abuse is particularly important today. The number of teenagers using marijuana, heroin, cocaine and other illicit drugs has doubled since 1992.

Charles LeMaistre, *Dallas Morning News* (1996)

The antitobacco, antialcohol, and antidrug crusades of the third Clean Living Movement became intertwined as they matured. The overall movement began with antismoking agitation in the mid-1960s, followed about ten years later by campaigns against alcohol and drugs. These crusades exhibited the classic phases of health-reform movements. After a perceived increase in problems associated with the use of various substances, reformers began with *moral suasive* (social-pressure and educational) campaigns that included recommendations for abstinence and the demonization of the substance in an effort to change attitudes about its use. When these activities were not entirely successful, the *coercive* (negative-sanctions) phase of the movement evolved. At the end of the century, a *backlash* against restrictions on certain behaviors began to emerge.

During the millennial Clean Living Movement, grassroots, not-for-profit, and government groups led the crusade. Coalitions between these associations spurred increased legislation to control individual behavior regarding the use of these substances. An undercurrent of the movement, as was found in the previous movements, was fear and hostility toward a particular group that was perceived as exhibiting deviant behaviors by the established middle class. In the late twentieth century, baby-boomer "hippies" and "flower children" became the dangerous class. During the Vietnam War years, many youth rebelled against the war and the "establishment's" values. As part of this rebellion, many young people smoked marijuana and used other drugs. However, alcohol and tobacco were still found to be the drugs of choice. Restrictive laws began to be passed against youthful drinking and other substances as a method to control what were considered to be dangerous and unhealthy activities (Engs 1978, 200; Gusfield 1986, 200–201).

THE ANTITOBACCO MOVEMENT

The antitobacco movement, the initial spark of the third Clean Living Movement, predated other health-reform agitations by about a decade. The antismoking movement was the most successful health campaign of the late twentieth century. After twenty years of reform activity, the crusade was successful in reducing a behavior perceived as harmful by a majority of middle-class Americans.[1] This could be compared to the anti–TB movement earlier in the century, when much of the nation adopted the reformers' position and took action to eliminate the problem from their lives. In contrast, other issues of the late twentieth-century movement were not necessarily embraced by large segments of the population.

From tobacco's peak consumption around 1980, when almost 50 percent of the population smoked, there was a decline to about 24 percent of the population over the age of twelve in 1993. Tobacco use increased to about 29 percent and remained at this level through 1996.

By the early 1990s, smoking was primarily a habit among the poor, uneducated, and disenfranchised. Burnham (1993, 110–111) noted that "smoking continued as a symbolic, often defiant, act among many young and non-middle-class and female population[s]." In the mid-1990s, after a decline for over a decade, an increase in smoking began among teenagers.[2] The January 20, 1997 *New York Times* suggested this was because youth were "embracing the dangerous habit as hip."

The Smoking Years, 1940s–1970s

Prohibitory laws against cigarette smoking that had been passed during the second movement were repealed by the early 1930s. After this time, there was a steady increase in the percentage of smokers. During World War II, tobacco—in this war, cigarettes—as had been found in previous wars, was considered an essential commodity for soldiers. The postwar economic boom, rapid urbanization, and glamorous advertising by cigarette manufacturers led to increased smoking among both males and females. Smoking was popularly depicted in many films, heavily advertised in the news media, and became chic and urbane among nationally known politicians, newsmen, and other high-profile individuals, as well as among the upwardly mobile. By the early 1970s, advertising targeted "liberated women" and "rebels" against the establishment, and cigarette smoking increased over the decade (Heimann 1960, 241–249; Burnham 1993, 99–111; Brandt 1998, 165; Troyer and Markle 1983, 124).

Reformers and Health Concerns about Smoking

For the most part, reformers appeared as members of organizations rather than individuals. Individual reformers of the second movement were replaced by various governmental and private advocacy groups. The antismoking movement had its symbolic beginning in 1964, with what became known as the "Surgeon General's Report" issued by the federal government.

The Government as Reformer

Some federal government officials played a significant role as reformers in the antismoking movement. Goldstein (1992, 112) has argued that government involvement in antismoking efforts became so pervasive that these activities themselves became the catalysts for much of the movement's growth and activity. McGowan (1995, 12–48) has divided this government involvement with the cigarette industry and antismoking activism in the late twentieth century into two phases.[3]

From 1965 to 1985, antismoking bills and limited federal regulations on smoking and concern for the health of the smoker were prominent. The period between 1985 to the mid-1990s focused on the effects of smoking on nonsmokers. Numerous state and local regulations were suggested or enacted to eliminate smoking from society. A third stage began to emerge in the mid- to late 1990s. Negotiations ensued between various government levels and the tobacco industry to reach settlements on allowable industry activities in exchange for liability limits against the industry.

Not-for-Profit and Grassroots Reformers

Both well-established associations and new grassroots advocacy groups became antitobacco activists. Established organizations, such as the American Lung Association, the American Cancer Society (ACS), and the American Heart Association (AHA), tended to promote educational programs throughout the movement. However, new antismoking groups formed in the late 1960s and 1970s, including ASH (Action on Smoking and Health), ANR (Americans for Nonsmokers' Rights), and GASP (Group Against Smokers' Pollution), modeled themselves on environmental activist groups and were interested in litigation. They tended to eschew education in favor of severe sanctions against both the smoker and tobacco. These newer groups pushed to stigmatize tobacco and to protect the rights of the nonsmoker for a smoke-free environment. Their activism led to smoking being seen as increasingly deviant during the last three decades of the twentieth century (Goldstein 1992, 117; Troyer and Markle 1983, 124–125; Brandt 1998, 172).

The Health Consequences of Smoking

The health consequences of smoking focused first on the smoker then on nonsmokers affected by secondary environmental smoke. This led to concerns about pregnant women smoking and the effect of passive smoke on children.

Risk to Smokers. Health risks associated with smoking began to be published in a serious way in the 1950s. A widely distributed study in 1954 by the American Medical Association (AMA) showed the association of lung cancer and smoking (Hammond and Horn 1954). This led many physicians to quit the habit themselves, but there was more reluctance in recommending that their patients also quit. The media began to increasingly discuss the dangers of smoking. Due to the accumulating evidence of smoking's association with various health problem, in 1964, Surgeon General Luther Terry issued the *Report on Smoking and Health* and condemned the practice. For a few weeks after the release of this much-discussed report, cigarette sales fell 20 to 25 percent. However, after this brief period, their sale rebounded and increased for the next fifteen years (Burnham 1989, 22–27; Brandt 1998, 164–167).

The Nonsmoker. Research in the mid-1970s began to suggest that sidestream smoke, passive smoking, or secondhand smoke (that is, smoke inhaled by nonsmokers in confined areas), was associated with health problems. In 1986, Surgeon General Koop released two reports on the dangers of passive smoke, and during the mid- and late 1980s, action against environmental smoke flamed (Brandt 1998, 167–170; U.S. Department of Health and Human Services 1986; Iglehart 1986).

Women and Children. An increase in women smoking began around World War II. Studies in the mid-1960s began to suggest that women who smoked had babies with lower birth weight. An increase in lung cancer was also noticed for women, beginning in the late 1960s.[4] These dangers were presented to the public in *Smoking and Health: A Report of the Surgeon General* (U.S. Department of Health, Education, and Welfare 1979). Beginning in the 1980s, some research suggested a relationship between parental smoking and respiratory health problems in children (Tager 1986). By the mid-1990s, an association between smoking during pregnancy and sudden infant death syndrome and miscarriages became widely publicized (DiFranza and Lew 1995). These research findings reinforced not only the perceived dangers of sidestream smoke, but also the dangers of smoking for women and children. These reports increasingly stigmatized smoking, so that "smokers . . . became an oppressive and dangerous minority" (Brandt 1998, 172).

Moral-Suasive Measures against Smoking and Tobacco, 1965–1975

Throughout the 1960s, federal and local public-health officials primarily presented factual information and set broad policy goals to reduce the proportion of smokers and prevent nonsmokers from initiating the habit. These programs grew in the early 1970s. In this decade, the coercive phase of the antismoking movement also emerged. For the rest of the movement, both the coercive and moral-suasion phases were found simultaneously.

Smoking and Health: Still a Moral Issue?

A common late twentieth-century misconception suggested that earlier antitobacco efforts were based solely on "morality" inasmuch as there was little evidence to suggest harm from smoking. This was opposed to late twentieth-century activism that was supposedly based purely on scientific evidence. Tate (1995, 6) has suggested that, with the notable exception of lung cancer, which was relatively unknown until the early 1930s, reformers in the two previous antismoking movements identified cigarettes as a cause of every health problem now linked to smoking, including heart disease, emphysema, and birth defects. This can be seen in publications from both the first and second Clean Living Movements (see Chapters 3 and 8). Tate argued that the late twentieth-century campaign against smoking, while focused more on public health than on private morality, still remained entangled in moralism. Goldstein (1992, 115) contends this might be due to the fact that "Throughout American history . . . addiction was considered a grave moral failing." As the movement surged over the last three decades of the century, moral suasion was often difficult to differentiate from prevention and education programming. This synthesis of morality and personal health behavior was suggested by the title of a popular work critical of antitobacco advocates' tactics: *For Your Own Good: The Anti-Smoking Crusade and the Tyranny of Public Health* (Sullum 1998).

Demonization of Tobacco

As has been found in previous movements, demonization of cigarettes, tobacco, and the tobacco companies emerged. The act of smoking and smokers themselves began to be stigmatized in the mid-1970s. By the mid-1980s, hostility toward smokers had increased to the point that they were often forced to smoke outside buildings where they worked. Smoking and smokers began to be increasingly associated with marginal and deviant social groups. By the late 1980s, not only tobacco and smokers, but also the tobacco companies were branded as evil (Goldstein 1992, 116–118). Larry White (1988) dubbed the tobacco industry the "Merchants of Death" in his book by that title.

Prevention Programs

During the late 1960s, various advocacy and even religious groups, such as the Seventh-Day Adventists, along with branches of the federal government, encouraged or sponsored smoking-cessation programs. In 1977, the American Cancer Society launched its first national "Great American Smokeout," a designated day on which smokers were requested not to smoke (*New York Times*, November 17, 1977). This event became an annual campaign throughout the rest of the century.

Numerous legislative and public-policy measures from the mid-1960s to the mid-1980s also attempted to dissuade individuals from using tobacco. The first major policy was the Cigarette Warning Label Act of 1966, which mandated labels on cigarettes to inform the public about the dangers of smoking. In 1972, the tar and nicotine content of cigarettes were required on packaging. In 1984, cigarette warning labels were replaced by four disease-specific warnings as part of the Comprehensive Smoking Education Act. In 1986, Congress legislated warning labels on smokeless tobacco (Troyer and Markel 1983, 133–135; Kluger 1996, 510, 563–564). These and other prevention programs occurred simultaneously with social sanctions against smoking, smokers, and the tobacco industry.

Coercive Legislation and Mandates: 1975–2000?

By the 1970s, various government levels began to take a more direct and restrictive approach to eliminate smoking. Major thrusts of the coercive phase of the movement were laws to create smoke-free environments, curtailment of advertisements, measures to prevent youth from smoking, and litigation against the tobacco industry (Goldstein 1992, 112–113).

Creating Smoke-Free Environments and a Smoke-Free Society

Legislation to ban smoking in public places began to appear in the 1970s. By the end of 1975, thirty-one states had approved legislation supporting smoking restrictions. Communities began to pass ordinances that required employers to insure that nonsmoking office workers were given special accommodations in the 1980s (Goldstein 1992, 113–114; Kluger 1996, 681–682; Sullum 1998, 145–152). These regulations were vigorously fought by the tobacco industry to prevent implementation.

In 1989, smoking was prohibited on all domestic flights of two hours or less. This was expanded to flights of up to six hours in 1990. By 1989, at least forty-four states had passed comprehensive laws limiting smoking, and 80 percent of American corporations had implemented companywide restrictions on smoking. Beginning in the mid-1990s, antismoking advocates were no longer content with separation of smokers from nonsmokers. They began to crusade for "zero tolerance" and elimination of smoking from all public places, including parks, outdoor stadiums, and even bars, the traditional establishment for smoking, drinking, and other "vices." California was the first state to pass legislation prohibiting smoking in bars, which took effect January 1, 1998. As of the turn of the twenty-first century, activists continue to press to eliminate all smoking from all public places (Goldstein 1992, 114–115; Sullum 1998, 151–153).

Tobacco Advertisement and the Death of Joe Camel

Over the duration of the movement, increasing social and legal sanctions were taken against cigarette advertising. In 1971, all cigarette ads were banned from radio and television by the federal Cigarette Labeling and Advertising Act. During the 1980s and early 1990s, activists advocated the elimination of tobacco advertisements in sports stadiums and sports events. The Justice Department ruled that positioning ads in sports stadiums visible by TV audiences was a violation of the 1971 ban. R. J. Reynolds, the largest tobacco company, agreed to remove its Marlboro Man ads after the ruling (*Los Angeles Times*, June 7, 1995).

In the late 1980s and early 1990s, antitobacco activists claimed that the cigarette industry was targeting children and youth through the use of cartoon characters. Joe Camel, a cleverly drawn cartoon, symbolized this catchy appeal to youth. Because children recognized the logo, activists were concerned they might be enticed to start smoking. The July 11, 1997 *Los Angeles Times* reported, "Joe became a lightning rod for complaints about cigarette makers targeting minors to replace the millions of smokers who quit or die." Health and antismoking groups blamed this cartoon for increased smoking among teenagers, "despite the country's deepening anti-smoking mood." Because of public pressure against the use of this cartoon, it was discontinued in 1997.

Legislation to Prohibit Tobacco Use among Youth

Concern about the increase in smoking among youth resulted in the FDA declaring in 1995 that cigarettes were an addictive drug. The FDA recommended sweeping regulations to curb smoking among youth. President Clinton (*New York Times*, August 11, 1995) endorsed the FDA's claim that cigarettes were essentially a "nicotine delivery device" and therefore a drug. If nicotine was a drug, it could be controlled by the FDA. Some of the proposed regulations by the agency included a ban on cigarette sales to anyone under eighteen and requiring photo identification as proof of age; the abolition of cigarette sales by vending machines and mail order; prohibition of cigarette billboards within 1,000 feet of schools; and a halt to tobacco brand-name sponsorship of sports and entertainment events and the sale or giveaway to youngsters of promotional merchandise bearing tobacco brand names or logos.

Litigation against Tobacco Companies

In the mid-1980s, relatives of individuals who had died from smoking-associated causes began to sue the tobacco companies. In the 1950s, suits had also been filed but they were not successful. However, in the early 1990s, some settlements were made between these individuals and the cigarette industry. In the mid-1990s, states and insurance companies also began to sue the tobacco industry to regain costs for treating smoking-related illnesses. Successful settlements were negotiated in Florida, Mississippi, Texas, and Minnesota. Minnesota, as reported in the May 9, 1998 *Sacramento Bee*, was an example of a typical agreement. The industry, besides paying the state millions of dollars in reimbursed health costs, agreed to cease marketing to minors in the state, restrict the sale of promotional merchandise such as caps, remove cigarette billboards in the state, and stop placing "tobacco products in movies or on television." In 1997, the tobacco industry, government bodies, and Congress negotiated for "a national settlement that would halt most pending lawsuits, supersede state settlements, and limit the companies' future liability" (*USA Today*, August 27, 1997). A national settlement was defeated by Congress in 1998. However, near the end of that year, all states had reached a settlement (*USA Today*, November 17, 1998). As of the turn of this century, it is not yet clear what effect further litigation or settlements would have on the duration of the late twentieth-century antitobacco movement or the trend in tobacco use.

Backlash against Antismoking Reforms

A backlash against antismoking reform began in the early 1990s among some upper-middle-class individuals and celebrities. Sullum (1998, 11) suggests that the "cigar boom of the 1990s can be seen as a rebellion against this attempt to redefine smoking." Sales of premium cigars began to rise in the late 1980s and continued through the 1990s. Smoking cigars after fashionable dinner events and the sale of emerging expensive cigars became de rigeur. A report in the January 7, 1997 *Washington Post* suggested that not only was there a backlash against tobacco, but also against low-fat diets, exercise, alcohol, and other aspects of the late twentieth-century Clean Living Movement. The report described trendy cigar and martini "retro" bars, reminiscent of 1950s settings, filled with smoke and martinis.

The increase in smoking among adolescents in the mid-1990s may also have signaled the beginning of a backlash phase of the antismoking movement. David Wagner (1997, 101), in a popular book concerning the movement, for example, suggested that "for many adolescents today, smoking serves as a symbol of growing up and, at least among working-class and poor kids, often as a common group activity intended to kill time and perhaps *arouse the ire of adults*" (italics added). As of the turn of the twenty-first century, it is not possible to tell if the backlash symbolized by an increase in smoking expensive cigars among the rich will continue. Likewise, it is not known if the increasing trend in cigarette consumption among youth will continue.

THE NEO-PROHIBITION MOVEMENT

Repeal of national prohibition in 1933 returned alcoholic beverages to the states' control. Some states continued to remain dry for several decades, while others had drinking-purchase laws that varied from eighteen to twenty-one years; some states had local-option laws. During the Depression, little change was seen in per capita consumption, which may have been due to the economic condition. After World War II, alcohol use began to climb. There have been many theories as to the reasons behind this increase, including the results of rapid urbanization, expanded wealth, public-relations efforts by the alcohol-beverage industry, positive media reports and advertisements, increased psychological stress, and growth of a youthful population arising out of the postwar baby boom (Engs 1992a; 1995, 227; Burnham 1993, 73–75; Lender and Martin 1987, 191, 206; Blocker 1989, 138). Some of these same factors had also precipitated increased consumption prior to the two earlier antialcohol movements, as discussed in Chapters 3 and 8.

The Wet Years, 1950s–1970s

During the 1950s and through the mid-1970s, "the bar" became the archetypal setting in most movies, business deals were made over a "two-martini lunch," and cocktail parties were considered the socially acceptable way of entertaining: Alcohol acceptance was at its peak. By the end of this period, about one-third of Americans abstained from alcohol, while many adolescents frequently became intoxicated. A clash of attitudes toward drinking, with little consensus on what constituted moderate and responsible consumption, became an undercurrent ready to explode again in another temperance era.[5]

At its peak in 1980, per capita consumption was about 2.9 gallons absolute alcohol per person per year; by the mid-1990s this had fallen about 15 percent. This decrease was attributed to many factors, particularly the aging of the baby-boom population. This trend was also seen in Europe. Nonalcoholic brews, similar to "near beer" during prohibition, increased in popularity, along with bottled water and soft drinks (USDC 1996, 148). Drinking among youth, especially college youth, declined, reflecting the overall decrease. However, among collegians, the decrease came from an increase in abstainers and a decrease in light to moderate drinkers. Heavier or at-risk drinkers remained stable (Engs and Hanson 1994, 2000).

Setting the Stage for Reform:
AA and the Disease Concept of Alcoholism

The roots of the late twentieth-century Clean Living Movement can be traced to the formation of Alcoholics Anonymous (AA) on the eve of World War II. This organization strove to help the problem drinker stay sober, similar to the Washingtonians and the Reform Clubs in two earlier eras. AA forces in the early 1940s joined with E. M. Jellinek (1890–1963), an alcoholism researcher at Yale, and suggested that alcoholism was a "progressive disease" that could be treated, rather than a "moral" problem. Part of the treatment regime was total abstinence for life. By the late 1960s, AA participation was built into most rehabilitation programs (Lender and Martin 1987, 185; Blocker 1989, 148–155; Peele and Brodsky 1991, 35–36).[6]

By the late 1960s, the federal government began to fund treatment programs. In 1970, a federal agency, the National Institute of Alcohol Abuse and Alcoholism (NIAAA), was created, with the mission to fund and coordinate alcoholism research. As the national consciousness increasingly accepted alcoholism as a treatable disease, public drunkenness was decriminalized and employers were encouraged to identify workers with drinking problems in order to refer them to treatment. Intervention was used to persuade workers to accept treatment or be fired from their jobs, an activity reminiscent of programs to eliminate smoking and drinking during the second movement. By the early 1980s, hundreds of treatment facilities had sprung up after Betty Ford (b. 1918), the wife of President Ford, acknowledged treatment for alcoholism in 1978. However, in the late 1980s and early 1990s, curtailment of hospitalization costs forced many of these centers to close or treat other problems (Blocker 1989, 150–153; *Washington Post*, April 22, 1978; Peele and Brodsky 1991, 35–40).

Perceived Social and Health Problems Related to Drinking

Increased public awareness of and attention to alcohol use and abuse in the late 1960s and 1970s led to a focus on other alcohol-related issues. These included drunken driving, youthful drinking, and alcohol consumption by pregnant women.

Drunken Driving and Youthful Drinking

In 1971, during the Vietnam War, the voting age was lowered to eighteen. Eighteen states also lowered the minimum drinking age. However, by the late 1970s some research suggested that this lower drinking age led to increased fatal motor-vehicle crashes among youth

(General Accounting Office 1987; Wagenaar 1989). Articles with titles such as "A New Prohibition for Teenagers" (Beck and Malamund 1979) in *Newsweek* began to appear, proposing changes in the law to prevent drunken driving. Drunken driving, especially among youth, began to be perceived as the major health and social problem related to drinking. Efforts to curtail this behavior provided the spark that ignited a new temperance movement.

Fetal Alcohol Syndrome (FAS) and "Hidden" Women Alcoholics

In the previous two temperance movements, social condemnation of women who abused alcohol emerged—in particular, women who drank even a small amount during pregnancy. David Musto (b. 1936), a drug and alcohol historian, has suggested that "belief in alcohol's ability to damage the fetus is a hallmark of American temperance movements in this and the past century" (Musto 1996, 80). In the early 1970s, researchers in Seattle had found Fetal Alcohol Syndrome among infants whose mothers had heavily consumed alcohol during pregnancy (Jones and Smith 1973). By the late 1970s, some researchers claimed that even a small amount of alcohol could cause the disorder (Sterling 1990). Not everyone agreed with these findings, however (Rosett and Weiner 1984; Abel and Sokol 1990). After media reports about FAS, an increase in reported cases occurred. This may have been because of more awareness concerning the problem rather than an actual increase in incidence.

During the late 1970s, increased public concern about alcoholism among women also emerged. Some professionals were concerned that there had been a dramatic increase in drinking and "hidden" alcoholism among women; by the late 1980s, this had extended to other alcohol-related health problems among women (Wilsnack and Beckman 1984, ix).[7]

Moral Suasion and the Beginning of the Coercive Phase, 1970–1980

Morris Chafetz (b. 1924), founding director of NIAAA, advocated teaching responsible drinking to both adults and young people. However, opposition to this position quickly emerged, and, in 1978, the NIAAA adopted the "public-health" or "control of consumption" model to reduce consumption. Responsible drinking was no longer an acceptable position (Sullum 1990, 32; Engs and Fors 1988, 26–27). Blocker (1989, 156) has noted that the new antialcohol rhetoric "echoed arguments first made in the 1830s . . . aimed at increasing the number of total abstainers and reducing overall consumption by invoking social controls." As part of this antidrinking attitude, federal agencies destroyed numerous government publications concerning methods for responsible drinking.[8] This "new-temperance" philosophy grew over the 1980s, and by the early 1990s, Stanton Peele (1993, 805), a critic of the movement, noted that the concept of moderation had been "completely expunged from the American scene."

Demonization of Alcohol and Moderate Drinking

The process of elimination of any concept of healthy or moderate drinking came from the demonization of alcohol, the beverage industry, and advocates of responsible drinking. Jacob Sullum (b. 1965), a social-policy critic deeply concerned about government intrusion into personal behavior, suggested that "Temperance advocates, both in and out of government, have set as their goal a reduction in per-capita alcohol consumption. They seek to achieve this goal . . . by stigmatizing beer, wine, and liquor as inherently bad" (Sullum 1990, 27). As part of the scapegoating process, reformers fostered a blurring of a distinction between alcohol use and abuse (Engs and Fors 1988; Peele and Brodsky 1998; Peele 1993).[9]

The Rise of Grassroots Organizations

Drunken driving became the catalyst for the formation of advocacy groups against alcohol, just as ardent spirits had been during the first movement and saloons during the second. Mothers Against Drunk Driving (MADD) and Rid Intoxicated Drivers (RID) organized around 1980. Both groups attacked weak drunken-driving laws and repeat offenders. The Center for Science in the Public Interest (CSPI), a consumer advocacy group formed in 1971, began to advocate the public-health model. In 1981, Students Against Driving Drunk (SADD) was formed to reduce drunken driving among youth. This group promoted a contract between parents and children. Children were obligated to phone their parents for transportation if they had been drinking. A "designated-driver" program also was encouraged. Over the 1980s and into the 1990s, government agencies, professional health organizations, and other special-interest groups, as a coalition, began to advocate stiffer laws. By the mid-1990s, these groups rated states according to "efforts to combat alcohol-impaired driving" (Russell et al. 1995, 240–241; Musto 1996, 79). By the early 1990s, many antialcohol groups began to flirt with a prohibitionary position. Sullum (1990, 27), for example, observed that these groups "argue that drinkers must be saved from themselves, lest their health suffer as a result of excessive consumption. Further, pointing to the role played by alcohol in violence and traffic accidents, they maintain that drinking endangers public safety."

OSAP: A Government Agency as a Reformer

Political action by grassroots organizations and others concerned about youthful alcohol consumption encouraged Congress in 1988 to establish the Office of Substance Abuse Prevention under the Department of Health and Human Services. However, this federal agency began to act as a reformer, advocating change in public policy through both moral suasive and negative social and legal sanctions. OSAP provided the media "editorial guidelines" to encourage new ways of describing alcohol. This included eliminating the term "responsible" and promoting "clear massages" of "no use." Designated-driver programs were also unacceptable (Office of Substance Abuse Prevention 1991; Engs 1991a). Under OSAP's guidelines, "safe, responsible, or low risk" drinking could not be discussed in schools or by teachers who received federal funding; only abstinence-based programs were acceptable. OSAP began to advocate for more coercive measures, such as higher taxes, methods to decrease availability, and even how to pressure politicians. However, in 1992, OSAP was challenged by some politicians for their advocacy activities, as they were a tax-supported agency (Office of Substance Abuse Prevention 1989, 1990, 1991; "Alcohol Industry Reps Demand GAO Report on OSAP Lobbying," *Alcoholism and Drug Abuse Week*, June 17, 1992; Engs 1991a).

Warning Labels: A Symbol of Moral Suasion

In 1981, the Surgeon General advised women who were pregnant, or considering pregnancy, to abstain from alcoholic beverages; over the 1980s, this campaign intensified. At the urging of various consumer and antialcohol groups, it was federally mandated in 1989 that all alcoholic beverages bear a warning label advising pregnant women not to drink. Kinsley (1991) noted that, by 1991, ten states also required taverns, restaurants, or distributors to post signs with this warning. The beverage label also contained other messages, such as a warning that alcohol impairs ability to drive or causes health problems. Research in the 1990s, however, found only "limited evidence of a positive impact on consumer knowledge, attitudes and behavior" due to these warning labels (Engs 1989, 116; Mosher 1997, 791).

The Coercive Phase, 1980s–2005?

Beginning in the late 1970s, government bodies and private advocacy groups, such as CSPI, the NCA (National Council on Alcoholism), and other temperance organizations, began to advocate for stricter laws to control consumption. Recommended measures included the elimination of alcohol advertising in campus media, elimination of electronic advertising for alcohol, and state-mandated "zero-tolerance" laws, which would automatically suspend driving licenses for under-age youth who had consumed any alcohol. Measures were suggested that were reminiscent of the two previous antialcohol movements, including a limit on the number of beverage outlets and their hours of operation, and "dram shop" laws in which hosts, bartenders, and taverns would be made liable for problems caused by an intoxicated persons (Scirvo 1998; Sullum 1990; Engs 1989, 1991b; Blocker 1989; Office of Substance Abuse Prevention 1991).

Raising the Drinking Age

In the late 1970s, some states began to raise the drinking age. From 1976 to 1984, twenty-eight states increased their drinking age. Pressure on Congress from grassroots and government coalitions resulted in the Federal Uniform Drinking Age Act of 1984, which threatened states with loss of highway funds if they did not raise their minimum drinking age to twenty-one by 1987; all states complied by 1988 ("Drinking Laws Come of Age" 1986; Engs and Hanson 1988). Introduction of more restrictive measures against alcohol, even though the problems related to its abuse had begun to wane, was also found in the previous movements.

Other Restrictions

There were restrictive sanctions against alcohol in the 1990s. Several state legislatures in this decade mandated lowering the blood alcohol concentration for driving from 0.10 to 0.08 percent. Others imposed zero-tolerance laws for underage drinkers. Federal excise taxes on alcoholic beverages were increased in 1991. Some state legislators also recommended mandatory treatment. For example, an article entitled "Pregnant Women Face Detention" (1998), in an international journal of alcohol news, reported that pregnant women in South Dakota and Wisconsin could be placed in treatment centers against their will "if they are judged to be drinking too heavily."

Results of the Countermeasures against Drunk Driving and Underage Drinking

After 1980, both per capita consumption of alcohol and fatal motor vehicle accidents related to drunken driving declined. The decrease in consumption mirrored the trend among adults. Some researchers claimed that the new higher-drinking-age laws were effective in reducing these fatalities (U.S. General Accounting Office 1987; Wagenaar 1989). Others suggested that safer automobiles, mandatory seat-belt laws, and lower speed limits also may have been factors in this decline. In addition, the decline had begun prior to any massive change in the drinking-age laws (Asch and Levy 1987; Engs and Hanson 1994; Whorton 1982). Collegiate programming spawned greater awareness concerning alcohol, but at the same time did not result in decreasing the problems related to irresponsible drinking (Wechsler et al. 1995; Engs and Hanson 1988, 1994, 2000).

The Beginning of the Backlash Phase, 1993–?

As has been found in other movements, conflicting activities were often found simultaneously. This has been particularly true for a reform issue that has not been acceptable to a large segment of the population or when people perceived that reformers were intruding on their personal behavior. The consumption of alcohol, as opposed to smoking, was still acceptable to the majority of Americans. This included a high proportion of youth under twenty-one years of age. This acceptance of alcohol resulted in signs of a burgeoning Backlash.

Backlash against the Temperance Movement

After the mandated twenty-one-year-old purchase laws in 1987, problems related to alcohol abuse among young adults increased. In the late 1980s and 1990s, increased violent behaviors and personal, social, and legal problems among collegians related to alcohol abuse were reported. This was because underage students were drinking in "underground" situations without adult social sanctions (Engs and Hanson 1989, 2000). *Newsweek* (Alder and Rosenberg 1994), for example, described this backlash behavior of collegians. Besides drunken behavior and deaths from overdrinking, various infractions of the twenty-one-year-old purchase laws, including use of fake or borrowed identification cards and a student black market to supply alcohol, thrived on most college campuses.

One of the first signs of a backlash against the demonization of alcohol was a "60 Minutes" television program in 1991 entitled the "French Paradox." The program reported that even though the French had a very high-fat diet, they had a lower prevalence of heart disease due to their wine consumption. Over the 1990s, there was an acceleration of research and reports related to the health benefits of moderate drinking or the lack of health consequences for small amounts of alcohol, such as "a drink a day to keep the heart attack away" (Fuchs 1995; Grønbaek et al. 1995; Rimm and Ellison 1995; Engs and Aldo-Benson 1995; Engs 1996a).

Another symbol of waning demonization and changes in attitudes toward alcohol was a change in the wording of the federal government's *Dietary Guidelines for Americans* (USDA 1990). The 1990 publication stated, "Alcohol has no net health benefit, is linked with many health problems, is the cause of many accidents, and can lead to addiction, their consumption is not recommended." The 1996 guidelines changed to the following: "Alcoholic beverages have been used to enhance the enjoyment of meals by many societies throughout human history . . . [and] when used in moderation may be safe and pleasurable." The later guideline recommended no more than a drink a day for women or two drinks a day for men. Legislative attempts and debate over changing the minimum drinking age ensued in Colorado, Wisconsin, and some other states in the late 1990s. Although they were not successful, discussions continued for possible future changes (Scirvo 1998).

Continuation of the Temperance Movement

In the mid- and late 1990s, the focus of alcohol problems shifted to college-student drinking. All alcohol use on campus was denounced on grounds it could produce "second-hand drinking" problems—an analogy to second-hand smoke—such as drunken roommates disturbing a dorm. Lurid tales of heavy drinking resulting in rapes and deaths and other problems, widely depicted in the media, flamed the antialcohol fire on the college campuses. Some government bodies pressured colleges to curtail drinking on campuses. In 1997, a few national fraternities announced they would ban alcohol from their chapter houses beginning in the year 2000 (Engs 2000; Scirvo 1998, 251).

The late twentieth-century temperance movement had many similarities to the previous movements. By the end of the 1990s, it was unclear whether the coercive phase of the movement was waning or to what extent the nation had entered the backlash phase of the cycle.

THE WAR ON DRUGS

The antidrug movement emerged in the early 1970s when the Nixon Administration created new agencies charged with halting the spread of heroin and providing treatment to addicts. In the late 1970s, a grassroots "parents movement" burst forth and, by the late 1980s, the focus of the movement began to shift to prevention of alcohol and tobacco use among youth on grounds these substances were gateway drugs. A backlash then erupted among the middle class over efforts to legalize marijuana for medical purposes in the 1990s.[10]

The "High" Years, 1965–1980

The nadir of drug use for pleasure in the United States was during World War II and the decade following it. Drug use was considered a deviant behavior by most Americans, and users were primarily blacks and Latinos in large urban cities. During the 1950s and early 1960s, users emerged among younger, antiestablishment ranks and also from more adventurous middle-class "slummers" (Engs 1978, 200–201; Burnham 1993, 113, 119–121). Journalists began to discuss this shift. Burnham (1993, 120) has suggested that media coverage of drug use among youth "was the first step in the process of . . . transforming it into a new kind of middle-class concern."

In the 1960s, marijuana and LSD use blossomed among intellectuals and "flower children." They also became widely used among Vietnam soldiers—some of whom actually went into battle "stoned"—and among other youth, who defiantly smoked illegally in public as a badge of rebellion (Engs 1978, 200). During the Kennedy era, the political climate and attitudes toward drugs began to shift. The "summer of love" in San Francisco's Haight–Ashbury district in 1967 symbolized the emerging counterculture's embrace of drug use among many middle-class youth. Acceptance of drugs reached a peak in 1978, when 65 percent of high school seniors did not consider regular marijuana use harmful. This positive attitude decreased to 23 percent ten years later. The increased use of marijuana, opiates, and hallucinogens, like alcohol and tobacco, rose over the 1970s and peaked around 1979–1980. At that point, about 60 percent of high school seniors had used marijuana and 33 percent "any illicit drug" (Johnston et al. 1989, 54, 129; 1998, 94, 98).

The Decline of Recreational Drug Use, 1980–1992

Over the 1980s recreational—nonmedical—drug use began to decline. However, cocaine became fashionable among some increasingly prosperous baby boomer or "yuppies" and did not reach its peak until the mid-1980s. Among youth, marijuana was the most common drug after alcohol and tobacco. By 1992 marijuana use among high school seniors had declined to 33 percent. However, after this date there was an increase in marijuana, cocaine, tobacco, and alcohol consumption. In 1997, about 50 percent of high school seniors had used marijuana, tobacco was used by 65 percent, cocaine by 9 percent, and alcohol by 82 percent (Gold 1993, 3–7; Johnston et al. 1998, 94).

The Beginnings of the Antidrug Movement, 1970–1980

Drug use among troops in Vietnam and rebellious youth alarmed many middle-class Americans in the late 1960s. War protests and liberal marijuana use were seen by older Americans as a rejection of traditional values and patriotism (Musto 1987, 254). Fear of these behaviors precipitated concrete antidrug measures in 1971, when President Richard

Nixon declared a "war" on drug abuse to stem the rising "narcotic trade."[11] The federal government, as it had for the antitobacco and antialcohol movements, helped to shape the antidrug movement.

The Federal Government as a Reformer

In the early 1970s, the government began to clamp down on drug use. Richard Schroeder (1980, 6), a critic of American drug policies, remarked that, after 1971, "The federal government mounted an energetic campaign to drive all kinds of drugs off the street." The Comprehensive Drug Abuse Prevention and Control act of 1970 instituted "no knock" house searches. Several federal agencies were created out of older agencies in 1973, including the Drug Enforcement Agency (DEA) and the National Institute of Drug Abuse (NIDA). The DEA's function was to eliminate drugs by law enforcement on the "supply side," while NIDA's mission was to implement prevention, treatment, and rehabilitation efforts on the "demand side" (Schroeder 1980, 6–9; Musto 1987, 263; Engs 1978, 274–276).[12]

Over the 1970s, the federal government spent several billion dollars on drug enforcement and prevention programs. Following Nixon's resignation, rhetoric relaxed against drugs and discussion of decriminalization emerged during the Carter administration in the late 1970s (Schroeder 1980, 6–9; Musto 1987, 257–267). Beginning with the Reagan administration, the war on drugs resumed and escalated.

The Rise of Grassroots Parents Movements

In 1978, Americans' attitudes toward drugs began to shift in a negative direction. Musto (1987, 270) observed that the decline in drug use was "associated, as it was in the 1920s and 1930s, not with indifference but with a positive antagonism to drugs, their effects, and (to some degree) those who use them." Parents, in particular, became increasingly concerned in the late 1970s about drug use among their children, which led to the formation of several antidrug organizations. PRIDE (Parents Resources Institute on Drug Education) was founded in 1978 by Georgia parents Ron and Marsha Manatt, concerned about possible damage to health smoking marijuana might have on teenagers. In 1980, they formed a national umbrella organization for other parents' groups, the National Federation of Parents for Drug-Free Youth (NFP). This highly organized antidrug group wielded much power over the 1980s in shaping drug policy (Musto 1987, 270–271; Schlosser 1994, 1, 10).

Prior to the formation of the conservative parents' groups, a promarijuana organization, NORML (National Organization for the Reform of Marijuana Laws), was formed around 1971. This group regarded marijuana as a benign recreational drug, a form of herbal medicine, and a product with industrial applications; they lobbied for a reduction in severe jail sentences for marijuana possession. NORML, along with some drug experts in the Carter Administration, pushed for the decriminalization of marijuana and more accurate information regarding drugs in official government literature. More objective literature began to be published in the mid- and late 1970s. However, these publications were seen by the increasingly powerful antidrug coalition as being "soft on drugs" and contributing to its use. Members of these groups began to monitor federal publications with an eye toward editing out comments favorable to drug use. As a result of their efforts, many government publications were removed from circulation (Burnham 1993, 138–139; Schlosser 1994, 2; Engs and Fors 1988; Musto 1987, 270–272; Bertram et al. 1996, 96–98).

Moral Suasion: "Just Say No to Drugs," 1980s

Nancy Reagan (b. 1923), wife of President Ronald Reagan, was the symbolic leader of the moral-suasive crusade to prevent drug use among children. She helped popularize the "just say no to drugs" campaign. This catchy phrase became a generalized abstinence-oriented message found in many health-reform campaigns during this era (just say no to sex, fat, tobacco, etc.). Mrs. Reagan spearheaded a personalized campaign against drugs by speaking to student groups, visiting drug-treatment centers, persuading the media to criticize drug use, and striving toward an atmosphere of intolerance for drug use in the nation (Reagan 1983; Musto 1987, 272–273; Engs and Fors 1988, 26–27).

Coercion: The Renewed War against Drugs, 1980s–2000?

Negative social and legal sanctions against drugs accelerated in the mid-1980s. The Comprehensive Crime Control Act of 1984 increased funding for enforcement. In 1985, emergence of crack cocaine, a cheap smokeable form of cocaine, prompted a new wave of fear, resulting in enormous media and public attention to a new "drug problem." At the height of public furor over this substance, the Anti-Drug Abuse Act of 1986 (amended in 1988) instituted a vast increase in funding for law enforcement. The U.S. customs office, under a zero-tolerance policy, was now allowed to seize property if any evidence of illegal drugs were found (Musto 1987, 274–275; Schlosser 1994, 10; *San Diego Union-Tribune*, November 12, 1988).

In the mid-1980s, urine testing for drugs was instituted, not only for safety-related jobs, such as airline pilots and nuclear power plant operators, but also for many other workers. Urine testing was strongly recommended by a number of reformers. High school students began being drug tested in the 1990s. These policies were challenged by civil libertarians, who fiercely contended that drug testing was an invasion of privacy, particularly for high school students. However, a challenge to random drug testing of students participating in extracurricular activities was upheld by the U.S. court of appeals in 1998 (*USA Today*, October 6, 1998).

Gateway Drugs and the Merging of Movements

In the late 1980s, the antidrug movement merged with and allied with many aspects of the antitobacco and antialcohol movements. Activists perceived that stemming the use of alcohol, tobacco, and marijuana—the drugs of choice among youth—was integral to preventing other drug use. This was illustrated by press reports of the era. For example, the August 13, 1985 *Chicago Tribune* reported, "Carlton Turner, Ronald Reagan's chief drug policy adviser, links any discussion of drug abuse to marijuana and alcohol," inasmuch as both were thought to lead to heroin and cocaine addiction. The intense focus upon illicit drugs such as cocaine and heroin now began to shift to alcohol and tobacco.

By 1990, an antidrug reform group, the National Commission on Drug-Free Schools, called alcohol and tobacco the most misused drugs in the country and criticized the alcohol and tobacco industries for "targeting youth" by using cartoon characters as part of their advertising.[13] During the mid-1990s, the gateway drug theory became a rallying point for many activists. In 1997, a zero-tolerance policy toward youthful alcohol, tobacco, and marijuana use was unveiled by the federal drug czar. Part of this program included the immediate suspension of driver's licenses for youth who tested positive for any substances. As of the turn of this century, many states are attempting to pass zero-tolerance laws (Peele and Brodsky 1998).

Backlash to the War on Drugs, 1985–2010?

The emergence of a backlash against antidrug laws slowly emerged in the mid-1980s. An era of increased crime began that may have been related to increased drug trafficking and battle for the control of drug territories in urban areas ("Why the Rise in Crime?" 1996). The U.S. Department of Justice's (1997) yearly report showed an increase in violent crime, which peaked in 1992 and then started to decrease. The decline may have been indicative of stable distribution territories for organized-crime syndicates.

After a decade of decline in marijuana use among youth, there was an upturn in use of this drug beginning in early 1992. Since the early 1990s, increasingly favorable attitudes toward marijuana have been found among college and high school youth (Johnston et al. 1998, 94).

Burnham (1993, 14–16) has implied that increasingly positive attitudes toward marijuana have largely been due to a concerted effort on the part of the media and economic interests. He suggested that drug-advocacy forces utilized the same economic and crime arguments as used by the alcohol industry and the media during prohibition.

A backlash among middle-class adults emerged in the late 1990s against marijuana laws in some states. It came in the guise of increased advocacy of marijuana for medical purposes. Sullum and Szasz (1998) suggested that medicalization of marijuana was the "most frequently endorsed alternative to the war on drugs," an idea that gained acceptance among voters in the late 1990s. In 1996, both Arizona and California passed initiatives allowing marijuana use for medical purposes. This trend appears to be continuing in other states.

SUMMARY

The antitobacco, antialcohol, and antidrug movements, as major components of the third Clean Living Movement, became intertwined as they did in the previous reform eras. Use of these substances rose and fell during this period. At the end of the 1990s, a backlash against some aspects of these health crusades began to emerge. However, it is still too early to know the lasting effects of the antisubstances crusades of the late twentieth-century movement.

NOTES

1. Many works have been published concerning the late twentieth-century antismoking movement from a variety of perspectives. See, for example, Brandt (1998), Burnham (1993), McGowan (1995), Tate (1995), and Troyer and Markle (1983). For more popular works, see Kluger (1996), Sullum (1998), and White (1998).

2. Smoking rates are from the National Household Survey, 1993 to 1996 (http://www.health.org/pubs/, last visited October 30, 1998).

3. McGowan suggests that, from 1911 to 1965, the role of government was the breaking of trusts and the regulation of the industry.

4. *Cancer Facts & Figures* (1999) showed that death from lung cancer among males began to decrease in the early 1990s. Among females it was still continuing to rise.

5. There have been a host of publications discussing the late twentieth-century temperance movement from various prospectives. See, in particular, Burnham (1993), Blocker (1989), Musto (1996), Lender and Martin (1987), and Wagner (1997).

6. See Kurtz (1979) for a detailed history of AA, and Jellinek (1961) for the development of the disease concept.

7. Most studies over the last thirty years of the twentieth century found little evidence for a dramatic increase in drinking or alcoholism among women. In reality, a decrease in consumption was found. Beginning in the late 1980s,

some research began to suggest an association of breast cancer with moderate consumption. See Engs (1996b) for an overview of mid-1990s literature that both supports and refutes the association of breast cancer and alcohol consumption. See, in particular, Wilsnack and Wilsnack (1997) for more information with regard to gender differences concerning alcohol consumption.

8. Edward Sands, a former NIDA/NIAAA official, in a private conversation at the August 1986 White House Conference for a Drug Free America, sponsored by those agencies, mentioned that millions of tax dollars worth of pamphlets and publications concerning responsible use of alcohol and other substances had been destroyed because they were "soft on drugs." Only materials describing the dangers of alcohol and other drugs along with a no-use message were now allowed to be distributed.

9. Throughout the 1980s and 1990s, most media reports did not differentiate between alcohol use and abuse. In articles where nonproblematic or even possibly healthy drinking were mentioned, the next paragraph often described alcohol-abuse problems or implied that all alcohol use led to abuse. This was even found in more scientific popular magazines. For example, the *Science News* (Raloff 1996) reported that one researcher "believes the data are now strong enough for physicians to begin recommending *a drink* with dinner for most patients at high risk of heart disease. On that point, Marion Nestle of New York University disagrees heartily. Citing 'the enormous social impacts of alcohol on society'—including drunk driving, violence against women and children, and gun-related accidents—she says that 'under no circumstances should people who aren't drinking be encouraged to do so'" (italics added).

10. Numerous works have addressed the antidrug movement since the early 1970s. A few selected sources offering different perspectives include Bertram et al. (1996), Burnham (1993), Gold (1993), Jonnes (1996), Musto (1987), and Schroeder (1980).

11. Musto (1987, 252) notes that the renewed popularity of drugs came about a lifetime after the previous surge of interest. Because the issue had faded from popular memory, the general population had little accurate firsthand knowledge of the effects of illicit drugs. This led to the exaggerations of their effects and "perceptions so extreme as to be laughable to the new drug users." As previously discussed, lack of accurate information about substances and little popular memory of past health crusades may figure into the resurgence of Clean Living Movements every eighty years or so. In the 1970s, misinformation concerning exaggerated dangerous effects of marijuana that were not experienced by youthful pot users may have led them to experiment with other substances on grounds they felt the establishment was generally lying to them. During this era, the film *Reefer Madness* from the 1930s, which depicts gross inaccuracies about marijuana, became a popular spoof of the ignorance of parents and other authority figures.

12. Details of drug-abuse legislation can be found in numerous NIDA and U.S. government publications.

13. See Burnham (1993) for details concerning advertising and public-relations campaigns by alcohol, tobacco, gambling, and other "bad habit" or "vice" interests to change public attitudes toward drinking, smoking, and so on.

14

Women's Lib, Neo-Purity, and AIDS

The poor homosexuals—they have declared war on Nature and now Nature is exacting an awful retribution.
Patrick Buchanan, *Washington Post* (1987)

There are few issues in the history of women's movements that have aroused such bitter and divisive controversy as abortion. . . . The battle between "prochoice" and "prolife" activists has embraced numerous other social changes and their impact on women's lives: the birth-control pill, the urgent need for more child-care centers, women's expanding presence in the workplace, and the place of motherhood in a woman's life, among others.
Rita J. Simon and Gloria Danziger,
Women's Movements in America (1991)

Once a disease becomes "fashionable," it generates its own establishment and vested interests. Aided by politicians, lobbyists and the media, the money and attention focused on AIDS in the United States since mid-1983 have ensured the development of an AIDS industry.
Dennis Altman, *AIDS in the Mind of America* (1986)

In the late 1960s, a feminist movement began to smolder. Similar to the two previous religious revitalization and reform cycles, this new feminist awakening championed many health and social reforms, including reproductive choices. Simultaneously, a campaign for lesbian and gay rights emerged. However, a backlash from the Christian Right opposed to these attitudes sprang to life in the 1970s. This neo-purity movement, which opposed abortion, sex education in the schools, and promoted "traditional" family values, continued through the 1990s. The most divisive health issue of the era was abortion. Venomous conflicts erupted between groups who supported the legal right of a woman to have a safe and legal abortion and those who considered it murder. Into the fervor of this millennial Clean Living Movement, a deadly new disease, acquired immune deficiency syndrome (AIDS), began to ravage the gay community as well as intravenous drug users, and added fuel to the movement's fire.

THE WOMEN'S LIBERATION MOVEMENT

Jo Freeman (1971, 1), a feminist scholar, suggested that "Sometime in the nineteen twenties, feminism died in the United States."[1] Organized feminism declined after women were finally granted the right to vote and remained dormant until the early 1950s. In the immediate postwar era, "feminism" became a negative epitaph. Women had worked at traditional male jobs during World War II but were often forced back home when their wartime jobs were given to returning men. However, in the postwar years, married women began to reinhabit the workplace, often in part-time or low-wage jobs. In addition, more women obtained university degrees, although the percentage compared to men had declined. These educated women were often underemployed and underpaid (Ryan 1992, 41–42; Freeman 1971, 7). Frustration among these highly educated but underemployed women led to a reawakening of a feminist instinct.

The Rebirth of Feminism, 1965–1975

The Feminine Mystique, published in 1963 by Betty Friedan (b. 1921), a freelance writer and housewife with three children, was the symbolic beginning of the modern women's liberation movement.[2] This book attacked domesticity, defined as the conditioning of women to accept passive roles and depend on male dominance similar to the nineteenth century "cult of true womanhood" (Davis 1991, 50–52).

In 1961, President Kennedy created the Commission on the Status of Women. Two years later it issued a report, *American Women*, which showed discrimination against women in every facet of American life. Of notable mention was wage discrimination; women earned up to 40 percent less than men on the same job. Title VII of the Civil Rights Act of 1964 provided for "affirmative action," which theoretically required equal opportunity in employment, benefits, and pay to women, whatever the nature of their employment. However, this law was only marginally enforced. In 1966, Friedan and other feminists founded the National Organization for Women when they became frustrated with lack of enforcement of this law (Ryan 1992, 43; Davis 1991, 45–47, 50–54; Flexner 1975, 341).[3]

When feminists began to organize at the end of the 1960s, two main factions emerged. These included a "mass movement" sector of older women who wished to reform the system, and several smaller groups of more radical young women who tended toward revolutionary changes. Both these groups contributed to change (Freeman 1971, 2–3; Flexner 1975, ix–x, 344–345; Ryan 1992, 40–45).

Feminism and Health, 1970s–1980s

Sheryl Ruzek (1978, 18–19), a sociologist, suggested that as women began in the 1960s to discuss their problems in "conscious raising" and "rap" sessions, they realized that equal rights in education, politics, and employment were seen as impossible unless women could control their own reproduction. The burden of child rearing sometimes made it difficult to leave repressive marital situations. In addition, during the late 1950s most physicians were male; patients were expected to be deferential and "obey" the authoritarian "orders" of their physicians and not ask questions or details about their health care. Because women were often not fully informed about reproduction and other health issues, the feminist movement spawned a separate women's health movement. This movement "emerged as a result of changes both in women's values and in the objective conditions of health care during the late 1960s and 1970s" (Ruzek 1978, 9). As women became more assertive, they "rejected the stereotypical passive feminine role supporting the traditional authoritarian medical–professional model, particularly in obstetrics and gynecology." This health movement began to alter expectations and definitions of what constituted quality care (Ruzek 1978, 218).

The Women's Health Movement

The publication of *Our Bodies Ourselves* by the Boston Women's Health Book Collective (1973) was the symbolic beginning of the women's health movement. The book was written by a feminist collective concerned with gaining control over all aspects of their lives, including health. In 1975, the National Women's Health Network was founded and became an umbrella for the burgeoning women's health movement. Interest in health issues spread to major universities and courses on women's health were offered, women of color organized their own health groups, and self-help groups and feminist health centers that focused on reproductive health emerged (Davis 1991, 228–235).[4]

This demand for more information and better healthcare included women questioning the safety of various birth-control devices, such as the Dalkon Shield, or powerful hormones, such as birth-control pills and DES (used to prevent miscarriage and as a "morning-after pill"). They questioned the need for total hysterectomies, radical mastectomies, and the use of forceps and drugs to hasten delivery. Home birthing, natural childbirth, more home-like hospital labor and delivery rooms, female midwives, and breast-feeding were advocated. In many cases, male physicians fought against or were bewildered by these demands of women patients. However, over the 1970s and 1980s changes were made in the healthcare system (Davis 1991, 228–242; Ruzek 1978, 33–52; Kaiser and Kaiser 1974, 652–655).

The Abortion Rights and Pro-Choice Movements

The major health issue of the women's rights movement was the right to a safe and legal abortion. Ruzek (1978, 18–19) argued that the abortion campaign became "crucial not only to women's freedom, but, also, to the growth of the women's movement itself." Despite restrictions on abortion during the late 1950s and early 1960s, it was estimated that about 1 million abortions—most of them illegal—were performed each year. *Newsweek*, in an article entitled "Abortion: Mercy or Murder" (1963), reported "American women who want abortions find illegal ones— often at considerable expense and often at considerable danger." Abortions were sought not only by single women but also by married women who had all the children they wanted or could support. By the mid-1960s, a growing number of Americans were calling for liberalization of the restrictive laws (Lee 1969, 5–6; Ruzek 1978, 19–20).

Rise of Grassroots Pro-Choice Organizations. In the late 1960s and early 1970s, several national grassroots organizations arose, including the National Association for Repeal of Abortion Laws and the Abortion Rights Association. These groups later coalesced into the National Abortion Reproductive Action League (NARAL). The purpose of this organization was to "develop and sustain a pro-choice political constituency in order to maintain the right to legal abortion for all women" (Gale Research 1998). This group lobbied, supported pro-choice candidates, and fought against laws attempting to take away the choice for safe, legal abortions throughout the rest of the century.

Legislative Reforms. Legislative reform was first enacted in Colorado in 1967, and by 1970, eleven other states had passed reform laws; Hawaii, Alaska, and New York repealed their restrictive laws.[5] In January 1973, the Supreme Court handed down a landmark decision in *Roe v. Wade*. This decision affirmed the legal right for women anywhere in the United States to legally receive an abortion in the first trimester of pregnancy. This Supreme Court decision precipitated a strong backlash against abortion by the Religious Right that continued throughout the rest of the century.

The Decline of the Women's Rights Movement, 1980s

The dynamic growth of feminist consciousness and organizing occurred between 1966 and the early 1970s. After defeat of the Equal Rights Amendment in 1982, the vibrancy of the women's liberation movement began to fade and change course.

An Equal Rights Amendment was first introduced in the 1920s. Although it was repeatedly submitted, it had been continuously ignored over succeeding decades. In 1970, it was introduced again by a group of activists from the newly reinvigorated women's movement. The amendment was passed by the House in 1970 and by the Senate in 1972 (Flexner 1975, 342). This amendment to the U.S. Constitution would have allowed equality for women in every facet of society. However, after a long struggle, it was defeated in 1982, falling short of the required two-thirds majority by three states (Ryan 1992, 69). The defeat of the ERA was credited to a well-organized antifeminist/new-right coalition that emerged as a backlash against the women's liberation movement. This countermovement included Stop ERA, the Mormon Church, political conservatives, antiabortion groups, and the hierarchy of the Roman Catholic Church, as reported in "What Killed Equal Rights?" (1982) by *Time*. This backlash coalition emerging out of the Christian Right became the core constituency of the third Clean Living Movement.

Effects of the Women's Liberation Movement

The symbolic decline of the women's liberation movement was the failure to ratify the Equal Rights Amendment. However, the movement had achieved success in the years it was most active. This is illustrated by an article found in *People* titled, "E.R.A. Is Dead, but the 10-Year Fight for It Brought Women a Long, Long Way" (1982). Many jobs traditionally held by males, such as airline pilot, astronaut, attorney, military commander, physician, and Supreme Court judge, or even the opportunity to play Little League baseball, were now open to females. Although the percentage of women in managerial, executive, and professional specialties increased, only modest gains had been made in salary (Simon and Danziger 1991, 78–81). In the 1990s, in many areas women still made less then men in equal positions.[6]

Similar to the two previous reform cycles, the women's movement ebbed after only a few of its many goals had been reached.[7] By the 1990s, young women took for granted their freedom to choose any job or career, not wholly realizing that their mother's generation had fought for that right. This is similar to young women in the decades after the Nineteenth Amendment taking for granted the right to vote and not being interested in other equity issues. By the 1990s, most educated women worked outside the home in meaningful jobs, and enrollment at colleges and universities was higher for women than for men. There was still pressure by groups such as NOW to keep the hard-earned rights for choice in reproductive health and to monitor against discrimination. Many of the smaller feminist groups evolved into single-issue organizations that helped women on a local level. Radical lesbian groups also turned many women away from the movement. This feminist movement, however, spurred a backlash from more traditional Americans with clashing agendas.

THE NEO-PURITY MOVEMENT

During the 1970s, the revitalized Religious Right waged a volatile countermovement against women's liberation and everything it seemed to represent. This backlash included antipathy toward feminists, sex education, pornography, unmarried sexual activity, and, in particular, abortion. The Religious Right considered these activities, along with homosexuality, factors in the disintegration of the "traditional family." A campaign against these behaviors constituted a major part of the late twentieth-century Clean Living Movement and was the main concern of the pro-family, or neo-purity movement.[8] Some reformers imbued with religious enthusiasm attempted to eliminate, by any means necessary, behaviors they perceived as being immoral. A few resorted to violence.

Change in Sexual Standards

The neo-purity movement was a reaction against a change in sexual standards that emerged after World War II. An aspect of the feminist movement was the "sexual revolution," where many women of the baby-boom generation strove for independence that also included equality with men in terms of sexual activities. There was an increase in the proportion of women having sexual intercourse outside of marriage. Burnham (1993, 193–194) has suggested that during the 1960s, "an incredible amount of commentary about standards and behavior began to appear in print" that was a factor in changing attitudes, standards, and behaviors of sexuality.

For generations, tensions had persisted between dominant middle-class standards that had emphasized fulfillment within marriage and other standards that did not. Some middle-class youth began to engage in behavior that had previously been associated with other segments of the population, including "impulsive coupling, and various types of nonmarital serial monogamy" (Burnham 1993, 184). The activities also included cohabitation and birthing children without benefit of marriage or a stable male partner. Preventing unwanted births was now easier due to the use of the "pill," which began to be marketed in the early 1960s. On the other hand, not all women, especially younger ones, used contraceptives which was reflected in statistics for increased out-of-wedlock pregnancy and the birth rate of the nation.[9]

The Antifeminism Backlash

The antifeminism backlash was a reaction to these sexual changes that were perceived as immoral by many older and more religious Americans. One of the most powerful reformers of this movement was Phyllis Schlafly. Not only did she spearhead the drive against the passage of ERA, she also crusaded against various aspects of more open sexuality.

Phyllis Schlafly

Phyllis Stewart Schlafly (b. 1924) grew up in a conservative Roman Catholic family and was educated in Catholic schools and at Radcliffe College. She did research for several Congressmen, including Senator Joseph R. McCarthy, and met and married John Schlafly, a lawyer, and devoted the next few years to community activities, her children, and Republican politics.

In 1964, Schlafly published *A Choice Not an Echo*, which became one of the "10 best-selling conservative books of all time." The book is credited with helping launch a political agenda that was adopted by the new religious right. Schlafly organized the defeat of the sweeping Equal Rights Amendment that had been swiftly passed by Congress and then ratified by thirty states within only the first year. She crusaded to defeat the amendment by suggesting that women would be drafted into combat, would be equally responsible in providing family financial support, and that homosexual marriages would be legalized (Morite 1978, 360–363).

Schlafly and her newly organized Eagle Forum also crusaded against sex education in the public schools, pornography, abortion, and homosexuality. The Eagle Forum sponsored antigay bills in many states to prevent public colleges and schools from funding gay and lesbian student groups and to make homosexual conduct a criminal offense (Minkowitz 1992).

Rise of Grassroots Pro-Family Associations, 1970s

Besides the Eagle Forum, several other ultraconservative grassroots associations organized in the 1970s and 1980s to champion purity reform causes. Beverly LaHaye, on the urging of her husband Tim, a conservative minister, founded an antifeminist group, Concerned Women for America (CWA), in 1979. The purpose of the group was to "restore the family to its traditional purpose" through education and lobbying. Other groups were also founded that focused on one or more "sexual morality" issues. Together, they constituted the pro-family movement.

"Just Say No to Everything Concerning Sex"

Reminiscent of the previous purity movement, pro-family crusaders fought against many aspects of sexuality in an effort to bring back "traditional sexuality." There were numerous examples of "just say no to everything" campaigns throughout the 1980s and 1990s, when the purity aspect of the Clean Living Movement was at its height.

Antipornography

Burnham (1993, 198–203) has argued that as sexual standards changed, a commercial pornography industry began to expand. *Playboy*, other "men's" magazines, and various commercial interests began to develop a mass market over the 1960s and 1970s. This market became increasingly involved with aggressive sexuality and other material that began to creep into more public places and the electronic media. A reaction against this increased commercialization helped precipitate an antipornography movement.

Although there had always been local groups against adult bookstores and erotic materials, a national movement against perceived objectional material emerged in the late 1970s. The National Federation for Decency—now called American Family Association (AFA)—was founded in 1977 by Rev. Donald Wildmon (b. 1938). Wildmon, a fundamentalist Methodist minister, led the fight against "violence, immorality, profanity and vulgarity," particularly in the electronic media, over the last two decades of the century (Gale Research 1998).

Anti-Art. Similar to the nineteenth-century purity campaigns, pro-family groups initiated attacks upon works of art. As reported by the *St. Louis Post-Dispatch*, August 3, 1989, Senator Jesse Helms introduced a bill to restrict funding to publicly funded art galleries that showed art that depicted themes of "sadomasochism, homoeroticism, the exploitation of children, or individuals engaged in sex acts" or works which denigrated a religious belief. Purity forces singled out photographers Robert Mapplethorpe and Andres Serrano, whose works were shown at some museums (*Washington Post*, June 7, 1989).

Anti–Electronic Media Pornography. The electronic media also came under attack by purity reformers. In the 1980s and 1990s, various groups attempted to force cable companies to eliminate or block channels that showed "erotica" ("Cable Blues in the Night" 1981; *Los Angeles Times*, February 14, 1993). Through the Communications Decency Act of 1996, an effort was made to ban pornographic material from the new 1990s medium, the Internet. However, the U.S. Supreme Court found this act to be a violation of the First Amendment right to free speech (*Atlanta Journal and Constitution*, July 3, 1997). Reformers pushed some libraries to block pornographic sites on their Internet resources. Libraries that took this action were sued by other parties. As of the turn of the twenty-first century, legal battles concerning this issue are still in process (*Orange County Register*, July 26, 1998).

Opposition to Sex Education

In the mid-1940s, family life education included anatomy and physiology, growth and development, puberty, marriage, and family living. In the late 1960s and 1970s, family life and health-education professionals began to recommend expansion of these topics and introduced more comprehensive curricula. This more broad-based approach, in addition to factual information concerning anatomy and physiology, favored strategies for clarification of values, the concept of responsible behavior, and topics such as masturbation, abortion, sexual excitement, and contraception.[10] However, these new comprehensive school-based health-education programs were quickly attacked by the emerging Christian Right. Anti-sex-education became another aspect of the new-purity movement. In reaction to the new curriculum, a countermovement soon called for the elimination of sex education in the schools. By the early 1980s, groups such as Concerned Women of America called for the elimination of what they considered three threats to family life. These were "global education" (a teaching approach that stresses a world view or global interdependence); sex education in the public schools, including school-based health clinics; and child pornography (*Los Angeles Times*, June 25, 1986).

Abstinence-Based Education. In the late 1980s, when there was fear that the new deadly disease AIDS would become epidemic and teen pregnancies were reaching an all-time high, public schools began to make the case for safe sex, including instruction in the use of condoms. Some conservative advocacy groups, like the Eagle Forum, which once opposed sex education, now rallied behind abstinence curriculums that taught slogans like "pet your dog, not your date." They were against safe-sex programs (*New York Times*, August 5, 1990).

The battle between conservative Christians pushing mandatory "chastity" education and groups advocating comprehensive sexuality education increased during the early and mid-1990s. Purity reformers launched curriculums such as *Sex Respect* and *Teen Aid*. These considered abstinence as the only choice outside of marriage and provided no objective information on methods to avoid sexually transmitted diseases or pregnancy. The federal Office of Adolescent Pregnancy Programs (OAPP) funded pilot testing of these programs. Under the Welfare Reform Act of 1996, federal funding for abstinence programs was allocated. In schools that received grants under this program, no discussion of birth control or disease prevention was allowed. Although all states applied for this funding, most attempted to find ways around the restrictions (*New York Times*, July 23, 1997; *USA Today*, July 14, 1997). Currently, at the turn of this century, the conflict over what should be taught in schools concerning sexuality still continues.

Demonization of Planned Parenthood. Since the 1940s, Planned Parenthood has provided contraceptive services and routine women's heathcare in addition to birth-control information to community and school groups (see Chapter 7 for the birth of the organization in the previous health-reform cycle). Some of the group's affiliates began to provide pregnancy-termination services after the *Roe* decision in 1973. Purity reformers in the late 1980s launched a crusade to prevent federal and community funding from being granted to Planned Parenthood on grounds it provided services to teenagers. The agency began to be presented as a sinister entity (Foege 1996, 201).

In some communities, the Christian Right pressured community-granting agencies, such as the United Way, to eliminate funding to Planned Parenthood on the threat of not donating to the agency. However, this strategy was not always successful. For example, in 1991 Christian Right groups in Bloomington, Indiana, as in many other parts of the United States at that time, attempted to force the United Way to drop Planned Parenthood from the list of agencies it funded. Some more moderate community members angry over this proposal designated all of their United Way donations exclusively to Planned Parenthood rather than the United Way's general fund. This resulted in more money mandated to Planned Parenthood than their scheduled allotment. The United Way did not eliminate Planned Parenthood, but required it to use its grant for purposes other than for abortion (Smith 1995, 67–72). However, funding for Planned Parenthood was eliminated in other communities.

The Pure or Chastity Campaign

In the mid-1990s, a chastity movement emerged, similar to the turn-of-the-century crusade, in which youths signed pledges to remain chaste until marriage. "Youth fests" and church services for purity began to be held in the Midwest. In 1997, the August 1, *Indianapolis Star*, for example, reported a church ceremony at which youths sealed their pledge of premarital chastity with a gold band to be given to their spouse upon marriage. Adolescents in this ceremony promised "to commit their lives to purity, save themselves for holy marriage, and give their bodies to Jesus."

THE PRO-LIFE OR ANTIABORTION MOVEMENT

The most emotionally fraught and venomous conflict of the late twentieth-century Clean Living Movement pitted those who advocated a woman's right to have access to safe and legal abortion against those who considered the voluntary termination of pregnancy murder. During the 1980s, abortion overshadowed all other issues for both feminists and conservatives alike. Davis (1991, 453) argued that "For both sides, it [abortion] stood for women's freedom and independence, especially the sexual freedom that conservatives found so threatening." The religious fervor of antiabortion crusaders recalled the reformist zeal of previous Clean Living Movements.[11]

Moral Suasion: Pressuring, Prayer Meetings, and Picketing, 1970s

The antiabortion movement started off as a moral-suasive campaign among Roman Catholics and conservative Christians to convince women to reject abortions and to persuade legislators not to further liberalize abortion laws. During the 1970s, these pro-life reformers began to alter attitudes about pregnancy and pregnant women. The feminist historian Flora Davis (1991, 243), suggested that "anti-abortion groups succeeded in personifying the fetus for many Americans, who had never before thought of it as an unborn baby." The term "baby" was applied to even the earliest stages of cellular development. Right-to-life forces in the late 1970s began referring to women undergoing abortions and physicians performing them as "murderers" who were "killing babies." Educational programs that included graphic films of abortion procedures, such as the *Silent Scream*, were shown to shock the public into rejecting abortion as part of the moral-suasion campaign (*Silent Scream* 1985).

The Rise of the NRLC and Other Grassroots Organizations

A crusade against abortion formed in the late 1960s when a few states began to repeal or reform their abortion laws. Grassroots groups calling themselves right-to-life or pro-life organizations formed under the authority and support of the Roman Catholic Church and other conservative religious groups. The National Right to Life Committee

(NRLC), one of the largest pro-life associations, was founded in 1973 by the Catholic Church as an umbrella organization for state and local groups. Its stated goal was the "protection of human life from abortion, euthanasia, and infanticide." It stressed lobbying and education and opposed violence. The NRLC and other national organizations formed a pro-life coalition that quickly began to gain power on the legislative front (Blanchard 1994, 62; "New York: Backlash on Abortion" 1972; Lowenthal 1978).

Coercion: Restrictive Legislation, Violence, and Murder, 1975–1990s

Both strident legislative efforts and violence earmarked the militant aspect of the third Clean Living Movement's antiabortion reform campaign. Reminiscent of earlier reformers, many pro-life crusaders believed that any position besides their own was not only wrong but also evil. These beliefs led to the demonization of abortion clinics, their workers, and pregnant women who wanted abortions. This hostility took the form of escalated violence precipitated by ultraradical elements of the movement.

Legislative and Court Decisions

After the *Roe* decision, pro-life forces pushed for legislation to eliminate abortions. These battles continued at both state and federal levels to the end of the century. By the end of 1978, thirteen states had passed resolutions calling for a constitutional convention to draft an amendment that would ban abortion and many contraceptives (Lowenthal 1978, 36; Davis 1991, 457–458; Segers and Byrnes 1995, 6–8). In the late 1970s, Congress eliminated federal funding for most abortions.

During the 1980s, state laws were passed that made it more difficult to obtain an abortion. This included permission of a husband or parental consent for a minor. By 1991, seventeen states had parental notification or consent laws in effect. However, in the late 1980s, some states began to reverse, or allow judicial bypass, after media reports of a teenager committing suicide, rather than informing her parents, and of another being shot by her father, who had impregnated her (Davis 1991, 458–460).[12]

In 1989, the *Webster v. Reproductive Health* decision marked a major turning point in the abortion conflict. This Supreme Court decision upheld a Missouri statute that banned abortion or even abortion counseling at any facility receiving public funding. Since most hospitals and clinics received some type of federal funding, this law would have eliminated almost all abortions. The *Webster* decision gave states new latitude to restrict abortion and many began to challenge the 1973 *Roe* decision. In the first year after *Webster*, more than forty states considered antiabortion laws (Segers and Byrnes 1995, 5–9; *New York Times*, June 27, 1990, October 25, 1989; "Pro-Choice Politicking" 1989).

"Partial-birth" or late-term abortions that were performed in only a very small percentage of pregnancy terminations was the next crusade of antiabortion forces. In the late 1990s, pro-life groups persuaded a number of states to pass bans on late-term abortions. However, the November 25, 1998 *USA Today* reported these laws were struck down in seven states, as the statutes were so vaguely written that "they effectively banned all abortions."[13]

Violence and War against Clinics and Clinic Workers

When Christian Rightists failed to pass a constitutional amendment against abortion, Davis (1991, 458) contends they attempted to restrict abortions in "any way they could." Lowenthal (1978) in *Newsweek* reported that antiabortion activists "backed by the authority and money of the Roman Catholic Church, [began] engaging in civil disobedience reminiscent of the antiwar movement and taking their case to legislators and courts." A more violent aspect of the pro-life movement evolved.

Joseph M. Scheidler (b. 1927), head of the Pro-Life Action League, in 1985 published *Closed: 99 Ways to Stop Abortion*. This handbook was a collection of methods that could be used to "successfully stop abortions." Randall Terry (b. 1959), influenced by this work, launched Operation Rescue with a week of clinic blockades in New York City during the spring of 1988. Terry carried this activity across the nation, reaching a peak in 1991. During this "summer of mercy," more than 2,600 protestors were arrested in Wichita, Kansas in six weeks.

When Operation Rescue became linked with several violent acts, including the shooting deaths of clinic workers, it lost support. By 1995, only a few dozen people attended Operation Rescue demonstrations. In the late 1990s, it began to expand into other areas of the purity movement.[14] In 1993, violence against abortion clinics escalated and, by 1999, seven clinic workers had been killed.

A Backlash against Abortion Restrictions

As pro-life groups instituted more challenges against abortion, pro-choice advocates rose up against these potential restrictions. In the 1980s and 1990s, there was a tug-of-war between passage and then repeal of various legislative efforts and Supreme Court decisions on both sides of the abortion issue.

NARAL and Other Grassroots Efforts to Keep Abortion Legal

The National Abortion and Reproductive Action League was founded in 1969 "to develop and sustain a pro-choice political constituency in order to maintain the right to legal abortion for all women" (Gale Research 1998). This organization attempted to keep abortion legal throughout the last decades of the century. In April 1989, when there was concern that *Roe* might be overturned, NARAL, NOW, and other feminist groups organized a "March on Washington" for abortion rights that drew more than 200,000 individuals from around the country. The potentially repressive *Webster* had paradoxically rejuvenated the women's and abortion-rights movements (Davis 1991, 466; "Pro-Choice: A Sleeping Giant Awakens" 1989; "The Family vs. the State" 1990).

Lawsuits against Violent Antiabortion Groups

In 1986, women's rights groups began to file lawsuits under the Racketeer Influence and Corrupt Organization Act (RICO) against Operation Rescue for intimidation, stalking, and damage to clinics. This act allowed huge fines, forfeiture of property, and prison terms (*New York Times*, June 11, 1986; Kelly 1995, 207). In 1998, a federal jury found the Pro-Life Action League and Operation Rescue liable for clinic damages under RICO, which opened the door for numerous class-action suits by clinics across the country (*USA Today*, April 21, 1998).

In 1990, the Supreme Court let stand a previous federal court order banning antiabortion protesters from blocking access to clinics and imposing heavy fines on anyone breaking the law ("Right to Lifers: New Tactics" 1990). In 1997, it ruled that protestors could confront patients on public sidewalks as long as they stayed at least fifteen feet away from clinic entrances and required "sidewalk counselors" to retreat if a patient indicated a desire not to be counseled (*Los Angeles Times*, May 21, 1990; *USA Today*, February 20, 1997).

Some New Drugs

In 1988, France began to market a new drug, RU-486, that would cause a pregnancy termination in the first three months of pregnancy when combined with a prostaglandin. Antiabortion groups threatened to boycott any pharmaceutical company marketing the drug. The FDA allowed the Population Council, a nonprofit biomedical research organization, to investigate the drug and clinical trials began in 1996. Simultaneously, two common drugs, methotrexate, used for the treatment of cancer, and misoprostol, an antiulcer medication, taken together were found to be an effective aborticide ("Battle over the Abortion Pill" 1988; "Abortion by Prescription" 1989; "Abortion in the Form of a Pill" 1995).

The Partial-Birth Abortion Rulings

Pro-life reformers attempted to push for laws against late-term or partial-birth abortions as a method of eventually eliminating all abortions. In the late 1990s, Congress passed a ban on these late-term abortions which was vetoed by President Clinton; the Senate failed to override the veto (Christian communities 1998). The conflict between reformers who crusaded for the elimination of abortions and those who supported the right for choice continued to the end of the twentieth century.

GAY RIGHTS, AIDS, AND A BACKLASH

Paralleling the 1960s civil rights and feminist surge, a "homophile" movement emerged to gain civil rights for homosexual women and men. As it gained ground, a deadly new disease took its greatest toll within the gay community. Fear of the disease led to increased hostility toward homosexuals on the part of the Religious Right. Antihomosexuality became a central theme of the neo-purity movement.

The Gay Rights Movement

Up to the late nineteenth century, homosexual acts were considered sinful and immoral like adultery or blasphemy; individuals who committed them were severely punished. However, after that time, attitudes changed regarding these behaviors. John D'Emilio (1983, 4), a historian, argued, "The [homosexual] label applied not merely to a particular sexual acts, as 'sodomite' once had, but to an entire person whose nature . . . was sharply distinguishable from the majority of 'normal' heterosexuals." This change in perception led to homosexuals being perceived as immoral and becoming second-class citizens if their status was known. For generations, they were fired from jobs, robbed, and beaten. Because of social taboos against their lifestyle, they often had little legal recourse against perpetrators of these acts and often did not report them. Gay bars, one of the few places they could openly congregate, were routinely raided by police and patrons were hauled off to jail. However, in the 1960s gay men and women began to perceive themselves "as members of an oppressed minority, sharing an identity that subjected them to systematic injustice" (D'Emilio 1983, 4). This led to the emergence of a gay liberation movement in the late 1960s.[15]

Ridinger (1996, xii–xiii) contendes this movement underwent three phases through the 1950s into the mid-1990s. The first phase began after World War II and included the foundation of the Mattachine Society and Daughters of Bilitis, associations for gays and lesbians, that laid the foundation for what came to be known as the homophile movement. The second, or activist phase, began with the Stonewall riots. In 1969, police raided the Stonewall Inn in New York City and met violent resistance from gay patrons of the bar. The weekend riot became the symbolic beginning of the gay liberation movement (D'Emilio 1983, 231–233). Various organizations subsequently formed, including the National Gay and Lesbian Task Force, to foster civil rights for gays as a minority group (Ridinger 1996, xiii). Ordinances and laws against gays began to be challenged and the repeal of various restrictions in housing, employment, and other activities were enacted in many states and communities. The third phase of the movement began in 1981 with the appearance of AIDS. When the federal government was perceived as being too slow to act against the deadly epidemic, anger and frustration surged out of the gay community. It expressed itself in the reemergence of combative activism through the street-theater militancy of groups such as ACT UP and Queer Nation that picketed and staged sit-ins (Ridinger 1996, xiii; "This Is Not a Scarecrow" 1998). A fourth phase in the movement began to emerge in the mid-1990s. Many Americans became more accepting of homosexuals. This is symbolized by the appearance of successful television sitcoms in which the main characters were lesbian or gay. After many years of pressure on the part of the gay movement, the American Medical Association in 1995 removed references to sexual orientation or homosexuality as a disease. The Human Right Commission (HRC), a middle-class gay lobbying organization founded in 1980, backed candidates who supported gay civil rights. Gays now became an "expected presence in politics" ("The New Gay Struggle" 1998).

The "Gay Plague"

In 1981, the July 3, *New York Times* headlined "Rare Cancer Seen in 41 Homosexuals." This was the first report of what became the AIDS epidemic. A rare pneumonia also began to be seen in gay men; researchers linked the two conditions to a common but unknown cause. By the end of 1983, the disease was also reported among intravenous drug users, heterosexual Haitian refugees, blood-transfusion patients, prostitutes, female sexual partners of infected men, and babies of infected mothers ("AIDS" 1985, 28–30; "Epidemiologic Notes and Reports" 1983, 1987; "Unexplained Immunodeficiency and Opportunistic Infections" 1982).[16]

In 1984, researchers from the Pasteur Institute in France and the National Cancer Institute in the United States simultaneously isolated the cause of AIDS, a variety of the t-cell leukemia virus which was later named the Human Immunodeficiency Virus. The disease became known as the HIV/AIDS complex or syndrome. Not everyone who became infected with the virus developed full-blown AIDS. However, about 50 percent of those diagnosed with AIDS died within a few years of developing the disease ("AIDS" 1985, 28–30). In 1985, an article, "The Great AIDS Race," in *Science News* announced that the first blood test for HIV infections had been approved by the FDA, which meant blood donors could be screened and infected individuals identified.

Preventing the Disease: Safe Sex, Needle Exchanges, and Condom Use

The distribution of latex condoms, teaching safe sex in schools, instructing drug addicts to use bleach to sterilize needles, and needle-exchange programs to prevent transmission of the disease were advocated by public-health educators. The first widely disseminated AIDS-education curriculum guide was published in 1987 (Yarber 1987). Various conservative religious groups, however, fought against all AIDS-prevention measures except abstinence, because they believed that the more comprehensive programs promoted "immoral behaviors" ("AIDS Becomes a Right-Wing Issue" 1987, 27; *San Francisco Chronicle*, November 10, 1989).

Although studies suggested that needle-exchange programs were effective in reducing the spread of AIDS, national funding for such programs was rejected by Congress in 1989 and again in 1998. Conservatives feared such a program would encourage drug use (*USA Today*, April 30, 1998).[17]

Arresting the Disease: New Drugs

Various drugs began to be developed during the late 1980s to attack HIV infections, including AZT. However, this drug proved to be toxic to many users and its effects often wore off (Grmek 1990, 185–186). In the mid-1990s, a new class of drugs called protease inhibitors became widely used in the United States. Beginning in 1995, deaths from AIDS decreased due to increased use of these medications among middle-class individuals with insurance. The CDC reported a 46-percent decline in deaths between 1996 and 1997, but HIV increased in poor and minority communities (Leland and Gordon 1996; Gideonese 1998).

The New Nativism and a Backlash against Gays

At the beginning of the AIDS epidemic, injecting drug users and Haitians were also stricken with AIDS. The disease was soon seen by the Religious Right as a moral, not a medical problem. Gays, drug users, and immigrants became scapegoated and a backlash against gay rights emerged.

Similar to moral reformers of the previous Clean Living Movement, who considered cholera and syphilis the result of immorality, the New Christian Right (NCR) condemned the "non-innocent" victims of AIDS and blamed their moral failure for the disease. Historian Erling Jorstad (1987, 202) remarked that "AIDS was considered by the NCR as God's punishment against homosexuals for their sinful and unrepentant behavior." It was proported to be "a sign from God that homosexuality is an 'abomination'" ("AIDS Becomes a Right-Wing Political Issue" 1987). This deep hostility toward gays with AIDS was reported by the popular press ("The Devil Did It" 1988). When a speaker at an ultra-conservative political-action conference mentioned that one-quarter to one-half of the gay population could be dead within five years, "a large chunk of the audience of 200 or so cheered and clapped." HIV/AIDS became a metaphor for evil and resulted in a cry from more militant reformers for more coercive public policies. In spite of this call for more coercive measures, the Supreme Court in 1987 "granted victims of communicable diseases the same rights in the work force as the handicapped . . . and the Centers for Disease Control advised against mandatory AIDS testing" ("AIDS Becomes a Right-Wing Political Issue" 1987).

HIV was also found in certain heterosexual immigrant populations. Early statistics showed that a disproportionate number of Haitian immigrants were affected with AIDS; they were thought to be "a bridge between Africa and the United States" for importation of the disease. Haitians visited Africa as workers, contracted HIV, had sex with American tourists, or immigrated into the United States, thus spreading the disease. However, since their strain of HIV resembled that of Americans and not of Africans, it was more likely that HIV was introduced to Haiti by gay tourists from the United States (Grmek 1990, 154). Conservatives campaigned to exclude Haitians and other immigrants from the United States if they tested positive for HIV. This attitude was reminiscent of Nativism in previous eras.

Blame, Hysteria, and the Cry for Tolerance

As deaths from the AIDS epidemic mounted, the homosexual community blamed the Reagan administration for not acting sooner to find a cause, prevention, and cure for AIDS. Dennis Altman (1986, 175), a gay-rights author, contended that "the White House has collaborated in fostering the idea that AIDS should be seen as a gay issue rather than a health emergency which should transcend the characteristics of those involved." The militant right, on the other hand, blamed the homosexual community for spreading the plague because they continued to "insist that they be allowed to continue their sexual practices undisturbed by public health officials . . . rather than submit themselves to the restrictions and procedures historically employed in treating sexually transmitted diseases" (Dannemeyer 1989, 188).

As a result of the media blitz concerning HIV/AIDS, many Americans became terrified they would acquire the disease through mere casual contact, such as handshakes from infected persons. However, numerous studies confirmed that only bodily fluids such as blood, semen, and vaginal secretions could transmit the virus ("The Devil Did It" 1988; Rushing 1995, 194–195). Because of AIDS hysteria, individuals with the infection began to be discriminated against for jobs, housing, medical insurance, and education. A symbol of the fight against this discrimination came from Ryan White, a hemophiliac Indiana boy, who had contracted the disease through a blood product. School officials prevented him from attending classes after being pressured by parents. White fought for the right to attend school and brought the fight for acceptance of those with HIV/AIDS to national attention. He died at age eighteen in 1990 (*Chicago Tribune*, April 27, 1986; *San Francisco Chronicle*, April 11, 1990).

During the 1990s, the hysteria waned. William Rushing (1995, xii), a sociologist, noted that "concerns about AIDS had begun to decline. The viral cause of AIDS is now known, the major types of high-risk behaviors have been identified, the rate of increase of new AIDS cases is slowing (at least in the United States), the ostracism of people with AIDS has become milder in tone, and the demonstrations and accusations by AIDS activists have been muted."

The Antigay Backlash

A backlash against gays as a result of the spread of AIDS spurred a revitalization of the Religious Right's antigay activism. Reformers began to wage legal battles against gays and attempted to convince the general public that homosexuals were immoral (Jorstad 1987, 201–202). Over the 1980s and 1990s, there was a legal tug-of-war between conservative reformers and gay-rights activists. Gays fought for the elimination of discrimination in housing, employment, and other arenas, while purity reformers attempted to prevent passage of laws giving them these rights (Adam 1995, 109–127; Button et al. 1997, 71–76, 175–184, 190–193).[18]

By the mid- to late 1990s, the Christian Coalition, along with anti-abortion and pro-family groups, became more vocal against gays. Hostility toward the Disney Company, long considered a family-film maker, emerged. A coalition of reform groups began to admonish, picket, or boycott Disney World and its products because of "Disney's rejection of family values and gay-friendly policies, such as insurance benefits for gay partners of employees." This pressure resulted in some states divesting themselves of Disney stock (*Orlando Sentinel*, August 31, 1997; *Dallas Morning News*, July 19, 1998).

There was a militant and violent aspect to the backlash. Minkowitz (1992) reported on the increase of "homophobic" incidences in the early 1990s, including "Operation Rescue-style tactics to blockade a gay and lesbian film festival" and an increase in violence against gays after campaigns to repeal antidiscrimination laws. In late 1998, a gay Wyoming student was beaten and killed. Focus on the Family, the Family Research Council, and the Christian Coalition began a national advertising campaign just before the killing, urging gays to convert to heterosexuality through religion. Some professionals blamed this killing on the conservative Christian's new antigay focus.[19] After the murder, in an article titled "To Be Young and Gay in Wyoming" (1998), *Time* reported the event a "lynching . . . to make a point." This murder sent a wave of public condemnation. It is too early to judge the effect of this death as a symbolic turning point in the antigay backlash on the part of purity reformers of the late twentieth-century Clean Living Movement.

SUMMARY

The rise of the women's rights movement in the late twentieth century, as it had in the earlier two awakenings, helped foster health reforms and gave more freedoms to women. Although the fervor of the movement declined, the National Organization for Women at the end of the century continued to defend women's rights. In contrast, a neopurity movement emerged out of the revivalism of the Religious Right. It crusaded against pornography, sex education, abortion, the homosexual lifestyle, and other sexuality issues. A gay rights movement began to emerge and was met with a backlash from the Religious Right, which intensified after the explosion of a new deadly disease, AIDS, initially discovered among gays. As the twentieth century closed, continued efforts to eliminate legal abortions and the new mood in favor of sexual abstinence before marriage continued.

NOTES

1. James Wilson (1980, 30), a political scientist, noted that women's movements, including the current one, have "acquired special visibility and influence in periods of social awakening. . . . Not since the volcanic struggles over prohibition and the suffrage sixty years ago have 'women's issues' so dominated the attention of political activists."

2. The late twentieth-century feminist movement encompassed both old and newly established reform associations, radical groups, and single-issue organizations devoted to a particular cause such as abortion rights. The term "women's liberation" serves as an umbrella term for the feminist revival of the

era. Over the last three decades of the twentieth century, a multitude of works concerning the feminist movement were published. A few selected references that touch on health aspects of the movement include Davis (1991), Ryan (1992), and Schneir (1994). The *Feminist Chronicles* by Carabillo et al. (1993) gives an encapsulation of the movement and the backlash to it.

3. In civil-rights groups, women were often relegated to clerical duties and other traditional "female activities" and not allowed leadership positions. This awoke women to their status as second-class citizens. As discussed in previous chapters, this also occurred during the pre–Civil War era, when women tried to become active in antislavery societies, as well as during the progressive era when they attempted to take leadership roles in the temperance movement. In all three reform cycles women broke off from the male-dominant groups and formed their own organizations.

4. During the peak of the self-help and women's clinics in 1976, Flora Davis (1991, 234–235), feminist historian, estimated they were about fifty feminist health centers in the United States.

5. States passing reform laws included Arkansas, California, Delaware, Georgia, Kansas, Maryland, New Mexico, North Carolina, Oregon, South Carolina, and Virginia (Hole and Levine 1971, 284–285). These laws followed the guidelines of the America Law Institute recommendations in 1959, which were endorsed in 1967 by the American Medical Association. These guidelines recommended that abortion should be available (1) when continuation of pregnancy would threaten either the life or health of the mother; (2) when the child might be born with a grave physical or mental defect; or (3) when pregnancy resulted from rape, incest, or other felonious intercourse, and threatened the mental or physical health of the mother (Lader 1967, 145–146; "Easing Abortion Rules" 1967).

6. *Time* magazine, in a feature entitled "Who's Come a Long Way Baby?" (1970), reported that in 1968 the "median wage for full-time women workers is 58.2% of that for men." Crampton and Hodge (1977) comment, "Three decades have passed but women's wages remain less than wages for men in equal positions." Women were now earning about 75 percent of what males earned.

7. *Time* ("Who's Come a Long Way Baby?" 1970) discussed the fifty-year anniversary of the Nineteenth Amendment, which gave women the right to vote. Many feminists marched in protest against this anniversary, as it had only won suffrage and not equality for women. The article reported that at the first women's rights convention at Seneca Falls in 1848, women "demanded the right to vote, to equal educational and vocational opportunities and to an ending of legal discrimination against women. Except for suffrage those demands have yet to be met."

8. Donald Meyer (1988, 358–359), a religious historian, suggested that "As evangelical preoccupation with abortion and homosexuality grew, it easily linked feminism to its targets." The antifeminist and antisexuality movements blended to form, by the late 1970s, a pro-family movement, or, as termed in this book, the neo-purity movement. One factor in this link was that feminism had increasingly became associated with lesbian radicalism.

9. "From 1950 to 1987, the proportion of out-of-wedlock births in the United States increased sixfold, from 4% to 24% of all births, respectively" ("Infant

Mortality by Marital Status of Mother" 1990). The Center for Disease Control (Ventura et al. 1999) reported that, between 1980 and 1990, teenage pregnancy rates remained relatively stable. In the late 1990s, they began to decrease.

10. These new curricula included *Family Life and Sex Education Curriculum and Instruction* (Schultz and Williams 1969) and *Sexuality and Human Values* (Calderone 1977). This comprehensive curriculum approach also began to appear in materials for teacher education, such as texts by Engs and Wantz (1978) and McCary (1973), during this era.

11. A number of works have been published over the last quarter century concerning both sides of the abortion issue. A few selected scholarly publications include Jacoby (1998), Craig and O'Brien (1993), and Segers and Byrnes (1995). Examples of popular works from opposing viewpoints include Sloan and Hartz (1992) and Glessner (1990). See, in particular, Blanchard (1994), who traces the antiabortion movement through the early 1990s.

12. These events were reported in various magazines. See, in particular, two articles: "The Right to Lifers New Tactics" (1990) and "Teenagers and Abortion" (1967), twenty years apart.

13. These states included Arkansas, Alaska, Arizona, Florida, Illinois, Michigan, and Montana.

14. Information concerning the rise and fall of Operation Rescue as a militant antiabortion group can be found in the *New York Times*, May 8, 1988; *New York Times*, February 28, 1990; "The Right to Lifers New Tactics" (1990); *Los Angeles Times*, March 2, 1989; *Orange County Register*, June 7, 1998; "Showdown in Atlanta," *Christianity Today*, September 16, 1988, 44–46.

15. Several works have been published in recent years concerning the gay rights movement. See, in particular, Adam (1995), Button et al. (1997), and Rutledge (1992). See Ridinger (1996) for a comprehensive list of references.

16. Hundreds of works were written in the last fifteen years of the twentieth century concerning the social, political, religious, medical, educational, and other aspects of AIDS for both popular and scholarly consumption. For a representative sample, see Altman (1986), Doka (1997), Grmek (1990), Fumento (1990), Shilts (1987), and Yarber (1987).

17. There were 110 needle-exchange programs in twenty-two states in 1998, as reported by the April 30, 1998 *USA Today*.

18. An antihomosexual and antigay-rights book, *Shadow in the Land: Homosexuality in America*, was written by Senator Dannemeyer in 1989. Dannemeyer argued that the homosexual lifestyle is dangerous to American society and its values and leads to the demise of traditional American values. Bull and Gallagher (1996, xi) chronicled "the emergence of gay rights as *the* social issue—and perhaps the most divisive political issue—of the 1990s" and discussed the "great battle" between the religious conservatives "who believe they are taking a last stand against moral decline . . . [and] gays and lesbians who believe they are fighting for the basic civil liberties guaranteed by the Constitution."

19. The *Associated Press*, December 11, 1998, quoted Nada Stotland, an American Psychiatric Association leader, who suggested that "spreading the idea that homosexuality is a disease or evil could make people 'feel less inhibited about beating up gays, or not giving them jobs.'"

15

Fitness, Health, and the New Eugenics

> That regular physical exercise promotes the general health is generally acknowledged.
>
> Kenneth H. Cooper, *Aerobics* (1968)

> I'm interested in food because what we're eating contributes to hundreds of thousands of deaths every year, about as many deaths as cigarette smoking.
>
> Michael Jacobson, *Progressive* (1994)

> Sex selection and, soon, cloning and genetic engineering will alter the very idea of parenthood. What happens to the intrinsic value of human life when choosing a baby becomes the ultimate "shopping experience"?
>
> Jeremy Rifkin, *USA Today* (1998)

In the late 1960s and early 1970s, a fitness, health, and dietary reform movement took shape that in many ways was similar to the fitness and health concerns of the previous two Clean Living Movements. By the mid-1980s, studies began to show that many middle- and upper-middle-class Americans had embraced a "healthier lifestyle." There was a noticeable decrease in consumption of high-fat diets and use of tobacco, and in the prevalence of heart disease and at the same time an increase in exercise among this population. Less-educated and poorer Americans were nevertheless found to have become less fit and more fat. In the late 1990s, some health professionals began to reason that since moral-suasion and coercive policies were often ineffective in changing "harmful health habits," the fault must lie in the genes.

This attitude was reminiscent of reformers in the previous reform movements. In the 1980s, methods were developed to allow previously infertile couples to conceive children, often with characteristics of their choosing. The search for "perfect" babies and a shift away from environmental to genetic causes of illness and behaviors evolved into a new eugenics movement.

THE FITNESS, HEALTH, AND DIET MOVEMENT

The crusade for fitness included exercise, health concerns, and diet interlinked over the course of the third Clean Living Movement. This health and fitness movement also became entwined with the antitobacco and antialcohol movements and took on the overtones of a religious ideology. The overall campaign for fitness and health took on many names, including the "healthy lifestyle," "wellness," and "health promotion" movement. With the development of antibiotics and other drugs and modern surgery in the post–World War II years, the chronic conditions of heart disease and cancer loomed as the most prevalent killers. Heightened interest slowly emerged in preventing these diseases, which were associated with a lack of exercise, poor diet, and other personal health habits.[1]

Birth of the Fitness and Wellness Movement, 1965–1975

In the 1930s, most Americas showed little interest in exercise. However, the federal government actively promoted sports through various depression-era work and social programs. When it was found that many American youth were unfit for military service in World War II, the armed forces sponsored sports activities. Mounting concern over a general lack of fitness resulted in President Dwight D. Eisenhower creating the Presidential Council on Physical Fitness in 1955. Concerned about flabby youth, he created the President's Council on Youth Fitness two years later. However, exercise and sports, for the most part, was something the average American considered important only for younger individuals or athletes. In 1979, adult physical fitness became of concern (Reiser 1985, 7–17; President's Council 1979).

In 1962, when it was found that one-quarter of American children "could not pass a simple physical test of pull-ups, sit-ups, and squat-thrusts," President John F. Kennedy and the Council on Physical Fitness campaigned to "focus attention on the physical education programs of public schools." Because many adults were also seen as unfit, "special 'exercises' for people who work at desks" were also championed. However, it was not until 1968, after Kenneth Cooper published *Aerobics*, that a new fitness movement took hold. Cooper's book represented the symbolic beginning of the late twentieth-century exercise and fitness movement.

Kenneth H. Cooper

Kenneth Cooper (b. 1931), a physician born in Ottawa, Ontario, was the son of a health professional who encouraged prevention. Early in his medical career, while exercising, he experienced a heart irregularity. Fear of lethal complications motivated him to volunteer as a subject in exercise physiology research. With a vigorous exercise regime, he found that his symptoms disappeared. Cooper began designing and testing an aerobics program for astronauts and U.S. Air Force pilots as a military physician.[2]

Cooper promoted this exercise system for overall fitness and well-being, and upon leaving the military in 1970, he founded the Aerobics Center in Dallas, Texas. In his early years, however, like many other health reformers in all three Clean Living Movements, he was considered a quack by orthodox physicians (*Washington Post*, February 24, 1983).

The Growth of the Fitness and Wellness Movement, 1970–1990

During the late 1960s, despite the lack of clear data as to the effects of exercise on health, running, jogging, aerobics, and other exercise began to increased in popularity. The quest for fitness over the 1970s and into the 1980s surged into a massive movement.

The Exercise and Fitness Craze, 1970s

In 1966, a magazine, *Runners World*, was founded. Symbolic of the explosion of the running and exercise movement, its circulation increased from roughly 28 thousand to over 300 thousand between 1978 and 1980, peaking in the late 1980s (*Ulrich's International Periodicals Directory* 1998). By the late 1970s, fitness was considered a "craze" or a "mania" by the news media. Exercise books took on religious overtones, with titles such as *Holistic Running* (Henning 1978) and *Zen Running* (Rohe 1974). Exercise was offered as a cure-all for practically everything and a path for self-improvement.

Accompanying the exercise craze was a boom in exercise clothing, shoes, health clubs, and equipment from the late 1970s into the 1990s. New exercise gadgets, in turn, became a fad as soon as they were introduced.[3] To meet the needs of millions of exercisers, numerous fitness clubs were established. The YMCA's activity statistics reflect this craze. Between 1970 and 1988, membership and participation in activities doubled from about 6 to 12 million (YMCA 1998). A popular movie star, Jane Fonda (b. 1937), brought out an aerobics video in 1982 which was purchased by millions and increased the popularity of aerobics routines. That same year, the Aerobics and Fitness Association of America was founded for fitness instructors, consultants, and trainers. The organization also started a magazine, *American Fitness*. Richard Simmons (b. 1948), a self-described former "fatty," launched a popular television diet and exercise show. By 1983, exercise was fully entrenched in the society, and Cooper's (1968) book, *Aerobics*, was "considered the bible of the fitness movement" as noted by the *Washington Post*, February 24, 1983. James Fixx (1932–1984), a runner, proselytized "running as a natural tranquilizer, an enhancer of sexual pleasure" in rhetoric similar to a religious conversion experience. *Runners World* became the "runner's cult magazine" (Fixx 1977, 239).

The Beginning of Balance, 1980s

By the early 1980s, Cooper developed a "wellness" approach to fitness that focused on disease prevention and health maintenance rather than disease management. He also began to advocate moderate, not strenuous exercise. Cooper's (1982) updated book recommended a balance between proper diet and exercise, as well as other lifestyle changes, such as the elimination of smoking, addictive drugs, and excessive alcohol, along with stress reduction and a regular physical examination. This integrative approach began to include other dimensions of health, including spiritual, mental, and social dimensions recommended by health-education specialists. This concept of balance and spirituality was likely influenced by the New Age eastern philosophy as discussed in Chapter 13. In the late 1980s, studies showed that more moderate exercise was as effective as vigorous exercise in reducing heart disease, cancer, and other chronic conditions. *Newsweek*, in an article titled "Learning to Harness the Power" (1989), noted that the "no pain, no gain" approach of the movement's earlier years began to be supplanted by encouragement of moderate exercise, such as "brisk leaf-raking, vigorous vacuuming," and walking.

Health Promotion and Wellness

Following World War II, a flurry of hospital and clinic construction came about as a result of the Hill–Burton Act. Personnel to staff these facilities were provided by the Health Manpower Act, which funded programs and the training of healthcare professionals. The philosophical orientation then was biomedical, rather than health education— cures rather than prevention. Beginning in the 1960s, initiatives were launched to generate greater equity in the distribution and the use of health resources between the rich and poor. Medicare and Medicaid allowed hospitals and physicians to service the aged and the poor. Although the gap between the rich and the poor was significantly reduced in terms of access to regular medical services, morbidity and mortality indicators continued to reflect strong social–economic disparities. This resulted in concern about cost containment and prevention. Over the 1980s and 1990s, dramatic change resulted in healthcare systems. Health maintenance organizations, an increase in outpatient procedures, and changes in insurance attempted to keep the cost of healthcare down. This led to a "health promotion" movement in the healthcare community that was more oriented toward prevention.[4]

In 1990, the federal government published *Healthy People 2000: National Health Promotion and Disease Prevention Objectives* (1990). This publication discussed health problems in the country, established goals for the reduction of specific problems, and proposed interventions to decrease the incidence of the problems. Over the 1990s, increased emphasis was placed on enhancing health and reducing "bad habits" (discussed in Chapter 13) to meet the "healthy 2000" goals to be acheived through education and legislative means.

Personal Responsibility for Health

In 1961, Halbert Dunn had published *High-Level Wellness*. This series of lectures discussed a balance between physical, mental, social, and spiritual aspects of health. His emphasis on prevention rather than treatment and maximizing potential health was adopted by the fitness and health movement and became an underlying concept of health promotion. During the growth of the fitness and wellness movement, personal responsibility for disease prevention began to be stressed. This philosophy became infused into campaigns against tobacco, drunk driving, and sexually transmitted and chronic diseases. It was up to the individual to prevent health problems by stopping smoking, changing dietary patterns, and exercising.

Reflecting middle-class concern with health and fitness, some publications launched health and fitness sections. For example, in 1984, *Newsweek* began a "Special Advertising Section: Health and Fitness." This section, which appeared every few months, contained information for healthy living and advertisements for various nostrums and prescription drugs to enhance well-being and to facilitate a long and healthy life. Metropolitan newspapers launched similar efforts.

Workplace Fitness and Health Movement

The fitness and wellness movement, like many other health crusades over the past 150 years, began with moral suasion and evolved into coercion when individuals did not change behaviors to meet the expectations of reformers. This was primarily seen in the workplace. Encouragement of fitness and lifestyle changes on the job began with health-promotion programs. In the early 1980s, a growing number of companies began to offer fitness activities for employees. Corporations found that employee sickness and medical-care costs for program participants decreased compared to nonparticipants.

However, in the 1990s, some companies began to use sanctions to force employees to exercise, lose weight, lower their cholesterol, and stop smoking in an effort to reduce company healthcare costs. Employees who did not take action to change their lifestyles began to be charged higher insurance premiums. *Newsweek* (Miller and Bradburn 1991) reported, in addition to increased premiums for unhealthy lifestyles and habits, some companies even fired employees for off-the-job habits such as smoking or did not hire smokers, reminiscent of Henry Ford during the second Clean Living Movement.

Diet and Nutrition

Along with fitness and health, a diet and nutrition movement grew over the last decades of the twentieth century. This movement included antagonism to new agricultural practices, including chemical fertilizers, as well as concerns about food safety, advocacy for organic food and vegetarianism, and strident crusades to eliminate sugar and fat from the diet. Similar to most health-reform movements, moral-suasive and coercive elements became entwined.

Changes in Eating Patterns

A change in American eating patterns emerged in the 1960s, which became the underlying basis for a nutrition reform movement. Up to this time, most Americans had eaten the majority of their meals at home. Dining out was for special occasions. The standard fare included meat and potatoes, supplemented by vegetables, dairy products, desserts, and fruits in season. After World War II, a stimulated economy and new technologies dramatically changed the food system (McIntosh 1995, 122, 127–128). One noticeable trend was a growth in home delivery of precooked items such as pizza and Chinese food. During the 1970s, drive-through windows at fast-food restaurants became popularized, and health and organic foods became readily available in retail outlets. Quick cooking of foods became possible in the early 1980s with microwave ovens. Fast-food restaurants, where customers had the choice of eating inside or taking food to go, mushroomed in number and scope. Most of these meals had high fat and caloric contents. By the end of the century, a large majority of Americans were eating their meals away from home or buying precooked meals from delis or supermarkets (*USA Today*, March 9, 1998). Snacking between meals became the norm for many Americans. This activity, along with several hours a day of sedentary activities such as TV watching and a lack of exercise, led to a high prevalence of poor nutrition and obesity. By the late 1980s, the USDA's (1999) *Healthy Eating Index* found that one-third or fewer of the people surveyed consumed the suggested number of servings from the five major food groups. From the 1970s through the rest of the century, Americans became fatter.

A fight against these poor nutritional trends became the undercurrent of the campaigns against fat, sugar, and junk food beginning in the 1970s. Nutrition reformers, as had been found for other personal health behaviors, attempted to change behavior through moral suasion and legal sanctions in order to get people to change "for their own good."[5]

Michael Jacobson and the Center for Science in the Public Interest

Michael Jacobson (b. 1943) and his Center for Science in the Public Interest became a leader in the nutrition reform area. Jacobson, raised in Chicago, had a graduate degree in microbiology from MIT. In 1970, he worked as a technical consultant for Ralph Nader's Center for the Study of Responsive Law in Washington. In this position he became concerned about fat, cholesterol, sodium, and sugar in foods ("Junk Food Enemy No. 1" 1996; Gale Research 1998; "Eschewing the Fat" 1994).

In the 1980s, fat became increasingly demonized. Jacobson and his CSPI began to wage war on the high fat content in various foods and, in particular, fast-food franchises. "To Jacobson, it seems, certain foods are simply evil, with no redeeming qualities worth noting," reported Jacob Sullum (1995), a public-policy critic. Because of pressure on the part of CSPI in the 1980s, fast-food restaurants began "cooking their french fries in vegetable oil instead of beef fat, providing nutrition facts to customers, and offering salads and other lighter choices" ("The Food Police" 1996).

In 1993, the CSPI began to attack ethnic foods for their high fat content. Stephen Glass (1996), a political commentator, wrote that a 25-percent decline in business at Chinese restaurants had ensued after the CSPI had pointed out the high amount of fat in one chicken dish. The center also attacked Italian and Mexican foods for their high fat contents, as reported by *Time* ("Chewing the Fat" 1994).

In "Junk Food Enemy No. 1" (1996), *U.S. News and World Report* commented that Jacobson "had profoundly altered the way America eats." CSPI led the fight for nutrition labels on every food item, convinced theaters to switch from saturated fats to less saturated oils on popcorn, and fought against whole milk and olestra (a synthetic fat), in addition to other foods. Similar to most other reformers, Jacobson attempted to convince individuals to give up their bad habits "for their own good." *USA Today*, February 21, 1996, quoted Jacobson as stating "CSPI's sole motivation is to save American lives by changing eating habits."

CSPI leaders also opposed alcohol. In the 1980s, they successfully lobbied to raise the drinking age and place warning labels on alcoholic-beverage containers. Throughout the 1990s, they continued to advocate increased taxes, elimination of advertisements in the electronic media, and other measures to decrease or eliminate alcohol consumption (see Chapter 13).

The Obesity Epidemic and Low-Fat Diets

Through the 1980s and 1990s, increased concern about a growing "obesity epidemic" emerged. By the mid-1990s, some individuals, such as Michael Fumento (b. 1960), a medical journalist, suggested that, based upon various studies, two-thirds of all Americans were too heavy for optimal health. He considered obesity a disease that appeared to be getting worse and advocated that Americans change their lifestyles. "Like any good convert, I'm standing on the rooftop and shouting my message to the people," he stated (Fumento 1997, xv–xix). Fumento (1997, xv), who had changed his lifestyle and lost twenty-five pounds, reminiscent of other reformers, exhibited a convert's zeal with rhetoric such as "its incidence is skyrocketing," and "there is no end in sight to this [obesity] epidemic." To reduce the problem, Fumento (p. 264) suggested "the best model for a societal campaign against obesity should resemble that of the antismoking campaign prior to late 1993. . . . We need to make overeating needs to be made gauche, uncouth, and nasty. We need to learn to sneer at twenty-four-ounce steaks, sixty-four-ounce sodas, monster muffins, and chocolate bars that pretend to be health foods."

The Low-Fat Diet. Over the last decades of the twentieth century, many special diets were developed to help Americans lose weight. Many who tried these diets did not change their lifestyles and often gained the weight back. In the late 1980s, some health professionals suggested that an extremely low-fat diet could reduce or even reverse some chronic diseases. Dean Ornish (b. 1953), a physician, published data in 1989 showing that atherosclerotic patients he had been treating without drugs or invasive surgery had reduced overall blockages in their arteries. An article in *Newsweek*, titled "Healer of Hearts" (1998), reported that patients were eating low-fat diets, exercising at least three hours a week, practicing stress management for one hour a day, and engaging in support groups to develop nurturing relationships and meditating (Ornish 1983, 1990).

A Food-Guidelines Fight

In the early 1990s, the USDA replaced the four food groups with a pyramidal guide, with grains at the base and sweets at the top, indicating that they should be eaten sparingly. By the mid-1990s, competing food pyramids were introduced. Rapaport (1996) discussed the new food guidelines, all diagramed as a pyramid. These guidelines included the Mediterranean, Asian, the Healthy-Eating Pyramid of the CSPI, along with the new USDA Food-Guide Pyramid. All contained different recommendations concerning alcohol, fat, and meat consumption. The only items agreed upon by the four competing classifications led to recommendations that Americans should eat more fruits, vegetables, and grains and less saturated fat. This competition for the recommended "right diet" was symbolic of the conflict concerning diet and nutrition in the 1990s.

The Plateau and Decline of the Health and Fitness Movement, 1990–?

Prevention (1950–1999), a health magazine, published *Prevention Index*, from 1983 until 1994, an annual survey that measured a broad range of health risks and healthy behavior. The results of this index and other surveys showed that, beginning in the late 1980s and continuing to the end of the century, little increased improvement was noted in exercise, nutrition, or weight control. In 1995, the index reported that Americans were getting fatter, drinking more, and driving too fast. Fewer Americans were limiting fat, exercising, and eating recommended amounts of fruits and vegetables accoording to *USA Today*, March 7, 1995. In 1997, the August 2 *Newsday* reported that use of rowing and cross-country ski machines and jogging had all declined. About 25 percent of Americans did not engage in any type of exercise. However, despite the decrease in frequent exercising, membership in health clubs was still on the upswing. YMCA membership and participation after the late 1980s had slower growth and began to plateau in the mid-1990s. This leveling off may be symbolic of the crest of the late twentieth-century fitness movement. In 1997, the YMCA had about 15 million members and participants.

Several studies showed a decrease in the proportion of youth engaging in healthy behaviors over the 1990s. This was found by the *Prevention Index* and the Center for Disease Control (1998) surveys. The proportion of overweight children and the use of various substances had increased. Those exercising and eating healthy diets had decreased.

The Emergence of a Backlash against
Fitness and Healthy Eating, 1990s

The decrease in fitness and increase in consumption of high-fat foods suggested the beginning of a backlash against the health and fitness crusade. In the 1990s, there also began to be an increase in portion sizes in food products. This was found in fast-food outlets and more fashionable sit-down restaurants. Some restaurants, for example, featured servings of steak so large that they could easily feed three or four people. Sizes of drinks, such as soda pop, also increased dramatically at food outlets (*USA Today*, February 20, 1996; March 31, 1997). In 1997, journalist Randi Epstein published an article, "Is There a Backlash Against Healthy Living?" in the January 7 *Washington Post*. Based upon interviews with a variety of individuals and statistics concerning increased consumption of high-fat foods and other "demonized" products, a backlash against the health movement appeared to be emerging. In the mid-1990s, there was an upturn in sales of classic cocktails, hamburgers and fries, high-fat cheeses, super premium ice cream, and cigars.[6]

One of the symbols of this backlash was increased hostility against the CSPI, not only on the part of food manufacturers and retailers, but also by political commentators and professionals. Reminiscent of other food and health reformers, the CSPI began to be increasingly seen as a fanatical "religion." For example, Stephen Glass (1996), a political commentator, quoted one FDA scientist as saying, "'The newsletter is a good read, but it's like a religion. They're a group of goody-two shoes too old for the playground. Just look at what they say about drinking. Like fat, alcohol is a CSPI taboo." The CSPI began to be referred to as the "national nag" in popular articles with titles such as "The Fat Police Go Wacky," "Junk Food Enemy No. 1," or "Attacked by a Killer Egg Roll." Glass (1996) expressed concern that the CSPI had "abandoned its commitment to sound science and is using media hype in its effort to improve nutrition in the U.S. and sell its newsletters." Glass concluded that the CSPI essentially pushed "a puritanical agenda against alcohol, meat, desserts, caffeine, wine, microwave ovens, and even flatulence."

Some commentators feared that there was too much government intrusion into private lives and behaviors. Jacob Sullum (1996), for example, expressed concern that official sanctions were now being used by public health interests to control behaviors associated with chronic illness or social problems. Sanctions included "raising alcohol taxes, restricting cigarette ads, banning guns, arresting marijuana growers, and forcing people to buckle their seat belts." Sullum further commented that "behavior cannot be transmitted to other people against their will and that people do not choose to be sick, but they do choose to engage in risky behavior. The choice implies that the behavior, unlike a viral or bacterial infection, has value. It also implies that attempts to control the behavior will be resisted."

Over the 1980s and 1990s, Americans became more and more likely to blame their health problems on forces outside themselves, rather than accept responsibility directly for their own behaviors. Because a large majority of the population did not change lifestyle behaviors that contributed to obesity, high cholesterol, hypertension, and other chronic conditions, these and other behaviors slowly began to be perceived as having a genetic basis.

THE NEW EUGENICS MOVEMENT

A new eugenics movement began to surface near the end of the twentieth century. Like the heredity and eugenics movements of the first and second Clean Living Movements, it gained visibility during the crest of the third movement. Reminiscent of the first two movements, after reformers had attempted to shape behavior through moral suasion and coercion, albeit with minimal results, reformers and others concluded that social problems or diseases must somehow be due to heredity. The next step in the thought process became advocacy for the fittest individuals with the "best genes" to reproduce or, in the case of the turn of the twenty-first century, manipulating genes and eliminating defective embryos in an effort to eradicate diseases and other undesirable conditions. In the last decade of the twentieth century, genetic traits began to be seen as the cause for many chronic illnesses and behaviors. Biotechnological advances now made it possible to manipulate pregnancies, and a movement for "better babies" was born.

The Conception of the New Eugenics
Movement, 1950s–1960s

Eugenics in the post–World War II era became demonized because of its association with Nazi experimentation and death-camp efforts to create a "perfect race." It was rarely discussed in scientific and academic circles in western cultures. Troy Duster (1990, vii), a sociologist, suggested that by mid-century, "social scientists believed that they had won the battle with hereditarians over who could better explain the great human concerns." However, as the science of genetics was expanding, "gradually, almost imperceptibly, our thinking about human social life has shifted to accept a grater role for genetics."

In the 1950s, for a few disorders, genetic counselors could tell from biochemical tests whether either potential parent carried a deleterious recessive gene but, generally, could only provide estimates of the risk of a child being born with the disorder. Genetic counseling tended to be accomplished with parents who already had one affected child. In the 1950s, there were fewer than twenty genetic counseling clinics and genetics was not required in most medical schools. As genetics came to be seen as more important over the 1960s and 1970s, courses in genetics became required in many medical schools and there was an increase in genetic counseling centers around the nation (Kevles 1985, 253–254). These activities reflected a growing interest in producing mentally and physically fit children.

The Birth of the New Eugenics, 1970s

The symbolic birth of the new eugenics movement was the publication of an article by psychologist Arthur R. Jensen (b. 1923) titled, "How Much Can We Boost IQ and Scholastic Achievement" (Jensen 1969). Jensen, however, was verbally attacked and harassed by groups and individuals, both within and without the scientific community, when he suggested that differences in intelligence between black and white Americans might have a genetic basis. Daniel Kevles (1985, 270), a historian, suggested that "on both sides of the Atlantic, Jensen's writings invigorated the hereditarian school of thought on intelligence, including the wing that was little if at all concerned with race."

Although arguments in academia raged throughout the rest of the twentieth century, subtle eugenic thinking on the questions of IQ began to emerge in the 1970s. This included physicians favoring sterilization for welfare mothers who had borne many illegitimate children or testing prospective parents to see if they were carriers of genetic defects (Hubbard and Wald 1993, 25–27). This new thinking included the rights of the "unborn" and the obligation of mothers not to abuse the fetus by using alcohol, smoking, or transmitting genetic diseases.[7]

Growth and Development of the
New Eugenics, 1980s–1990s

As biotechnological advances became reality in the 1980s, the new eugenics began to evolve in a subtle manner. However, the term "eugenics" was rarely used, due to its previous negative associations. Donald Kevles (1985, 252) noted that scientists from different fields pursued one element or another of what he termed a "reform-eugenic program." Diane Paul (1995, 2), a political scientist, noted that the new eugenics arose in the "benevolent guise of medical genetics." As new technologies became more common, predicative tests created the need to make choices concerning prospective mates, whether or not to abort a fetus, or even the selection of the right sperm or egg for a "perfect baby."

In the last decade of the twentieth century, the new eugenics movement experienced a growth spurt. Genes began to be seen as the bases of most behaviors and diseases. Based upon research reports over the previous year, Sharon Begley (1999), a *Newsweek* journalist, pointed out that "eccentric personality traits" were suggested as "shadow" forms of genetic-based mental illness, a gene for "general intelligence [had] been discovered," and "religion and moral values" could now be inferred from genetics. In addition, "genetics will let parents choose their baby's traits and [let] scientists grow spare human parts." Although the term "eugenics" was not mentioned in the article, many would consider various procedures eugenic manipulations, such as couples looking through lists of donor eggs and sperm to "chose one based on his or her traits," or choosing the desired gender for their offspring.

In-Vitro Fertilization and Donor Egg and Sperm Selection

One of the biggest advances in the late twentieth-century eugenics movement was a new biomedical technique, in-vitro fertilization (IVF), the implantation of an embryo from a donor egg and sperm in the uterus after it had been fertilized in a petri dish. With IVF, a woman could have a choice of sperm, or even egg donors. This technique constituted the next step up from "artificial insemination" and "germinal choice"—storing semen of extraordinarily gifted men in sperm banks for future use. Germinal choice was first introduced in 1959 by Hermann Muller (1890–1967), a geneticist and eugenicist. Muller was concerned about the increase of potentially lethal genes in the human gene pool and the deterioration of the quality of the human race. Better health conditions kept more individuals alive so that "deleterious genes were no longer being eliminated," and radioactive fallout from the nuclear testing of the era was causing increased mutations (Kevles 1985, 259–260). To solve this problem, Muller reasoned, frozen sperm of outstanding men, or those with minimum genetic problems, could be used to maintain evolution to the highest level. A "sperm bank," the California Repository for Germinal Choice, was established for this purpose using sperm from distinguished scientists and Nobel laureates (Kevles 1985, 263–264).

In the late 1960s and early 1970s, genetic engineering began to be discussed by the news media. For example, Albert Rosenfeld, a respected science reporter, proclaimed in the June 13, 1969 issue of *Life*, "We are now entering an era when, as a result of new scientific discoveries, some mind-boggling things are likely to happen. Children may routinely be born of geographically separated or even long-dead parents, virgin births may become relatively common, women may give birth to other women's children." His predictions proved to be accurate.

Less than a decade later, in 1978, the first test tube baby, Louise Brown in England, was born using the in-vitro fertilization process. This technique also allowed for possible elimination of defective embryos prior to implantation (Kevles 1985, 265). The United States lagged behind other nations in this technique: "Because of the ethical sensitivity of the issue, no government funds were available for IVF research" (Singer and Wells 1985, 3). The first clinic did not open until 1980, and the first IVF child was born in 1981 (Singer and Wells 1985, 3). Despite the initial controversies, these techniques became common and grew in demand, not only for couples but also for single women.

The "Designer" or "Better" Baby

The "right" to have a physically and mentally sound infant led to the search for a "better baby" in the last decade of the century through the use of greater technological advances. Kevles and Hood, in the November 8, 1992 *Los Angeles Times*, for example, remarked that parents already chose to abort fetuses with certain disabilities or diseases and were interested in choosing the sex of their child.

By the end of the 1990s, sperm banks were advertising over the Internet urging consumers to buy their sperm donated by highly educated or athletically gifted men. The November 2, 1997 *St. Petersburg Times*, for example, reported that one advertisement urged parents to "Give your child a genetically advantaged start in life" and "put more of our best genes into the human gene pool." Some scientists even attempted to patten new genes to produce perfect babies. In 1994, the April 8 *Chicago Tribune* reported that "Two U.S. scientists have applied for a European patent for genetically engineered 'designer sperm' that would allow a father to pass down only 'healthy' genes to his children." However, this patent application "provoked outrage and concern on both sides of the Atlantic as it raised the specter of eugenics-using science to 'improve' the human race to some subjective standard." An article in the *Chicago Sun-Times*, May 5, 1998, noted that "leading molecular biologists and geneticists met to discuss the prospect of making genetic changes in the human 'germ line'—sperm and eggs—that would be passed on to future generations. The ability to alter genes before conception raises the possibility that we might be able to re-engineer our genetic blueprints and redirect the course of our biological evolution."

Genetic Testing and Screening

Prenatal testing became increasingly common over the last two decades of the century. Amniocentesis—the examination of fetal cells discarded in the surrounding anionic fluid—and legalized abortion together stimulated a major boom in prenatal genetic diagnosis. By the mid-1970s, a hundred or so known chromosomal disorders, along with twenty-three inborn errors of metabolism, could be detected in utero. By the early 1980s, amniocentesis could detect the high probability of the neural tube defects anencephaly and spina bifida (Kevles 1985, 256–257, 294). Middle-class women began to elect prenatal testing and many physicians recommended this procedure for women over the age of thirty-five in order to determine the possibility of Down's syndrome—a type of mental retardation caused by an extra chromosome—which is more common among this age group. Many women elected an abortion for this and other conditions.

Genetic screening of prospective parents and infants also became increasingly common. In the early 1960s, a test for PKU, a recessive condition found in one out of eighty Euro-Americans, was developed and infants began to be screened for this disease. By the early 1970s, adult carriers of at least fifty genetic disorders could be identified. Few argued for screening everyone, but some favored screening people from groups at comparatively high risk for a particular recessive disorder (Hubbard and Wald 1993, 24, 34–36; Kevles 1985, 255–256).

In 1976, Congress passed the National Genetic Diseases Act, which provided funding for research, screening, counseling, and professional education for several diseases in which genetic mutation were implicated. Assisted by federal funding, many states enlarged their postnatal screening programs (Hubbard and Wald 1993, 34–35; Kevles 1985, 256). The number of genetic counseling centers had jumped to about 400, many of them supported by the March of Dimes which had launched an effort in the 1970s to eliminate birth defects when the battle against polio had been won (Kevles 1985, 257).

Human Genome Project

The Human Genome Project (HGP) was an international scientific quest to decipher the genetic code of human heredity. The project began in 1987 in the United States with the support of two federal agencies, the National Institutes of Health and the Department of Energy. In 1987, the November 8 *Los Angeles Times* reported that "With work proceeding at dozens of laboratories across the country and in Japan and Europe, researchers hope to complete their basic task by 2005." Over the 1990s, various genes associated with a variety of conditions and behaviors were frequently announced by the news media from this project. HGP had a profound impact on medicine due to the fact that when a gene for a particular disease, such as ovarian cancer, had been detected, a test could be developed. Gene therapy now became a reality in providing whatever protein the body failed to provide, such as genetically engineering bacteria to produce insulin, or changing patients' own cells or reproductive cells to eliminate the defective gene being passed on to potential descendants (McGee 1997, 17–19).

Because of ethical, legal, and social implications of research resulting from the project, the Human Genome Privacy Act developed guidelines for safeguarding the personal privacy of genetic information. This included providing individuals access to their records. However, the bill allowed access to information by various agencies and did not address the problems of intended use. Research such as manipulating reproductive cells—"germ line engineering"—was put on hold. These issues were still being discussed at the turn of the twenty-first century (Hubbard and Wald, 1993, 153; McGee 1997, 17–19).

DNA Identification Systems

Law enforcement began to use DNA testing to match a suspect's genetic profile with evidence. This "fingerprinting technique" is based upon the premise that DNA is unique for each individual. However, due to political considerations and the fact that DNA can be contaminated, this option has been refuted in some court cases. The most highly profiled case was a California jury finding O. J. Simpson, a football celebrity, innocent in the alleged murder of his wife, based upon "faulty" DNA evidence in the late 1990s. Hubbard and Wald (1993, 151–153) reported that despite problems with this technique, several states began to take blood samples from more violent criminals to be stored in databanks for police use across the United States. In 1992, the Defense Department announced plans to establish a repository of genetic information on all American service members as a new way of identifying future war casualties.

Inherited Tendencies and Traits: Chronic Diseases and Behaviors

Human Genome Project researchers attempted to find predictive genetic markers for genetic causes of disease. Over the last decade of the century, various conditions were increasingly attributed to genes. Every few weeks, a new media announcement reported a correlation between a cluster of genes and a certain disease. These included a genetic predisposition for a number of chronic diseases, such as Type

Two diabetes, heart disease, and cancer. It was further postulated that if an individual with the trait had certain environmental factors, such as lack of exercise, smoking, being overweight, or having a poor diet, he or she would be more likely to succumb to the condition, compared to individuals who did not have these negative lifestyle factors (Hubbard and Wald 1993, 76–92).

Besides diseases, some researchers began to suggest that various behaviors and characteristics resulted from genetic tendencies or traits. This had also been suggested by hereditarian and eugenic reformers in the previous eras. Hubbard and Wald (1993, 93) point out that genetic links were often correlated with some stigmatized segment of society. They implied that social, political, or religious reasons, along with flaws in the studies, may have accounted for many of these associations (Hubbard and Wald 1993, 93–107). Over the late 1980s and 1990s, researchers began to suggest genetic tendencies for alcoholism, mental illness, homosexuality, shyness, racial differences in IQ beyond the usual assumptions of intellectual diversity, and criminality (Duster 1990, vii). Some groups with these conditions grasped at these results, as their behavior could now be explained as a disease, such as alcoholism, or as biologically determined, such as homosexuality. Other groups vehemently opposed these possible associations on grounds they were racist.

Cloning

The most science-fiction aspect of the new eugenics movements appeared to be taken from the 1978 film, *The Boys from Brazil*, in which clones of Hitler were produced. Cloning is the process of reproducing the exact genetic makeup of the donor. The cloned organism is an "identical twin" to the donor. By the end of the 1960s, only a frog had been successfully cloned. However, in 1997, due to biotechnology advances, the first cloned adult mammal—Dolly, the sheep—was produced in Britain. The December 30 *USA Today* considered this development "by far the biggest scientific breakthrough of the year." After this successful mammalian cloning, most Western cultures put a moratorium on human cloning. However, the December 17, 1998 *Washington Post* reported, "Researchers in South Korea, say they have created a cloned human embryo that was a genetic replica of a 30-year-old woman. If true, it would be the first known cloning of a human embryo, and vivid evidence that while nations around the world contemplate the ethics of human cloning, there is little to stop scientists from pursuing the controversial technology." As of the turn of the twenty-first century, a cloned human infant is yet to be realized through biotechnology.

Concerns about the New Eugenics Movement

As technology marched forward, eugenics under the banner of biotechnology began to become operational. Increased research and new procedures elected by many caused alarm among both professionals and nonprofessionals. Hubbard and Wald (1993, 24–25) point out that although "race purity" or "building a strain of supermen may have died," the eugenic ideal that "it is more beneficial for certain people to have children than others, and that a vast range of human problems can be cured once we learn how to manipulate our genes, remains very much with us." These scholars expressed concern about the revolution of bioscience and the effects of the new eugenics on society.[8]

A Brave New World?

Aldous Huxley's (1971) *Brave New World*, which broached the subject of cloning and other genetic manipulation to create a perfect society, was published 1932 at the peak of the previous eugenics movement. Fear that this type of genetically engineered society could actually emerge began to be expressed over the 1990s in several forms. Professionals discussed concern about the social ramifications of the new biotechnology, entertainment offered fictionalized accounts of repressive eugenic-based societies, the media featured articles and programming concerning the topic, and active opposition to research conclusions or to procedures such as pregnancy termination surfaced. Duster (1990, 113) asserted that a new eugenics movement with political overtones was very much in evidence. This was indicated by increased prenatal detection of inherited disorders and the search for genetic markers for multifactorial disorders such as heart disease, diabetes, and mental illness.

The association of genes with some certain characteristics, however, was denounced or criticized in some cases. When one Human Genome Project researcher group suggested there might be a genetic factor in crime, their funding for a conference to discuss the topic was eliminated on grounds it was not considered a "politically correct" hypotheses (Hilts 1992). Herrnstein and Murray (1994), in *The Bell Curve*, suggested that African-Americans as a group appeared to score lower on standard IQ tests, whereas Asian-Americans scored higher compared to Euro-Americans. This work was immediately branded as "racist" and considered to be based upon "flawed research" methodology by many (Jacoby and Glauberman 1995).

At the beginning of 2000, demand for new eugenic technology for curing disease and increasing the probability for better babies is still on the upsurge. At the same time, hostility and fear of the social ramifications of the new eugenics is also increasing. Duster (1990, 112), in his *Backdoor to Eugenics*, concluded that the "front door to eugenics is closed," but that a "subtle and subliminally compelling idea is starting to penetrate the collective conscious, namely, that the 'defective fetus' can be eliminated." Near the beginning of the new biotechnological surge, however, Kevles (1985, 296) did suggest that the "most powerful restraint on the revival of eugenics has been nature itself. Single genes account for only a small fraction of human traits, disorders, and diseases. Like intelligence, most human characters are polygenic, and therefore not even genetically understood, let alone subject to manipulation."

SUMMARY

This chapter discussed the exercise, diet, and health movement, along with the emergences of eugenic activities. Although there is no overt connection between the new eugenics and the fitness movement, the desire to have fit and healthy babies could be an unconscious manifestation of the concern for good health. The new eugenics movement began to surge at the peak of health and fitness concerns in the early 1990s, as it had in the previous health-reform eras.

NOTES

1. During the upsurge of the health and fitness movement, Lewis Thomas (1977, 42), a physician, argued that, because of media "propaganda" that attempted to convince people they were sick, "there is a public preoccupation with disease that is assuming the dimension of a national obsession." The rise of health concerns and the wellness movement began during the years of increased mass mailings and television that brought "imminent perils posed by multiple sclerosis, kidney disease, cancer, heart disease, cystic fibrosis, asthma, muscular dystrophy, and the rest." Other observers reason that the health and fitness movement had its roots in the medicalization of social problems and life in general inasmuch as many conditions, including problem drinking, drug addictions, and obesity, began to be called "diseases." See Goldstein (1992, 2–14) and Peele (1989) for more information concerning this topic.

2. Biographical information on Kenneth Cooper can be found in the *Gale Literary Data Bases* (1998), http://www.galenet.com, last visited on November 22, 1998; *Washington Post*, February 24, 1983; and *Denver Rocky Mountain News*, April 2, 1996.

3. See a sampling of a few *Newsweek* articles which suggest the development and popularization of fitness equipment and apparel beginning in the late 1970s: "Keeping Fit: America Tries to Shape Up" (1978); "Doing the Reebok Be-Bop" (1989); and "How High? How Fast?" (1996).

4. See Knowles (1977) for the changes in healthcare until the late 1970s. See, in addition, Green (1981), Greenberg and Raymond (1994), and Helms

(1993) for more information concerning health promotion in the latter decades of the century.

5. For hostile reactions against crusaders who attempted to coerce better eating behaviors and attacked the food and vitamins industry, see Wagner (1997) and Armstrong and Armstrong (1991).

6. The authors of several popular books poked fun at or discussed in detail the repressiveness of the "puritanical" or "new temperance" movement, and they could represent the beginning of a backlash. See Shaw (1996), Sullum (1998), and Wagner (1997).

7. See Chapter 13 for information about arrests and mandatory treatment of pregnant women with alcohol or cocaine addiction.

8. During the late 1980s and 1990s, many general and academic works began to be published concerning positive and negative aspects of the new eugenics. See Cranor (1994), Hubbard and Wald (1993), Paul (1995), and Singer and Wells (1985) for publications aimed at the general reader. See Duster (1990), Kevles (1985), McGee (1997), Neuhaus (1990), and VanDyck (1995) for more scholarly works on the subject. Earlier important works include Haller (1963) and Bajema (1976).

Epilogue

I have attempted to show that over the past 200 years a health-reform movement has emerged about every eighty years. These clean-living cycles surged with, or were tangential to, religious awakenings. Simultaneously with these awakenings, outgroups such as immigrants and/or youth were seen to exhibit behaviors that contributed to the undermining of society. Fear of these dangerous classes and a desire on the part of the middle classes to eliminate disease, crime, poverty, and other perceived health or social problems led to crusades in each of the three reform eras against alcohol, tobacco, drugs, meat or fat, impure food, and certain sexual behaviors. Reformers in each era claimed that, based upon the latest evidence, these activities were extremely detrimental to America's physical, mental, social, or spiritual health. The substances or behaviors were demonized and reformers claimed that it was now time to eliminate them completely from society.

The desire for improved health and social change also led to campaigns in favor of exercise, semivegetarian diets, women's rights, chastity, and eugenics. In each movement, alternative religions were founded that adopted some aspect of health reform as dogma. In the reform aspect of each cycle, a new infectious disease threatened the population, and alternative treatment modalities emerged, some of which were later incorporated into orthodox medicine and public-health interests. Over each succeeding cycle, reformers became more likely to represent grassroots beliefs, or even to be state or federal officials, rather than independent activists.

The reform aspect of each submovement within the overall Clean Living Movement lasted approximately twenty-five to forty years. Antialcohol and antitobacco campaigns tended to have longer durations compared to pro-exercise or dietary-change crusades. Both moral suasion and sanctions of various kinds were used to convince people to adopt certain modes of behavior. Eugenics surged as other issues crested or were on the wane. A backlash emerged among some segments of the population against reform efforts when the crusades were most strident. After the reform surge of the movement had dissipated, laws made during the reform era were often ignored or repealed. During the thirty- to forty-year ebb of the cycle, with a few exceptions, the memory of the movement disappeared from public awareness.

Today, at the turn of the twenty-first century, many submovements within the millennial Clean Living Movement have crested and are beginning to wane. However, it still too early to know what ramifications these movements may have for the future or when they will cease to be important to society. Based upon the patterns of the waxing and waning of the different health reform issues presented in this work, I would like to offer a few speculative guesses as to the courses of certain issues.

I anticipate that eugenic concerns will continue to increase and may reach a peak about 2020. There will be increasing controversy concerning genetic background and biotechnology in terms of jobs, insurance, and healthcare expenditures. Concerns about diet and exercise will continue to wane and will be of little interest to today's youth as they age. This, in turn, will result in an upturn of chronic diseases before 2020. By 2010, the legal purchase age for alcohol will be lowered in certain circumstances, and marijuana will increasingly be allowed for medical purposes and will be legal for sale in some states for recreational use. By 2020, tobacco use, in some form, will again become fashionable. The neo-purity movement will continue to surge and reach a peak about 2015, youthful chastity will be an accepted norm among the middle class, and increasing numbers of middle-class women will work out of their homes in order to care for their children. Some of the New Age religions will become mainstream by 2030. A new religious awakening and, in its wake, the fourth Clean Living Movement, will rise around 2040.

References and Bibliography

Aaron, Paul, and David Musto. 1981. Temperance and prohibition in America: A historical overview. In *Alcohol and public policy: Beyond the shadow of prohibition*, ed. Mark H. Moore and Dean R. Gerstein, 127–181. Washington, D.C.: National Academy Press.

Abbott, Twyman O. 1910. The rights of the non-smoker. *Outlook* 94: 763.

Abel, Ernest, and Robert Sokol. 1990. Is occasional light drinking during pregnancy harmful? In *Controversies in the addictions field*, ed. Ruth C. Engs, 158–166. Dubuque, Iowa: Kendall/Hunt.

Abortion by prescription. 1989. *Newsweek*, 17 April, 61.

Abortion in the form of a pill. 1995. *Newsweek*, 11 September, 76.

Abortion: mercy or murder. 1963. *Newsweek*, 13 August, 54.

Adam, Barry D. 1995. *The rise of a gay and lesbian movement*. Rev. ed. New York: Twayne; London: Prentice Hall International.

Adler, Margot. 1979. *Drawing down the moon: Witches, druids, goddess-worshipers and other pagans in America today*. New York: Viking.

———. 1996. Why I am a UU pagan. *UU World* 10: 14–18.

AIDS. 1985. *Newsweek*, 12 August, 28–30.

AIDS becomes a right-wing political issue. 1987. *Time*, 23 March, 24.

Alcott, William A. 1972a. *The physiology of marriage*. 1855. Reprint. New York: Arno Press and New York Times.

———. 1972b. *The young husband, or duties of man in the marriage relation*. 5th stereotype ed. 1851. Reprint. New York: Arno Press and New York Times.

———. 1844. *The house I live in; or, the human body. For the use of families and schools*. Boston: D. S. King.

———. 1835. *The young man's guide*. 4th ed. Boston: S. Coleman.

———. 1833. *The young man's guide*. Boston: Lilly, Wait, Colman, and Holden.

Alder, Jerry, and Debra Rosenberg. 1994. The endless binge. *Newsweek*, 19 December, 72.

Alexander, Kay. 1992. Roots of the New Age. In *Perspectives on the New Age*, ed. James R. Lewis and J. Gordon Melton, 30–47. Albany: State University of New York Press.

Alexander, Thomas G. 1981. The word of wisdom: From principle to requirement. *Dialogue: A Journal of Mormon Thought* 14 (Autumn): 78–88.

Allen, Nathan. 1853. *The opium trade*. Lowell, Mass.: James P. Walker.

Allsop, Kenneth. 1961. *The bootleggers: The story of prohibition*. New Rochelle, N.Y.: Arlington House.

Altman, Dennis. 1986. *AIDS in the mind of America*. New York: Anchor/Doubleday.

American Academy of Political and Social Science (AAPSS). 1909. *Race improvement in the United States*. Philadelphia: AAPSS.

Anderson, J. E., and L. L. Dahlberg. 1992. High-risk sexual behavior in the general population: Results from a national survey, 1988–1990. *Sexually Transmitted Diseases* 17: 320–325.

Anderson, Robert M. 1979. *Vision of the disinherited: The making of American Pentecostalism*. New York: Oxford University Press.

Anti-Cigarette Crusade. 1901. *The Outlook* 67: 607–608.

Armstrong, David, and Elizabeth Metzger Armstrong. 1991. *The great American medicine show*. New York: Prentice Hall.

Arrington, Leonard J. 1959. An economic interpretation of the word of wisdom. *BYU Studies* 1 (Winter): 37–49.

Asch, P., and D. T. Levy. 1987. Does the minimum drinking age affect traffic fatalities? *Journal of Policy Analysis and Management* 6: 180–192.

Ash, Roberta. 1972. *Social movements in America*. Chicago: Markham.

Ashley, Richard. 1976. *Cocaine: Its history, uses and effects*. New York: Warner Books.

Asimov, Isaac. 1988. *Prelude to foundation*. New York: Bantam Books.

Aspiz, Harold. 1987. Sexuality and the pseudo-sciences. In *Pseudo-science and society in nineteenth-century America*, ed. Arthur Wrobel, 144–165. Lexington: University of Kentucky Press.

Atkins, Gaius Glenn. 1932. *Religion in our times*. New York: Round Table Press.
———. 1923. *Modern religious cults and movements*. New York: Fleming H. Revell.

Bajema, Carl Jay, ed. 1976. *Eugenics then and now*. Stroudburg, Pa.: Dowden, Hutchingson, and Ross.

Baker, La Reine Helen. 1912. *Race improvement or eugenics, a little book on a great subject*. New York: Dodd, Mead.

Baldwin, Dwight. 1855. *Prize essay: Evils of tobacco as they affect body, mind and morals*. New York: Fowlers and Wells.

Banfield, Maude. 1903. The journal's trained nurse. *Ladies' Home Journal*, 20 May, 26.

Barnesby, Norman. 1913. Eugenics and the child. *Forum* 49: 341–348.

Barrett, David V. 1996. *Sects, "cults" and alternative religions: A world survey and sourcebook*. London: Blanford.

Barry, Kathleen. 1988. *Susan B. Anthony: A biography of a singular feminist*. New York: New York University Press.

Bartlett, John. 1980. *Familiar quotations: A collection of passages, phrases, and proverbs traced to their sources in ancient and modern literature*, 346. 15th and 125th Anniversary edition. Boston: Little, Brown.

Bates, Anna Louise. 1995. *Weeder in the garden of the lord: Anthony Comstock's life and career*. New York: University Press of American.

Bates, Barbara. 1992. *Bargaining for life: A social history of tuberculosis, 1876–1938*. Philadelphia: University of Pennsylvania Press.

Battle over the abortion pill. 1988. *Newsweek*, 7 November, 10.

Beck, Melinda, and Phyllis Malamund. 1979. A new prohibition for teenagers. *Newsweek*, 2 April, 38.

Beecher, Catherine. 1856. *Physiology and calisthenics for schools and families*. New York: Harper and Brothers.

Beecher, Lyman. 1846. *Six sermons on the nature, occasions, signs, evils & remedy of intemperance*. With preface by the Rev. William Reid. Glasgow: Office of the Scottish Temperance League.

Beeton, Beverly. 1995. How the West was won for woman suffrage. In *One woman one vote: Rediscovering the woman suffrage movement*, ed. Marjorie Wheeler, 99–116. Troutdale, Ore.: New Sage Press.

Begley, Sharon. 1999. Into the gene pool. *Newsweek*, 4 January, 68–74.

Behr, Edward. 1996. *Prohibition: Thirteen years that cleansed America*. New York: Arcade.

Beisel, Nicola Kay. 1997. *Imperiled Innocents: Anthony Comstock and family reproduction in Victorian America*. Princeton, N.J.: Princeton University Press.

Bennett, D.R.M. 1971. *Anthony Comstock: His career of cruelty and crime*. 1879. Reprint. New York: Da Capo Press.

Bennion, Lowell "Ben." 1984. Incidence of Mormon polygamy in 1880: Dixie versus Davis Stake. *Journal of Mormon History* 11: 27–42.

Benson, Herbert. 1997. *Timeless healing: The power and biology of belief*. New York: Simon and Schuster.

———. 1975. *The relaxation response*. New York: Avon Books.

Berman, Brian M., and David B. Larson. 1994. *Alternative medicine: Expanding medical horizons*. Washington, D.C.: Office of Alternative Medicine, NIH.

Bertram, Eva, Morris Blachman, Kenneth Sharpe, and Peter Andreas. 1996. *Drug war politics: The price of denial*. Berkeley and Los Angeles: University of California Press.

Betts, John Rickards. 1971. American medical thought on exercise as the road to health, 1820–1860. *Bulletin of the History of Medicine* 45: 138–152.

Beveridge, William I. 1977. *Influenza: The last great plague, an unfinished story of discovery*. New York: Prodist.

Billings, John S. 1893. Municipal sanitation: Defects in American cities. *Forum* 15: 304–310.

Billington, Ray Allen. 1974. *The origins of Nativism in the United States 1800–1844*. New York: Arno Press.

Bisland, Elizabeth. 1899. New law of health. *North American Review*, 168: 458.

Blackwell, Elizabeth. 1852. *Popular and practical science: The laws of life, with special reference to the physical education of girls*. Vol. 2. New York: George P. Putnam.

Blair, Hugh. 1830. Opium eaters and snuff chewers. *Journal of Health* 1: 296–299.

Blake, John B. 1974. Health reform. In *The rise of Adventism: Religion and society in mid-nineteenth-century America*, ed. Edwin S. Gaustand, 30–49. New York: Harper and Row.

————. 1962. Mary Gove Nichols, prophetess of health. *Proceedings of the American Philosophical Society* 106: 219–234.

Blanchard, Dallas A. 1994. *The anti-abortion movement and the rise of the religious right: From polite to fiery protest.* New York: Twayne.

Blane, Howard T., and Morris E. Chafetz, eds. 1979. *Youth, alcohol, and social policy.* New York: Plenum Press.

Blocker, Jack S., Jr. 1989. *American temperance movements: Cycles of reform.* Boston: Twayne.

————. 1985. *"Give to the winds thy fears": The women's temperance crusade, 1873–1874.* Westport, Conn.: Greenwood.

————. 1976. *Retreat from reform: The prohibition movement in the United States 1890–1913.* Contributions in American History 51. Westport, Conn.: Greenwood Press.

Blustein, Bonnie Ellen. 1991. *Preserve your love for science.* New York: Cambridge University Press.

Boas, Franz. 1894. Human faculty as determined by race. *Proceedings* 43: 301–327.

Boffeta, P., and L. Garfinkel. 1990. Alcohol drinking and mortality among men enrolled in an American Cancer Society prospective study. *Epidemiology* 1: 342–348.

Bok, Edward. 1904. The "patent medicine" curse. *Ladies Home Journal*, May, 18.

Booth, Martin. 1996. *Opium: A history.* New York: Simon and Schuster.

Bordin, Ruth. 1981. *Woman and temperance: The quest for power and liberty, 1873–1900.* Philadelphia: Temple University Press.

Borish, Linda J. 1990. Farm females, fitness, and the ideology of physical health in antebellum New England. *Agricultural History* 64: 17–30.

Boston, Alex. 1996. *The most dangerous man in America? Pat Robertson and the rise of the Christian Coalition.* Amherst, N.Y.: Prometheus Books.

Boston Women's Health Book Collective. 1973. *Our bodies, ourselves: A book by and for women.* New York: Simon and Schuster.

Boyer, Paul S. 1968. *Purity in print: The vice-society movement and book censorship in America.* New York: Charles Scribner's Sons.

Boyle, T. Coraghessan. 1993. *The Road to Wellville.* New York: Viking.

Brandt, Allan M. 1998. Blow some my way: Passive smoking, risk and American culture. In *Ashes to ashes: The history of smoking and health*, ed. S. Lock, L. A. Reynolds, and E. M. Tansey, 164–191. Amsterdam and Atlanta: Rodopi.

Brecher, Edward M. 1972. *Licit and illicit drugs: The Consumers Union report on narcotics, stimulants, depressants, inhalants, hallucinogens, and marijuana—including caffeine, nicotine, and alcohol by Edward M. Brecher and the editors of Consumer Reports.* Boston: Little, Brown.

Bromley, David G., and Phillip E. Hammond. 1987. *The future of new religious movements*, Macon, Ga.: Mercer University Press

Broun, Heywood C., and Margaret Leech. 1927. *Anthony Comstock, Roundsman of the Lord.* New York: Albert and Charles Boni.

Brown, L. Ames. 1916. Suffrage and prohibition. *North American Review* 203 (January): 93–100.

Brown, Susan Love. 1992. Baby boomers, American character, and the New Age: A synthesis. In *Perspectives on the New Age*, ed. James R. Lewis and J. Gordon Melton, 87–96. Albany: State University of New York Press.

Bruce, Steve. 1988. *The rise and fall of the new Christian right: Conservative Protestant politics in America 1978–1988.* Oxford: Clarendon Press.

Bruehl, Charles P. 1928. *Birth control and eugenics: In the light of fundamental ethical principles.* New York: Joseph F. Wagner.

Bryant, Lucinda L. 1992. TB: The white plague returns. *State Legislatures* 18 (September): 29–31.

Buchan, William. 1838. *Domestic medicine: Or, a treatise on the prevention and cure of diseases, by regimen and simple medicines: With directions for the management of common cases in surgery, etc.* Cincinnati: U. P. James.

Buchanan, Patrick. 1987. Quoted in the *Washington Post*, 4 February, 1, 21.

Buenker, John D. 1973. *Urban liberalism and progressive reform.* New York: Charles Scribner's Sons.

Buhle, Mari Jo, and Paul Buhle, eds. 1978. *The concise history of woman suffrage: Selections from the classic work of Stanton, Anthony, Gage and Harper.* Urbana: University of Illinois Press.

Bull, Chris, and John Gallagher. 1996. *Perfect enemies: The religious right, the gay movement, and the politics of the 1900s.* New York: Crown.

Bullough, Vern L., and Martha Voght. 1973. Homosexuality and its confusion with the "secret sin" in pre-Freudian America. *Journal of the History of Medicine and Allied Sciences* 27: 143–155.

Burnham, John C. 1993. *Bad habits: Drinking, smoking, taking drugs, gambling, sexual misbehavior, and swearing in American history.* New York: New York University Press.

———. 1989. American physicians and tobacco use: Two surgeons general, 1929 and 1964. *Bulletin of the History of Medicine* 63: 1–31.

———. 1984. Change in the popularization of health in the United States. *Bulletin of the History of Medicine* 58: 183–187.

———. 1972. Medical specialists and movements toward social control in the progressive era: Three examples. In *Building the organizational society: Essays on association activities in modern America,* ed. Jerry Israel, 19–30, notes 249–251. New York: Free Press.

Burt, John J., and Linda Brower Meeks. 1975. *Education for sexuality: Concepts and programs for teaching.* Philadelphia: Saunders.

Bush, Lester E., Jr. 1992. *Health and medicine among the Latter-Day Saints: Science, sense and scripture.* New York: Crossroad.

———. 1982. Mormon "physiology," 1850–1875. *Bulletin of the History of Medicine* 56: 218–237.

———. 1981. The word of wisdom in early nineteenth century perspective. *Dialogue: A Journal of Mormon Thought* 14 (Autumn): 46–65.

———. 1976. Birth control among the Mormons: Introduction to an insistent question. *Dialogue: A Journal of Mormon Thought* 10 (Autumn): 12–44.

Bushman, Richard L. 1984. *Joseph Smith and the beginnings of Mormonism.* Urbana: University of Illinois Press.

Butler, Jonathan M. 1974. Adventism and the American experience. In *The rise of Adventism: Religion and society in mid-nineteenth-century America,* ed. Edwin S. Gaustad, 173–206. New York: Harper and Row.

Button, James W., Barbara A. Rienzo, and Kenneth D. Wald. 1997. *Private lives, public conflicts: Battles over gay rights in American communities.* Washington, D.C.: Congressional Quarterly.

Cable blues in the night. 1981. *Newsweek*, 24 August, 48.

Calderone, Mary, ed. 1977. *Sexuality and human values: The personal dimension of sexual experience.* New York: Association Press.

Calkins, Raymond. 1901. *Substitutes for the saloon.* Boston: Houghton Mifflin.

Campbell, Eileen, and J. H. Brennan. 1994. *Body, mind and spirit: A dictionary of new age ideas, people, places, and terms.* Rutland, Vt.: Charles E. Tuttle Company.

Cancer facts and figures. 1999. American Cancer Society. http://www.cancer.org/statistics/index.html. Last visited August 19, 1999.

Carabillo, Toni, June Bundy Csida, and Judith Meuli. 1993. *Feminist chronicles 1953–1993.* Los Angeles: Women's Graphics.

Carson, Gerald. 1957. *Cornflake crusade.* New York: Rinehart.

Carter, Charles Frederick. 1907. The rising tide of Temperance. *Harper's Weekly Magazine* 51, 7 December, 1790–1791.

Carter, R. B. 1906. Alcohol and tobacco. *Cornhill* 94 (July): 101–120.

Carwardine, R. 1978. *Trans-Atlantic revivalism: Popular Evangelicalism in Britain and America, 1790–1865.* Westport, Conn.: Greenwood Press.

Catt, Carrie Chapmann, ed. 1940. *Victory: How women won it: A centennial symposium 1840–1940.* New York: H. W. Wilson.

Cayleff, Susan E. 1988. Gender, ideology, and the water-cure movement. In *Other healers: Orthodox medicine in America*, ed. Norman Gevitz, 82–98. Baltimore: Johns Hopkins University Press.

Center for Disease Control and Prevention. 1998. Youth risk behavior surveillance. *MMWR* 47: 1–31.

———. 1997. Tuberculosis morbidity—United States. *MMWR* 46: 695–700.

———. 1994. Expanded tuberculosis surveillance and tuberculosis morbidity—United States, 1993. 1994. *MMRW* 43: 361–365.

Charity Organization Society. 1903. *A handbook on the prevention of tuberculosis being the first annual report of the committee on the prevention of tuberculosis.* New York: Charity Organization Society.

Cherrington, Ernest H. 1920. *The evolution of prohibition in the United States of America.* Westerville, Ohio: American Issue Press.

Chesler, Ellen. 1992. *Woman of valor: Margaret Sanger and the birth control movement in America.* New York: Simon and Schuster.

Chesterton, Gilbert Keith. 1922. *Eugenics and other evils.* London: Cassell and Co.

Chewing the fat. 1994. *Time*, 1 August, 12.

Christian communities. 1998. *Christian century*, 7 October, 894–896.

The cigarette and its users. 1910. *Harper's Weekly*, 17 September, 25.

Clark, Norman. 1976. *Deliver us from evil: An interpretation of American prohibition.* New York: W. W. Norton.

———. 1965. *The dry years: Prohibition and social change in Washington.* Seattle: University of Washington Press.

Close, Ellis. 1997. Promise keepers: Here to pray for the nation. *Newsweek*, 13 October, 28–32.

Cole, Edith Walters. 1975. Sylvester Graham, lecturer on the science of human life: The rhetoric of a dietary reformer. Ph.D. diss., Indiana University.

Coles, Larkin B. 1855. *The beauties and deformities of tobacco-using: Or its ludicrous and its solemn realities.* 45th ed. Boston: Ticknor, Reed, and Fields.

————. 1854. *Philosophy of health: Natural principles of health and cure: Or, health and cure without drugs: Also, the moral bearings of erroneous appetites.* 37th ed. Boston: Ticknor, Reed, and Fields.

Collier, Richard. 1974. *The plague of the Spanish Lady: The influenza pandemic of 1918–1919.* New York: Atheneum.

Committee of Fifty: 1893–1903. 1905. Boston: Houghton Mifflin.

Cooper, Kenneth H. 1982. *The aerobics program for total well-being: Exercise, diet, emotional balance.* New York: M. Evans.

————. 1968. *Aerobics.* New York: Bantam Books.

Cordasco, Francesco. 1991. *Homeopathy in the United States: A bibliography of homeopathic medical imprints, 1825–1925.* Fairview, N.J.: Junius-Vaugn Press.

————. 1985. *American medical imprints, 1820–1910: A checklist of publications illustrating the history and progress of medical science, medical education, and the healing arts in the United States—A preliminary contribution.* Vols. 1 and 2. Totowa, N.J.: Rowman and Littlefield; Fairview, N.J.: Junius-Vaughn Press.

Courtwright, David T. 1982a. *Dark paradise: Opiate addiction in America before 1940.* Cambridge: Harvard University Press.

————. 1982b. Opiate addiction in the American West, 1850–1890. *Journal of the West* 21 (July): 23–31.

Craig, Barbara Hinkson, and David M. O'Brien. 1993. *Abortion and American politics.* Chatham, N.J.: Chatham House.

Craig, Winston J. 1991. In the pink of health: William Alcott, Sylvester Graham and dietary reforms in New England, 1830–1870. *Adventist Heritage* 14 (Fall): 34–41.

Crampton, Charles A. 1900. A food label. *Current Literature* 28: 308.

Crampton, Suzanne M., and John Hodge. 1997. The equal pay act: The first 30 years. *Public Personnel Management* 26: 335–338.

Cranor, Carl F. 1994. *Are genes us?* New Brunswick, N.J.: Rutgers University Press.

Creel, George. 1915. Poisoners of the public health. *Harper's Weekly,* 2 January, 4–6.

Crell, A. F., and W. M. Wallace. 1823–1824. *The family oracle of health or, magazine of domestic economy, medicine, and good living, adapted to all ranks of society, from the palace to the cottage.* London: J. Walker.

Crosby, Alfred W. 1989. *America's forgotten pandemic: The influenza of 1918.* Cambridge: Cambridge University Press.

————. 1976. *Epidemic and peace, 1918.* Westport, Conn.: Greenwood Press.

Cross, W. R. 1965. *The burned over district: The social and intellectual history of enthusiastic religion in western New York, 1800–1850.* New York: Harper and Row.

Crowley, Geoffrey. 1997. How to live to 100. *Newsweek,* 30 June, 56–67.

Daggett, Mabel Poitter. 1912. Women building a better race. *World Work* 25: 228–234.

Dai, Bingham. 1937. *Opium addiction in Chicago.* Shanghai: Commercial Press Limited.

Dakin, Edwin F. 1929. *Mrs. Eddy: The biography of a virginal mind.* New York: Charles Scribner's Sons.

Daniels, W. H. 1878. *The temperance reform and its great reformers.* New York: Nelson and Phillips.

Dannemeyer, William. 1989. *Shadow in the land: Homosexuality in America.* San Francisco: Ignatius Press.

Dannenbaum, Jed. 1981. Origins of temperance activism and militancy among American women. *Journal of Social History* 15: 235–252.

D'Antonio, Michael. 1992. *Heaven on earth.* New York: Crown.

Danziger, Gloria, and Rita J. Simon. 1991. *Women's movements in America: Their successes, disappointments, and aspirations.* Westport, Conn.: Praeger.

Darwin, Charles. 1871. *The descent of man, and selection in relation to sex.* Vol. 2. London: John Murray.

———. 1859. *Origins of the species by means of natural selection, or the preservation of favoured races in the struggle for life.* London: John Murray.

Dass, Baba Ram. 1971. *Be here now.* Cristabol, N.M.: Lama Foundation.

Davenport, Charles Benedict. 1914. The eugenics programme and progress in its achievement. In *Eugenics: Twelve university lectures*, ed. Lucy James Wilson, 1–14. New York: Dodd, Mead.

———. 1911. *Heredity in relation to eugenics.* New York: Holt and Co.

———. 1909. Influence of heredity on human society. In *Race improvement in the United States*, ed. American Academy of Political and Social Science, 16–21. Philadelphia: American Academy of Political and Social Science.

Davis, David B. 1967. *Ante-bellum reform.* New York: Harper and Row.

Davis, Flora. 1991. *Moving the mountain: The women's movement in America since 1960.* New York: Simon and Schuster.

Daynes, Kathryn M. 1991. Plural wives and the nineteenth-century Mormon marriage system. Ph.D. diss., Indiana University.

Dayton, Donald W. 1987. *Theological roots of Pentecostalism.* Grand Rapids: Francis Asbury.

A defense of the Graham system of living: Or, remarks on diet and regimen. Dedicated to the rising generation. 1835. New York: William Applegate.

D'Emilio, John. 1983. Sexual politics, sexual communities: The making of homosexual minority in the United States 1940–1970. Chicago: University of Chicago Press.

Dennett, Mary Ware. 1926. *Birth control laws: Shall we keep them, change them or abolish them.* New York: Frederick H. Hitchcock.

De Quincy, Thomas. 1821. *Confessions of an English opium-eater.* New York: Crowell.

DeVilbiss, Lydia Allen. 1923. *Birth control: What is it?* Boston: Small, Maynard.

The devil did it. 1988. *Nation,* 5 March, 291.

De Witt, Benjamin Parke. 1968. *The Progressive Movement.* 1915. Reprint. Seattle: University of Washington Press.

Diem, Andrea Grace, and James R. Lewis. 1992. Imagining India: The Influence of Hinduism on the New Age movement. In *Perspectives on the New Age*, ed. James R. Lewis and J. Gordon Melton, 48–58. Albany: State University of New York Press.

DiFranza, Joseph R., and Robert A. Lew. 1995. Effect of maternal cigarette smoking on pregnancy complications and sudden infant death syndrome. *Journal of Family Practice* 40: 385–394.

Dillon, Mary Earhart. 1944. *Frances Willard from prayers to politics.* Chicago: University of Chicago Press.

Dillow, Gordon L. 1981. Thank you for not smoking. *American Heritage* 32: 94–107.

Divett, Robert T. 1979. Medicine and the Mormons. *Dialogue: A Journal of Mormon Thought* 12: 16–25.

Doing the Reebok be-bop. 1989. *Newsweek,* 17 June, 79.

Doka, Kenneth J. 1997. *AIDS, fear, and society: Challenging the dreaded disease.* Bristol, Pa.: Taylor & Francis.

Dosch, Nancy Cole. 1993. Exploring alternatives: The use of exercise as a medical therapeutic in mid-nineteenth-century America, 1830–1870. Ph.D. diss., University of Maryland.

Dossey, Larry, and James P. Sawyers. 1994. Introduction. In *Alternative medicine: Expanding medical horizons,* ed. Brian M. Berman and David B. Larson, xxxvii–xiviii. Washington, D.C.: U.S. Government Printing Office.

Doty, Alvah H. 1898. The federal government and the public health. *North American Review* 166: 543–551.

Dougdale, Richard L. 1910. *The Jukes: A study in crime, pauperism, disease, and heredity.* New York: G. P. Putnam's Sons.

Douglas, Mary, and Steven Tipton, eds. 1983. *Religion and America: Spiritual life in a secular age.* Boston: Beacon Press.

Dowbiggin, Ian Robert. 1997. *Keeping America sane: Psychiatry and eugenics in the United States and Canada, 1880–1940.* Ithaca, N.Y.: Cornell University Press.

Drake, Daniel. 1832a. Epidemic cholera in Cincinnati. *Western Journal of Medical and Physical Sciences* 6: 321–364.

———. 1832b. *Practical treatise on the history, prevention, and treatment of epidemic cholera designed both for the profession and the people.* Cincinnati: Corey and Fairbank.

Dresser, Horatio W. 1919. *A history of new thought movement.* New York: Crowell.

Drinking laws come of age. 1986. *U.S. News and World Report,* 9 June, 21.

Drotlet, J. Godias, and Anthony M. Lowell. 1952. *A half century's progress against tuberculosis in New York City, 1900–1950.* New York: New York Tuberculosis and Health Association.

The drug-endangered nation. 1914. *Literary Digest,* 28 March, 678–688.

DuBois, Ellen C. 1997. *Harriot Stanton Blatch and the winning of woman suffrage.* New Haven: Yale University Press.

Dubois, Jean. 1974. Marriage: Physiology discussed, trans. William Greenfield. In *Sex for the Common Man: Nineteenth-century Marriage Manuals.* New York: Arno Press and New York Times.

Dubos, Rene, and Jean Dubos. 1952. *The white plague tuberculosis, man and society.* Boston: Little, Brown.

Duffy, John. 1992. *The sanitarians.* Urbana and Chicago: University of Illinois Press.

Dunn, Halbert L. 1961. *High-level wellness.* Virginia: R. W. Beatty.

Duster, Troy. 1990. *Backdoor to eugenics.* New York: Routledge.

Easing abortion rules. 1967. *Newsweek,* 3 July, 51.

Eastman, Mary F. 1891. *Biography of Dio Lewis.* New York: Fowlers and Wells.

Eddy, Mary Baker. 1906. *Science and health with keys to the scriptures*. Boston: First Church of Christ Scientist.
Eisenberg, David, Ronald C. Kessler, Cindy Foster, Frances E. Norhock, David R. Calkins, and Thomas Delbanco. 1993. Unconventional medicine in the U.S.: prevalence, cost, and patterns of use. *New England Journal of Medicine* 328: 246–252.
Ekirch, Arthur A. 1974. *Progressivism in America. A study of the era from Theodore Roosevelt to Woodrow Wilson*. New York: New Viewpoints.
Eliot, Charles W. 1914. The American Social Hygiene Association. *Social Hygiene* 1 (December): 1–5.
Ellwood, Charles A. 1914. The eugenics movement from the standpoint of sociology. In *Eugenics: Twelve university lectures*, ed. Lucy James Wilson, 213–239. New York: Dodd, Mead.
Engelman, L. 1979. *Intemperance: The lost war against liquor*. New York: Free Press.
Engs, Ruth C. 2000. What should we be researching? Or how those pesky "barbarians" and sanguine "romans" influence research. In *Learning about drinking*, ed. Marcus Grant. Washington, D.C.: International Center for Alcohol Policies.
———. 1998. The relationship between smoking and low grades: Has much changed in a hundred years? Paper presented at the American School Health Association Annual Meeting, October, Colorado Springs, Colorado.
———. 1997. Cycles of social reform: Is the current anti-alcohol movement cresting? *Journal of Studies on Alcohol* 58: 223–224.
———. 1996a. Has the American clean living (anti-alcohol) movement crested? Paper presented at the Kettil-Bruun Epidemiology Conference, 7 June, Edinburgh, Scotland.
———. 1996b. Women, alcohol, and health: A drink a day keeps the heart attack away? *Current Opinion in Psychiatry* 9: 217–220.
———. 1995. Do traditional western European drinking practices have origins in antiquity? *Addiction Research* 2: 227–239.
———. 1992a. *American cycles of prohibition: Do they have origins in western European culture?* Paper presented at the Kettil-Bruun Epidemiology Conference, 4 June, Toronto, Canada.
———. 1992b. It is healthier to drink moderately than to abstain: A politically incorrect statement in America's third clean living cycle. Paper presented at the Nutrition Club, 15 October, Purdue University.
———. 1991a. Resurgence of a new "clean living" movement in the United States. *Journal of School Health* 61: 155–158.
———. 1991b. Romanization and drinking norms: A model to explain differences in Western society. Paper presented at the Society of American Archaeology Annual Meeting, 27 April, New Orleans.
———. 1989. Do warning labels on alcoholic beverages deter alcohol abuse? *Journal of School Health* 59 (March): 116–118.
———. 1981. Responsibility and alcohol. *Health Education* 12: 20–22.
———. 1979. *Alcohol and other drugs: Self-responsibility*. Bloomington, Ind.: Tichenor.
———. 1978. *Teaching health education in the elementary school*. Boston: Houghton Mifflin.

————, ed. 1990a. *Controversies in the addictions field*. Dubuque, Iowa: Kendall/ Hunt.

————, ed. 1990b. *Women: Alcohol and other drugs*. Washington, D.C.: Alcohol Drug Problems Association; Dubuque, Iowa: Kendall/Hunt.

Engs, Ruth C., and M. Aldo-Benson. 1995. The association of alcohol consumption with self-reported illness in university students. *Psychological Reports* 76: 727–736.

Engs, Ruth C., B. A. Diebold, and D. J. Hanson. 1996. The drinking patterns and problems of a national sample of college students, 1994. *Journal of Alcohol and Drug Education* 41: 13–33.

Engs, Ruth C., and Nancy Dosch. n.d. *The relationship of the temperance and other clean living movements: 1820–1870*. Unpublished.

Engs, Ruth C., and S. Fors. 1988. Drug abuse hysteria: The challenge of keeping perspective. *Journal of School Health* 58: 26–28.

Engs, Ruth C., and D. J. Hanson. 2000. Reduction of consumption theory: A test using the drinking patterns and practices of collegiates in the United States, 1983–1994. *College Student Journal*.

————. 1994. Boozing and brawling on campus: A national study of violent problems associated with drinking over the past decade. *Journal of Criminal Justice* 22: 171–180.

————. 1989. Reactance theory: A test with collegiate drinking. *Psychological Reports* 64: 1083–1086.

————. 1988. University students drinking patterns and problems: Examining the effects of raising the purchase age. *Public Health Reports* 1: 65–83.

Engs, Ruth C., and Edwin van Teijlingen. 1997. Correlates of alcohol, tobacco and marijuana use among Scottish postsecondary helping-profession students. *Journal of Studies on Alcohol* 58: 435–444.

Engs, Ruth C., and Molly Wantz. 1978. *Teaching health education in elementary school*. Boston: Houghton Mifflin.

Epidemiologic notes and reports: Antibody to human immunodeficiency virus in female prostitutes. 1987. *MMWR* 36: 157–161.

Epidemiologic notes and reports: Immunodeficiency among female sexual partners of males with acquired immune deficiency syndrome (AIDS)— New York. 1983. *MMWR* 31: 697–698.

Epstein, Barbara Leslie. 1981. *The politics of domesticity: Women, evangelism, and temperance in nineteenth-century America*. Middletown, Conn.: Wesleyan University Press.

E.R.A. is dead, but the 10-year fight for it brought women a long, long way. 1982. *People*, 5 July, 32.

Eriksen, S. 1990. Drunken Danes and sober Swedes? Religious revivalism and the temperance movements as keys to Danish and Swedish folk cultures. In *Language and construction of class identities: The struggle for discursive power in social organization*, ed. B. Strath, 1–10. Gottenburg: Department of History.

Ernst, Robert. 1991. *Weakness is a crime: The life of Bernarr Macfadden*. Syracuse: Syracuse University Press.

Eschewing the fat. 1994. *People*, 8 August, 81.

Eugenics and birth control. 1916. *Literary Digest*, 11 November, 1248.

Extensions of the Food and Drugs Act. 1914. *Scientific American*, 7 March, 194.

Fairholt, F. W. 1859. *Tobacco: Its history and associations*. London: Chapman and Hall.

Fall, Delos. 1897. A plea for the teaching of sanitary science in our schools. *Education* 17: 266–275.

The family vs. the state. 1990. *Newsweek*, 9 July, 22–23.

Faulkner, Harold U. 1939. *American political and social history*. New York: F. S. Crofts.

Fed dope bureau censors drug info. 1984. *High Times*, April, 19, 27.

Fehlandt, August F. 1904. *A century of drink reform in the United States*. Cincinnati: Jennings and Graham.

Ferree, Myra Marx, and Julia McQuillan. 1998. Gender-based pay gaps. *Gender & Society* 12: 7–40.

Fink, Arthur E. 1938. *Causes of crime, biological theories in the United States, 1800–1915*. Philadelphia: University of Pennsylvania Press.

Fisher-LaMay, Craig L. 1989. Testing the limits of free expression: Anthony Comstock and America's Victorian age. Ph.D. diss. University of North Carolina at Chapel Hill.

Fiske, John. 1869. *Tobacco and alcohol: It does pay to smoke; the coming man will drink wine*. New York: Leypoldt and Holt.

Fixx, James F. 1977. *The complete book of running*. New York: Random House.

Fletcher, Horace. 1898. *Happiness as found in forethought minus fearthought*. New York: Stokes.

Fletcher, Robert S. 1943. *A history of Oberlin College: From its foundation through the Civil War*. Oberlin, Ohio: Oberlin College Press.

Flexner, Eleanor. 1975. *Century of struggle: The woman's rights movement in the United States*. Cambridge: Harvard University Press.

Foege, Alec. 1996. *The empire God built: Inside Pat Robertson's media machine*. New York: John Wiley and Sons.

Fogarty, Robert S. 1980. *Dictionary of American communal and utopian history*. Westport, Conn.: Greenwood Press.

Fogel, Robert W. 1995. The fourth great awakening and the political realignment of the 1990s. *Brigham Young University Studies* 35 (3): 31–43.

The food police. 1996. *Health*, November–December, 77.

Foster, Jeffrey Clayton. 1996. The rocky road to a "drug free Tennessee": A history of the early regulation of cocaine and the opiates, 1897–1913. *Journal of Social History* 19: 547–564.

Foster, Lawrence. 1991. *Women, family and utopia: Communal experiments of the Shakers, the Oneida community, and the Mormons*. Syracuse: Syracuse University Press.

———. 1981. *Religion and sexuality: Three American communal experiments of the nineteenth century*. New York: Oxford University Press.

Fowler, Lorenzo N. 1850a. *The illustrated phrenological almanac*. New York: Fowlers and Wells.

———. 1850b. *Marriage: Its history and ceremonies with a phrenological and physiological exposition of the function and qualifications for happy marriages*. 21st ed. New York: Fowlers and Wells.

———. 1848. *Phrenological and physiological almanac for 1848*. New York: Fowlers and Wells.

———. 1844. *The phrenological alamanc*. New York: Lorenzo Fowler.

Fowler, Orson S. 1870. *Sexual science; including manhood, womanhood; and their mutual interrelations; love its laws, power etc.* Philadelphia: National.

———. 1869. *Supplement to "the family." Offspring, and their hereditary endowment: Or paternity, maternity, and infancy; including sexuality; its laws, facts, impairment, restoration, and perfection etc.* Boston: O. S. Fowler.

———. 1859a. *The family: In three volumes.* Vol. 1, *Matrimony;* Vol. 2, *Parentage;* Vol. 3, *Children and home.* New York: O. S. Fowler.

———. 1859b. *Matrimony: As taught by phrenology and physiology: In three parts.* Part I, *Love;* Part II, *Selection;* Part III, *Courtship and married life.* Boston: O. S. Fowler.

———. 1851a. *Amativeness: Or evils and remedies of excessive and perverted sexuality including warning and advice to the married and single, etc.* 13th ed. New York: Fowlers and Wells.

———. 1851b. *Love and parentage: Including important directions and suggestions to lovers and the married concerning strongest ties and the most sacred and momentous relations of life.* 13th ed. New York: Fowlers and Wells.

———. 1847a. *Hereditary descent: Its laws and facts applied to human improvement.* New York: Fowlers and Wells.

———. 1847b. *Love and parentage, applied to the improvement of offspring.* 13th ed. New York: Fowler and Wells.

———. 1841. *Fowler on matrimony: Or phrenology and physiology applied to the selection of suitable companions for life; including the analysis of the domestic faculties; and also directions to the married for living affectionately and happily together, etc.* Philadelphia: O. S. Fowler.

———. 1840. Laws of hereditary descent from "Combe on infancy." *American Phrenological Journal* 3 (October): 36–37.

Fox, Arnold, and Barry Fox. 1996. *Alternative healing.* Franklin Lakes, N.J.: Career Press.

Freeman, Jo. 1971. *The women's liberation movement: Its origin, structures and ideals.* Pittsburgh: Know, Inc. (Documents from the womens liberation movement an on-line archival collection, http://scriptorium.lib.duke.edu, last visited November 23, 1998).

Friedan, Betty. 1963. *The feminine mystique.* New York: Norton.

Fuchs, C. S. 1995. Alcohol consumption and mortality among women. *New England Journal of Medicine* 332: 1245–1250.

Fumento, Michael. 1997. *The fat of the land: The obesity epidemic and how overweight Americans can help themselves.* New York: Viking.

———. 1990. *The myth of heterosexual AIDS.* New York: Basic Books.

Galanter, Marc. 1989. *Cults: Faith, healing, and coercion.* New York: Oxford University Press.

Gale Research. 1998. *Assocations Unlimited* (http://galenet.gale.com, last visited November 28, 1998).

Galton, Francis. 1883. *Inquiries into human faculty and its development.* London: Macmillan.

———. 1869. *Hereditary genius: An inquiry into its laws and consequences.* London: Macmillian.

Gaustand, Edwin S., ed. 1974. *The rise of Adventism: Religion and society in mid-nineteenth-century America.* New York: Harper and Row.

Gavit, John Palmer. 1927. *Opium.* New York: Brentano's.

Gevitz, Norman. 1988. *Other healers: Orthodox medicine in America*. Baltimore: Johns Hopkins University Press.

Gibbons, Henry. 1865. *Tobacco, and its effects: A prize essay*. New York: Nelson and Philips.

Gideonese, Ted. 1998. Death drops but the plague continues. *Newsweek*, 19 October, 72.

Gienapp, William E. 1987. *The origins of the Republican party: 1852–1856*. New York: Oxford University Press.

———. 1985. Nativism and the creation of a republican majority in the north before the Civil War. *Journal of American History* 72: 529–559.

Gillick, M. R. 1984. Health promotion, jogging, and the pursuit of the moral life. *Journal of Health Politics, Policy and Law* 9: 369–387.

Gillispie, Charles C., ed. 1971. *Dictionary of scientific biography*. Vol. 3, *Charles Bendict Davenport*. New York: Charles Scribner's Sons.

Glass, Stephen. 1996. Hazardous to your mental health. *New Republic* 215: 16–18.

Glessner, Thomas A. 1990. *Achieving an abortion-free America by 2001*. Portland, Ore.: Multnomah.

Goddard, Henry H. 1913. *Sterilization and segregation*. New York: Russell Sage Foundation.

———. 1912. *The Kallikak family, a study in the heredity of feeble-mindedness*. New York: Macmillian.

Gold, Mark S. 1993. *Cocaine*. New York: Plenum Medical.

Goldstein, Michael S. 1992. *The health movement: Promoting fitness in America*. New York: Twayne.

Gordon, Anna A. 1898. *The beautiful life of Frances E. Willard*. Chicago: Woman's Temperance Publishing Association.

Gordon-McCutchan, R. C. 1981. The irony of evangelical history. *Journal for the Scientific Study of Religion* 20: 309–326.

Gosney, Ezra S., and Paul Popenoe. 1929. *Sterilization for human betterment: A summary of results of 6,000 operations in California, 1909–1929*. New York: Macmillian.

Gould, Lewis L., ed. 1974. *The progressive era*. Syracuse: Syracuse University Press.

Graham, Judith, ed. 1996. *Current biography yearbook 1996*. New York: H. W. Wilson.

Graham, Sara Hunter. 1996. *Women suffrage and the new democracy*. New Haven: Yale University Press.

Graham, Sylvester. 1848. *A lecture to young men on chastity intended also for the serious consideration of parents and guardians*. 10th ed. Boston: Charles H. Peirce.

———. 1839. *The science of human life*. London: William Lorsell.

———. 1837. *A treatise on bread and bread making*. Boston: Light and Stearns.

———. 1833. *A lecture on epidemic diseases generally, and particularly the spasmodic cholera. Delivered in the City of New York, March 1832*. New York: Day.

Grant, George. 1988. *Grand illusions: The legacy of Planned Parenthood*. Brentwood, Ind.: Wolgemuth and Hyatt.

Grant, Madison. 1970. *The passing of the great race*. New York: Arno Press.

Gray, H. S. 1909. The boy and the cigarette habit. *Education* 29: 294–315.

Gray, Madeline. 1979. *Margaret Sanger: A biography of the champion of birth control*. New York: Richard Marek.

Green, Lawrence W. 1981. *Emerging federal perspectives on health promotion*. New York: Teachers College Columbia University.

Green, Martin. 1992. *Prophets of a new age: The politics of hope from the eighteenth through the twenty-first centuries*. New York: Charles Scribner's Sons.

Greenberg, Daniel S. 1997. Rooting out quack medicine. *Journal of Commerce* 413: 9.

Greenberg, Henry M., and Susan U. Raymond, eds. 1994. *Beyond the crisis: Preserving the capacity for excellence in health care and medical science*. New York: New York Academy of Sciences.

Greene, Harvey. 1986. *Fit for America*. New York: Pantheon Books.

Grinspoon, Lester, and James B. Bakalar. 1985. *Cocaine: A drug and its social evolution*. Rev. ed. New York: Basic Books.

Griscom, John H. 1868. *The use of tobacco: And the evils, physical, mental, moral, and social, resulting therefrom*. New York: G. P. Putnam's Sons.

———. 1845. *The sanitary condition of the laboring population of New York*. New York: Harper and Brothers.

Grittner, Frederick K. 1990. *White slavery: Myth, ideology and American law*. New York: Garland Pub.

Grmek, Mirko D. 1990. *History of AIDS: Emergence and origin of a modern pandemic*. Princeton, N.J.: Princeton University Press.

Grønbaek M. A., T. Deis, U. P. Srensen, Schnohr Becker, and G. Jensen. 1995. Mortality associated with moderate intakes of wine, beer, or spirits. *British Medical Journal* 310: 1165–1169.

Gulick, Luther H. 1908. The high tide of physical conscience. *World's Work* 16: 10383–10386.

Gusfield, Joseph R. 1986. *Symbolic crusade: Status politics and the American temperance movement*. 2d ed. Urbana: University of Illinois Press.

———. 1962. Status conflicts and the changing ideologies of the American temperance movement. In *Society, culture, and drinking patterns*, ed. David J. Pittman and Charles R. Snyder, 101–120. New York: John Wiley and Sons.

Hague, W. Grant. 1914. *The eugenic marriage: A personal guide to the new science of better living and better babies*. Vol. 2. New York: Review of Reviews Company.

Hahnemann, Samuel. 1983. *Organon of medicine*, trans. Jost Khunzli. London: Gollancz.

Haley, Bruce. 1978. *The healthy body and victorian culture*. Cambridge: Harvard University Press.

Hall, Emmett Campbell. 1910. Deadly drugs and beverages. *Good Housekeeping Magazine*, November, 582–584.

Haller, Mark H. 1963. *Eugenics: Hereditarian attitudes in American thought*. New Brunswick, N.J.: Rutgers University Press.

Hambrick-Stowe, Charles E. 1996. *Charles Finney and the spirit of American evangelicalism*. Grand Rapids, Mich.: W. B. Eerdmans.

Hamm, Richard F. 1996. Administration and prison suasion: Law enforcement in the American temperance movement, 1880–1920. *Contemporary Drug Problems* 21: 375–399.

————. 1995. *Shaping of the Eighteenth Amendment: Temperance reform, legal culture, and the policy, 1880–1920.* Chapel Hill: University of North Carolina Press.

Hammond, E. Cuyler, and Daniel Horn. 1954. The relationship between human smoking habits and death rates: A follow-up study of 187,766 men. *Journal of the American Medical Association* 155: 1316–1328.

Handy, Robert T. 1966. *The social gospel in America 1870–1920.* New York: Oxford University Press.

Hanegraaff, Wouter J. 1996. *New age religion and Western culture: Esotericism in the mirror of secular thought.* New York: E. J. Brill.

Hansen, Klaus J. 1981. *Mormonism and the American experience.* Chicago: University of Chicago Press.

Hanson, David. J. 1995. *Preventing alcohol abuse.* Westport, Conn.: Praeger.

Hardman, Keith J. 1987. *Charles Grandison Finney, 1792–1875: Revivalist and reformer.* Syracuse, N.Y.: Syracuse University Press.

Harper, Ida H., ed. 1922. *The history of woman suffrage.* Vol. 5. New York: National American Women Suffrage Association.

Hart, Hastings H. 1912. Sterilization as a practical measure. New York: Department of Child Helping of the Russell Sage Foundation.

Hatch, Nathan O. 1984. Millennialism and popular religion in the early republic. In *The evangelical tradition in America*, ed. Leonard I. Sweet, 113–130. Macon, Ga.: Mercer University Press.

Healer of hearts. 1998. *Newsweek,* 16 March, 50.

Healthy people 2000: National health promotion and disease prevention objectives. 1990. Washington, D.C.: U.S. Department of Health and Human Services.

Heath, D. B. 1989. The new temperance movement: Through the looking glass. In *Current Issues in Alcohol/Drug Studies*, ed. Edith S. Liansky Gomberg, 143–168. New York: Haworth Press.

Hečlo, Hugh. 1996. The sixties' false dawn: Awakenings, movements and postmodern policy-making. *Journal of Policy History* 8: 34–63.

Heelas, Paul. 1996. *The new age movement: The celebration of the self and the sacralization of modernity.* Cambridge, Mass.: Blackwell.

Heimann, Robert K. 1960. *Tobacco and Americans.* New York: McGraw-Hill.

Hellman, Arthur D. 1975. *Laws against marijuana: The price we pay.* Urbana: University of Illinois Press.

Helms, Robert B., ed. 1993. *American health policy: Critical issues for reform.* Washington D.C.: AEI Press.

Hemmingway, William. 1913. Building men not champions. *Harper's Weekly,* 14 June, 11.

Henning, Joel F. 1978. *Holistic running: Beyond the threshold of fitness.* New York: Antheneum.

Henson, Graham E. 1909. Let us stop dying before we have to. *The World Today* 17: 1044–1047.

Herbst, Jurgen. 1963. Editor's introduction to *Our country*, by Josiah Strong. Cambridge, Mass.: Belknap Press of Harvard University Press.

Herrnstein, Richard J., and Charles Murray. 1994. *The bell curve: Intelligence and class structure in American life.* New York: Free Press.

Hicks, John D. 1931. *The populist revolt a history of the Farmers' Alliance and the People's Party.* Minneapolis: University of Minnesota Press.

Hill, Donna. 1983. *Joseph Smith, the first Mormon.* Midvale, Utah: Signature Books.

Hilts, Philip J. 1992. US puts a halt to talks tying genes to crime. *New York Times,* 5 September, 1.

Hirshberg, Leonard K. 1913. Marvelous preventives of disease. *Worlds Work,* 25 April, 684–694.

Hitchcock, Edward. 1831. *Dyspepsia forestalled and resisted: Or lectures on diet, regime, and employment.* Amherst, Mass.: J. S. and C. Adams.

———. 1830. Dyspepsia forestalled and resisted: Or lectures on diet, regimen, and employment. *Journal of Health* 1: 311–315.

Hitchcock, Edward, Jr. 1895. The gymnastic era and athletic era of our country. *Outlook,* 18 May, 816–818.

Hoffer, Eric. 1951. *The true believer: Thoughts on the nature of mass movements.* New York: Harper and Row.

Hofstadter, Richard. 1959a. *The age of reform: From Bryan to F.D.R.* New York: Alfred A. Knopf.

———. 1959b. *Social Darwinism in American thought.* New York: George Braziller.

———, ed. 1986. *The progressive movement: 1900–1915.* New York: Simon and Schuster.

Hole, Judith, and Ellen Levine. 1971. *Rebirth of feminism.* New York: Quadrangle Books.

Holt, Michael F. 1973. The politics of impatience: The origins of know nothingism. *Journal of American History* 60: 309–331.

Holt, William Leland. 1913. Economic factors in eugenics. *Popular Science Monthly* 83: 471–483.

Hopkins, Charles Howard. 1961. *The rise of the social gospel in American Protestantism, 1865–1915.* New Haven: Yale University Press.

Hopkins, Mary A. 1915. Birth control and public morals: An interview with Anthony Comstock. *Harper's Weekly,* 22 May, 489–490.

How high? How fast? 1996. *Newsweek,* 24 July, 22.

How much, if any, should we smoke? 1907. *American Monthly Review of Reviews* 35: 342–343.

How the new drug laws work. 1915. *Literary Digest,* 10 July, 57–58.

Hubbard, Ruth, and Elijah Wald. 1993. *Exploding the gene myth.* Boston: Beacon Press.

Hubbell, Charles B. 1904. The cigaret habit—a new peril. *The Independent,* 18 February, 375–378.

Huber, John B. 1913. Books: Preventive medicine. *Harper's Weekly,* 13 September, 29.

Hudson, Winthrop S. 1974. A time of religious ferment. In *The rise of Adventism: Religion and society in mid-nineteenth-century America,* ed. Edwin S. Gaustand, 1–17. New York: Harper and Row.

———. 1965. *Religion in America.* New York: Charles Scribner's Sons.

Hufford, David J. 1988. Contemporary folk medicine. In *Other healers: Unorthodox medicine in America,* ed. Norman Gevitz, 228–264. Baltimore: Johns Hopkins University Press.

Huxley, Aldous. 1971. *Brave new world.* London: Folio Society.

Iglehart, Ferdinand C. 1911. Voting out the liquor traffic. *Review of Reviews* 43: 215–218.

Iglehart, J. K. 1986. The campaign against smoking gains momentum. *New England Journal of Medicine* 314: 1059–1064.

Important facts for young men showing the destructive effects of masturbation and the frequency of hernia and rupture. 1844. West Brookfield: Charles A. Mirick.

Index. 1830. *Journal of Health* 2: 387–391.

———. 1829. *Journal of Health* 1: 385–390.

Inebriety—a disease. 1897. *Harper's Weekly*, 20 November, 1160.

Infant mortality by marital status of mother—United States, 1983. 1990. *MMWR* 39: 521–523.

Ingle, Dwight J. 1973. *Who should have children? An environmental and genetic approach.* Indianapolis: Bobbs-Merrill.

Jacobs, Philip P. 1908. *The campaign against tuberculosis in the United States.* New York: Charities Publication Committee.

Jacobson, Michael. 1994. Quoted by Linda Rocawich. Michael Jacobson. *Progressive* (September): 30–35.

Jacoby, Kerry N. 1998. *The drive to abolish abortion since 1973.* Westport, Conn.: Praeger.

Jacoby, Russell, and Naomi Glauberman, eds. 1995. *The bell curve debate: History, debate, opinions.* New York: Times Books.

Jellinek, Elvin M. 1961. *The disease concept of alcoholism.* New Haven: Hillhouse.

Jensen, Arthur R. 1969. How much can we boost IQ and scholastic achievement. *Harvard Educational Review* 39: 1–123.

Jessee, Dean C., ed. 1989. *The papers of Joseph Smith.* Vol. 2, *Journal, 1832–1842.* Salt Lake City: Deseret.

Johnson, Haynes. 1989. To war: Rhetoric and reality. *Washington Post*, 8 September, 2a.

Johnson, P. E. 1978. *A shopkeeper's millennium: Society and revivals in Rochester, New York 1815–1837.* New York: Hill and Wang.

Johnson, Richard Christian. 1973. *Anthony Comstock: Reform, vice and the American way.* Ph.D. diss. University of Wisconsin.

Johnston, Lloyd D., Patrick M. O'Malley, and Jerald G. Bachman. 1998. *National survey results on drug use from the Monitoring the Future study 1975–1997.* Vol. 1. Rockville, Md.: National Institute on Drug Abuse, U.S. Dept. of Heath and Human Services.

———. 1989. *Drug use, drinking, and smoking: National survey results from high school, college, and young adults populations: 1975–1988.* Rockville, Md.: U.S. Department of Health and Human Services.

———. 1987. *National trends in drug use and related factors among American high school students and young adults, 1987–1986.* Washington, D.C.: U.S. Department of Health and Human Services.

Jones, K. L., and D. W. Smith. 1973. Recognition of the fetal alcohol syndrome in early infancy. *Lancet* 2: 999–1001.

Jonnes, Jill. 1996. *Hep-cats, narcs, and pipe dreams: A history of America's romance with illegal drugs.* New York: Scribner.

Jordan, David Starr. 1902. *The blood of the nation: A study of the decay of races through the survival of the unfit.* Boston: American Unitarian Association.

Jordan, Harvey Ernest. 1914. Eugenics: Its data, scope and promise, as seen by the anatomist. In *Eugenics: Twelve university lectures,* ed. Lucy James Wilson, 107–138. New York: Dodd, Mead.

Jorstad, Erling. 1987. *The new Christian right, 1981–1988: Prospects for the post-Reagan decade.* Vol. 25, *Studies in American Religion.* Lewiston, N.Y.: Edwin Mellen Press.

Junk food, enemy no. 1. 1996. *U.S. News and World Report,* 13 May, 89.

Kaiser, Barbara, and Irwin Kaiser. 1974. The challenge of the women's movement to American gynecology. *American Journal of Obstertics and Gynecology* 120: 652–661.

Kaufman, Martin. 1988. Homeopathy in America: The rise and fall and persistence of a medical heresy. In *Other healers: Orthodox medicine in America,* ed. Norman Gevitz, 99–124. Baltimore: Johns Hopkins University Press.

Kazin, Michael. 1995. *The populist persuasion: An American history.* New York: Basic Books.

Keelor, Richard O. 1978. Quoted in John S. Long. The Fitness Mania. *U.S. News and World Report,* 27 February, 37–40.

Keeping fit: America tries to shape up. 1978. *Newsweek,* 23 May, 79.

Keller, Mark. 1979. Foreword, *Youth, alcohol, and social policy,* ed. Howard T. Blane and Morris E. Chafetz, ix–xi. New York: Plenum Press.

Keller, Morton. 1977. *Affairs of state.* Cambridge: Belknap Press of Harvard University Press.

Kelly, Aidan A. 1992. An update on neopagan witchcraft in America. In *Perspectives on the new age,* ed. James R. Lewis and J. Gordon Melton, 136–151. Albany: State University of New York Press.

Kelly, James R. 1995. Beyond compromise: Casey, common ground, and the pro-life movement. In *Abortion politics in the American states,* ed. Mary C. Segers and Timothy A. Byrnes, 205–224. Armonk, N.Y.: M. E. Sharpe.

Kennedy, David M. 1970. *Birth control in America: The career of Margaret Sanger.* New Haven: Yale University Press.

Kennedy, Joseph. 1985. *Coca exotica, The illustrated story of cocaine.* Cranbury, N.J.: Associated University Presses.

Kenny, Michael G. 1990. The democratic medicine of Dr. Elias Smith. *Annual Proceedings* 15: 133–141.

Kern, Louis J. 1981. *An ordered love: Sex roles and sexuality in Victorian Utopias— the Shakers, the Mormons, and the Oneida community.* Chapel Hill: University of North Carolina Press.

Kerr, Austin, K. 1985. *Organized for prohibition: A new history of the Anti-Saloon League.* New Haven: Yale University Press.

Kesselman, Amy. 1991. The "freedom suit": Feminism and dress reform in the United States, 1848–1875. *Gender and Society* 5: 495–510.

Kett, Joseph F. 1968. *The formation of the American medical profession.* New Haven: Yale University Press.

Kevles, Daniel J. 1985. *In the name of eugenics: Genetics and the uses of human heredity.* New York: Alfred A. Knoff.

Kevles, Daniel J., and Leroy Hood, ed. 1992. *The code of codes: Scientific and social issues in the human genome project.* Cambridge: Harvard University Press.

Kiger, Patrick J., and Lucy Page Gaston. 1997. *Discovery Channel Online* (http:/ /discovery.com, last visited June 23, 1999).

Kinsley, M. 1991. Cocktails for two. *New Republic*, 3 June, 6.

Kluger, Richard. 1996. *Ashes to ashes: America's hundred-year cigarette war, the public health, and the unabashed triumph of Philip Morris*. New York: Alfred A. Knopf.

Knopf, S. Adolphus. 1922. *A History of the National Tuberculosis Association: The anti-tuberculosis movement in the United States*. New York: National Tuberculosis Association.

———. 1914. The modern aspect of the tuberculosis problem in rural communities and the duty of the health officers. *American Journal of Public Health* 4: 1132.

Knowles, John H., ed. 1977. *Doing better and feeling worse: Health in the United States*. New York: W. W. Norton.

Kober, George M. 1897. The progress and achievements of hygiene. *Science* 6: 789–799.

Kobler, John. 1973. *Ardent spirits: The rise and fall of prohibition*. New York: Putnam.

Krout, John Allen. 1925. *The origins of prohibition*. New York: Russell and Russell.

Kselman, Thomas. 1983. *Miracles and prophecies in nineteenth-century France*. New Brunswick, N.J.: Rutgers University Press.

Kurtz, Ernest. 1979. *Not-God: A history of alcoholics anonymous*. Center City, Mich.: Hazelden Educational Services.

Lader, Lawrence. 1967. *Abortion*. Boston: Beacon Press.

Larson, Andrew Karl. 1946. *Agricultural pioneering in the Virgin River basin*. Provo, Utah: Brigham Young University Press.

Larson, Edward J. 1995. *Sex, race and science: Eugenics in the deep south*. Baltimore: Johns Hopkins University Press.

Laughlin, Harry Hamilton. 1922. *Eugenical sterilization in the United States*. Chicago: Psychopathic Laboratory of the Municipal Court of Chicago.

Lawrence, S. 1990. Keeping Employees Healthy. *Personnel Journal* 16: 14.

Learning to harness the power. 1989. *Newsweek*, 13 November, 50.

Lee, Mable, and Bruce L. Bennett. 1960. This is our heritage. *Journal of Health, Physical Education and Recreation* 31 (April): 25–33, 38–47.

Lee, Nancy Howell. 1969. *The search for an abortionist*. Chicago: University of Chicago Press.

Legan, Marshall S. 1987. Hydropathy, or water-cure. In *Pseudo-science and society in nineteenth-century America*, ed. Arthur Wrobel, 79–99. Lexington: University of Kentucky Press.

———. 1971. Hydropathy in America: A nineteenth century panacea. *Bulletin of the History of Medicine* 45: 267–280.

Leland, John, and Jeanne Gordon. 1996. The end of AIDS. *Newsweek*, 10 December, 62.

LeMaistre, Charles. 1996. Tobacco's role as gateway drug often ignored. *Dallas Morning News*, 21 October, 15A.

Lender, Mark E. 1984. *Dictionary of American temperance biography: From temperance reform to alcohol research, the 1600s to the 1980s*. Westport, Conn.: Greenwood Press.

Lender, Mark E., and J. K. Martin. 1987. *Drinking in America: A history*. Rev. and exp. ed. New York: Free Press.

Leonard, Priscilla. 1908. The Christmas stamp in America. *Outlook* 90: 265–268.

Levine, Harry Gene. 1992. Temperance cultures: Concern about alcohol problems in Nordic and English-speaking cultures. In *The nature of alcohol and drug related problems*, ed. M. Lader, G. Edwards, and D. C. Drummond, 15–36. Oxford: Oxford University Press.

———. 1984. The alcohol problem in America: From temperance to Alcoholism. *British Journal of Addiction* 79: 109–119.

———. 1978. The discovery of addiction. *Journal of Studies on Alcohol* 39: 147–151.

Lewis, Dio. 1871. *Our girls*. New York: Harper and Brothers.

———. 1862. *New Gymnastics*. Boston: Ticknor and Fields.

Lewis, James R., and J. Gordon Melton, eds. 1992. *Perspectives on the New Age*. Albany: State University of New York Press.

Lienesch, Michael. 1993. *Redeeming America: Piety and politics in the new Christian right*. Chapel Hill: University of North Carolina Press.

Lindsay, Thomas M. 1905. Revivals. *Contemporary Review* 88: 344–362.

Lissner, Edward. 1907. Dry days in the south. *Harper's Weekly*, 20 July, 1057.

Locke, David R. 1885. Prohibition. *North American Review* 143: 382–397.

Low, A. Maurice. 1913. To make opium contraband. *Harper's Weekly*, 31 May, 8.

Lowenthal, Jeff. 1978. Abortion under attack. *Newsweek*, 5 June, 36–47.

Lucas, Philip C. 1992. The new age movement and the Pentecostal/charismatic revival: Distinct yet parallel phases of a fourth great awakening? In *Perspectives on the New Age*, ed. James R. Lewis and J. Gordon Melton, 189–212. Albany: State University of New York Press.

Macfadden, Mary. 1956. *Dumbells and carrot strips: The story of Bernarr Macfadden*. London: Victor Gollancz.

Malone, Dumas, ed. 1957. *Dictionary of American biography*. Vols. 6 and 7. New York: Charles Scribner's Sons.

Mann, Arthur, ed. 1963. *The progressive era: Liberal renaissance or liberal failure?* New York: Holt, Rinehart and Winston.

Marcus, Alan I. 1979. Disease prevention in America: From a local to a national outlook, 1880–1910. *Bulletin of the History of Medicine* 53: 184–202.

Markel, Howard. 1997. *Quarantine! East European Jewish immigrants and the New York City epidemics of 1892*. Baltimore: Johns Hopkins University Press.

Marsden, George M. 1991. *Understanding fundamentalism and evangelicalism*. Grand Rapids, Mich.: William B. Eerdmans.

———. 1983. Preachers of paradox: The religious new right in historical perspective. In *Religion and America spiritual life in a secular age*, ed. Mary Tipton and Steven Tipton, 150–168. Boston: Beacon Press.

Martin, E. S. 1900. This busy world. *Harper's Weekly*, 7 July, 631.

Mason, Harry B. 1900. The urgent need of pure food reform. *Outlook* 65: 400–406.

Maxcy, Spencer J., and Terry Todd. 1987. The educational philosophy of a superman: Bernarr Macfadden and the physical culture movement. *Vitae Scholasticae* 6: 155–187.

McCall, Laura. 1994. "With all the wild, trembling, rapturous feelings of a lover": Men, women, and sexuality in American literature, 1820–1860. *Journal of the Early Republic* 14: 71–89.

———. 1989. "The reign of brute force is now over": A content analysis of Godey's Lady's Book, 1830–1860. *Journal of the Early Republic* 9: 217–236.

McCary, James Leslie. 1973. *Human sexuality*. New York: Van Nostrand.

McCue, Robert J. 1981. Did the word of wisdom become a commandment in 1851? *Dialogue: A Journal of Mormon Thought* 14 (Autumn): 66–77.

McCuen, Gary E., and David L. Bender, eds. 1972. *The sexual revolution: Traditional mores versus new values*. Minneapolis: Greenhaven Press.

McGee, Glenn. 1997. *The perfect baby: A pragmatic approach to genetics*. Lanham: Rowman & Littlefield.

McGowan, Richard. 1995. *Business, politics, and cigarettes: Multiple levels, multiple agendas*. Westport, Conn.: Quorum Books.

McIntosh, Elaine N. 1995. *American food habits in historical perspective*. Westport, Conn.: Praeger.

McLoughlin, William G. 1978. *Revivals, awakenings, and reform: An essay on religion and social change in America, 1607–1977*. Chicago: University of Chicago Press.

———. 1968. Introduction: How is America religious? In *Religion in America*, ed. William G. Mcloughlin and Robert N. Bellah, ix–xxiv. Boston: Houghton Mifflin.

McNeill, William Hardy. 1976. *Plagues and peoples*. Garden City, N.Y.: Anchor Press.

Melton, J. Gordon. 1992. New thought and the New Age. In *Perspectives on the New Age*, ed. James R. Lewis and J. Gordon Melton, 15–29. Albany: State University of New York Press.

———. 1986. *Encyclopedic handbook of cults in America*. New York: Garland.

Melton, J. Gordon, Phillip Charles Lucas, and Jon R. Stone. 1997. Prime-time religion: An encyclopedia of religious broadcasting. Phoenix: Oryx Press.

Meyer, Donald. 1988. *The positive thinkers: Popular religious psychology from Mary Baker Eddy to Norman Vincent Peale and Ronald Reagan*. Rev. ed. with a new introduction. Middletown, Conn.: Wesleyan University Press.

Miller, A., and E. Bradburn. 1991. Shape up—or else. *Newsweek*, 1 July, 42.

Miller, L. K., and Lawrence W. Fielding. 1995. The battle between the for-profit health club and the "commercial" YMCA. *Journal of Sport and Social Issues* 19: 76–107.

Mines, Flavel. 1891. Drunkenness is curable. *North American Review* 153: 442–449.

Minkowitz, Donna. 1992. Outlawing gays. *Nation*, 19 October, 420–422.

Money, John. 1985. *The destroying angel: Sex, fitness & food in the legacy of degeneracy theory, graham crackers, Kellogg's corn flakes & American health history*. Buffalo, N.Y.: Prometheus Books.

Moore, Mark. H., and Dean R. Gerstein, eds. 1981. *Alcohol and public policy: Beyond the shadow of prohibition*. Washington, D.C.: National Academy Press.

Morantz, Regina Markell. 1977. Nineteenth century health reform and women: A program of self help. In *Medicine without doctors: Home health care in American history*, ed. Gunder B. Risse, Ronald L. Numbers, and Judith Walyer Leavitt, 73–93. New York: Science History Publications.

Morite, Charles, ed. 1978. *Current biography*. New York: H. W. Wilson.

Mosher, James F. 1997. What place for alcoholic beverage container labels? A view from the United States. *Addiction* 92: 791.

Mott, Frank L. 1957. *History of the American magazine: 1741–1850*. Cambridge: Belknap Press of Harvard University Press.

———. 1930. *History of American magazines*. Vol. 5. Cambridge: Harvard University Press.

Must lady nicotine follow John Barleycorn? 1919. *The Literary Digest*, 15 March, 19–20.

Musto, David F. 1996. Alcohol in American history. *Scientific American* 274 (April): 78–83.

———. 1989a. America's first cocaine epidemic. *Wilson Quarterly* 13: 59–64.

———. 1989b. Evolution of American attitudes toward substance abuse. *Annals of the New York Academy of Science* 562: 3–7.

———. 1987. *The American disease: Origins of narcotic control*. New York: Oxford University Press.

National Institute of Alcohol Abuse (NIAAA). 1976. *Drinking etiquette for those who drink and those who don't*. Rockville, Md.: NIAAA.

Neuhaus, Richard John, ed. 1990. *Guaranteeing the good life: Medicine and the return of eugenics*. Grand Rapids, Mich.: William B. Eerdmans.

The new gay struggle. 1998. *Time*, 26 October, 32.

New York: Backlash on abortion. 1972. *Newsweek*, 22 May, 32.

NHSDA. 1998. *Office of applied studies, national household survey on drug abuse advance report #18*, http://www.samhsda.gov/oas/nhsda, last visited August 11, 1998.

Nissenbaum, Stephen. 1980. *Sex, diet and debility in Jacksonian America: Sylvester Graham and health reform*. Westport, Conn.: Greenwood Press.

Noyes, John Humphrey. 1872. *Male continence*. Oneida, N.Y.: Office of Oneida.

Numbers, Ronald L. 1976. *Prophetess of health: Ellen G. White*. New York: Harper and Row.

O'Donnell, John A., and R. R. Clayton. 1982. The stepping stone hypothesis: Marihuana, heroin and causality. *Chemical Dependency* 4: 229–241.

Office for Substance Abuse Prevention (OSAP). 1991. *OSAP Issue Forum: A response to societies mixed messages: Environmental strategies to reduce ATOD problems*. Philadelphia: U.S. Alcohol, Drug Abuse and Mental Health Administration (ADAMHA).

———. 1990. *Prevention Monograph 6–Youth and drugs: Societies's mixed messages*. Rockville, Md.: OSAP.

———. 1989. *Policy review guidelines: Message and material review process*. Rockville, Md.: OSAP.

Ogle, Maureen. 1993. Domestic reform and American household plumbing, 1840–1870. *Winterthur Portfolio* 28: 33–58.

O'Hara, Leo J. 1989. *An emerging profession: Philadelphia doctors 1860–1900*. New York: Garland.

Ornish, Dean. 1990. *Dr. Dean Ornish's program for reversing heart disease: The only system scientifically proven to reverse heart disease without drugs or surgery*. New York: Random House.

———. 1983. *Stress, diet, and your heart*. New York: Holt, Rinehart, and Winston.

O'Shea, Michael V. 1923. *Tobacco and mental efficiency*. New York: Macmillian.

Pace, Gene. 1982. Wives of nineteenth-century Mormon bishops: A quantitative analysis. *Journal of the West* 21 (3): 23–31.

Pacific coast social hygiene conference. 1914. *Survey,* 29 August, 554.

Park, Roberta J. 1977. The attitudes of leading New England transcendental-
    ists toward healthful exercise, active recreations and proper care of the
    body: 1830–1860. *Journal of Sport History* 4: 34–50.

Parmet, Robert D. 1966. Connecticut's know-nothings: A profile. *Connecticut
    Historical Society Bulletin* 31 (3): 84–90.

The "patent medicine" crusade. 1905. *The Nation,* 9 November, 376.

Paul, Diane B. 1995. *Controlling human heredity: 1865 to the present.* Atlantic
    Highlands, N.J.: Humanities Press International.

Paulson, Ross Evans. 1973. *Women's suffrage and prohibition: A comparative study
    of equality and social control.* Glenview, Ill.: Scott, Foresman.

Paulty, Philip J. 1985. The struggle for ignorance about alcohol: American physi-
    ologists, Wilbur Olin Atwater, and the Woman's Christian Temperance
    Union. *Bulletin of Historical Medicine* 64: 366–392.

Peabody, Francis G. 1905. *The liquor problem: A summary of investigations con-
    ducted by the Committee of Fifty, 1893–1903.* Boston: Houghton Mifflin.

Pearl, Raymond. 1908. Breeding better men. *World Work* 15: 9818–9824.

Peel, Robert. 1988. *Health and medicine in the Christian science tradition.* New
    York: Crossroad Press.

———. 1977. *Mary Baker Eddy: The years of authority.* New York: Holt, Rinehart
    and Winston.

———. 1971. *Mary Baker Eddy: The years of trial.* New York: Holt, Rinehart and
    Winston.

———. 1966. *Mary Baker Eddy: The years of discovery.* New York: Holt, Rinehart
    and Winston.

Peele, Stanton. 1993. The conflict between public health goals and the temper-
    ance mentality. *American Journal of Public Health* 83: 805–810.

———. 1989. *Diseasing of America: Addiction treatment out of control.* Lexington,
    Mass.: Lexington Books.

Peele, Stanton, and Archie Brodsky. 1998. Gateway to nowhere: How alcohol
    came to be scapegoated for drug abuse. *Addiction Research* 5: 419–426.

———. 1991. Abuse. *Reason,* November, 32–39.

Pernick, Martin S. 1997. Eugenics and public health in American history. *Ameri-
    can Journal of Public Health* 87: 1767–1772.

———. 1996. *The black stork: Eugenics and the death of "defective" babies in Ameri-
    can medicine and motion pictures since 1915.* New York: Oxford Univer-
    sity Press.

Perry, Lewis. 1983. Sex and communitas. *Queen's Quarterly* 90: 768–778.

Peterson, Paul H. 1972. An historical analysis of the word of wisdom. Master's
    thesis, Brigham Young University.

Phillips, Paul T. 1996. *A kingdom on earth: Anglo-American social Christianity,
    1880–1940.* University Park: Pennsylvania State University Press.

Phrenological Almanac. 1844. New York: Fowler and Wells.

Pickens, Donald. 1968. *Eugenics and the progressives.* Nashville, Tenn.: Vanderbilt
    University Press.

Pittman, David J. 1980. *Primary prevention of alcohol abuse and alcoholism: An
    evaluation of the control of consumption policy.* St. Louis, Mo.: Social Sci-
    ence Institute, Washington University Press.

Pittman, David J., and Charles R. Snyder. 1962. *Society, culture, and drinking patterns.* New York: John Wiley and Sons.

Pivar, David J. 1973. *Purity crusade: Sexual morality and social control, 1868–1900.* Westport, Conn.: Greenwood Press.

Pollack, Norman. 1967. *The populist mind.* Indianapolis: Bobbs-Merrill.

———. 1962. *The populist response to industrial America: Midwestern populist thought.* Cambridge: Harvard University Press.

Powell, Aaron Macy. 1976. *The National Purity Congress.* 1896. Reprint. New York: Arno Press.

Pregnant women face detention. 1998. *AIM* 7: 14.

President's Council on Physical Fitness. 1979. *Adult physical fitness: a program for men and women.* Washington, D.C.: U.S. Government Printing Office.

Prevention. 1950–1999. Emmaus, Pa.: Rodale Press.

Prevention Index. 1983–1993. Emmaus, Pa.: Rodale Press.

Pro-choice: A sleeping giant awakens. 1989. *Newsweek,* 24 April, 39–40.

Pro-choice politicking. 1989. *Newsweek,* 9 October, 34–36.

Prohibition or temperance—Which? 1903. *Outlook* 73: 857–859.

Purcell, N. 1985. Wine and wealth in ancient Italy. *Journal of Roman Studies* 75: 1–19.

Putney, Clifford. 1994a. Men and religion: Aspects of the church brotherhood movement, 1880–1920. *Anglican and Episcopal History* 58: 430–467.

———. 1994b. *Muscular Christianity: The strenuous mood in American Protestantism, 1880–1920.* Hanover, N.H.: Brandeis University Press.

———. 1991. Character building in the YMCA, 1880–1930. *Mid-America, An Historical Review* 73: 49–70.

Quebedeaux, Richard. 1983. *The new charismatics.* Rev. ed. San Francisco: Harper and Row.

Raloff, J. 1996. Have the Danes solved the French paradox? *Science News* 149: 197.

Rapaport, Jeniffer. 1996. Dueling pyramids. *Women's Sport and Fitness* 18: 95–97.

Rauschenbusch, Walter. 1904. The ideals of social reformers. *American Journal of Sociology* 2: 202–219.

Reagan, Nancy. 1983. Quoted in Carmody, John, "Now here's the news," *Washington Post,* 13 October 1983, D9.

Reed, Ralph. 1996. *Active faith: How Christians are changing the soul of American politics.* New York: Free Press.

Reed, W. James. 1978. *From private vice to public virtue: The birth control movement and American society since 1830.* New York: Basic Books.

Reich, David. 1996. Review. *UU World* 10: 52–55.

Reichley, A. James. 1992. *The life of the parties: A history of American political parties.* New York: Free Press.

Reid, George W. 1982. *A sound of trumpets: Americans, adventists, and health reform.* Washington, D.C.: Review and Herald.

Reiser, S. 1985. Responsibility for personal health. *Journal of Medicine and Philosophy* 10: 7–17.

Remini, Robert V. 1989. *The Jacksonian era.* Arlington Heights, Ill.: Harlan Davidson.

Remini, Robert V., and Edwin A. Miles. 1979. *The era of good feelings and the age of Jackson, 1816–1841.* Arlington Heights, Ill.: AHM.

Remley, Mary L. 1983. *Sport history in the United States: An overview.* Bloomington, Ind.: Organization of American Historians.

Rentoul, Robert Reid. 1906. *Race culture: Or, race suicide (a plea for the unborn).* New York: Walter Scott.

Richards, Edgar. 1890. Legislation on food adulteration. *Science,* 22 August, 101–104.

Ricketson, Shadrach. 1806. *Means of preserving health, and preventing diseases: Founded principally on an attention to air and climate, drink, food, sleep, exercise, clothing, passions of the mind, and retentions and excretions, etc.* New York: Collins Perkins.

Ridinger, Robert B. Marks. 1996. *The gay and lesbian movement: References and resources.* New York: G. K. Hall.

Rifkin, Jeremy. 1998. Avoid this dangerous path. *USA Today,* 11 September, 14A.

The right to lifers new tactics. 1990. *Newsweek,* 9 July, 23–28.

Rimm, E. B., and R. C. Ellison. 1995. Alcohol in the Mediterranean diet. *American Journal of Clinical Nutrition* 61: 1378S–1382S.

The rise of born-again politics: A profile of Jerry Falwell. 1980. *Newsweek,* 15 September, 28–32, 36, 37.

Robert, Joseph C. 1949. *The story of tobacco in America.* New York: Alfred A. Knopf.

Robertson, Constan. 1970. *The Oneida community: An autobiography, 1851–76.* Syracuse, N.Y.: Syracuse University Press.

Robertson, Pat. 1986. *America's date with destiny.* Nashville: Nelson.

Rochard, Jules M. 1892. Tobacco and the tobacco habit. *Popular Science Monthly* 41: 670–682.

Rockafellar, Nancy. 1986. In gauze we trust: Public health and the Spanish influenza on the home front. *Pacific Northwest Quarterly* 77 (3): 104–113.

Rohe, Fred. 1974. *The zen of running.* New York: Random House.

Rohrer, James R. 1990. The origins of the temperance movement: A reinterpretation. *Journal of American Studies* 24: 228–235.

Room, R. 1987. *Social dimensions of alcohol dependence.* Berkeley, Calif.: Medical Research Institute of San Francisco, Alcohol Research Group.

Rorabaugh, William J. 1991. Alcohol in America. *OAH Magazine of History* 6: 17–19.

———. 1979. *The alcoholic republic, an American tradition.* New York: Oxford University Press.

———. 1976. Estimated U.S. alcoholic beverage consumption, 1790–1860. *Journal of Studies on Alcohol* 37: 360–361.

Rosell, Garth M. 1984. Charles G. Finney: His place in the stream. In *The evangelical tradition in America,* ed. Leonard I. Sweet, 131–148. Macon, Ga.: Mercer University Press.

Rosenberg, Charles E. 1987. *The cholera years: The United States in 1832, 1849, and 1866.* Chicago: University of Chicago Press.

———. 1976. *No other gods: On science and American social thought.* Baltimore: Johns Hopkins University Press.

Rosenberg, Charles E., and Carroll Rosenberg. 1968. Pietism and the origins of the American public health movement: A note on John H. Griscom and Robert M. Hartley. *Journal of the History of Medicine and Allied Sciences* 23: 16–35.

Rosenfeld, Albert. 1969. Challenge to the miracle of life. *Life,* 13 June, 40.

Rosett, Henry, and Lyn Weiner. 1984. *Alcohol and the fetus: A clinical perspective.* New York: Oxford University Press.

Ross, Edward. 1901. The causes of race superiority. *Annals of the American Academy of Political and Social Science* 18 (July): 67–89.

Rossiter, W. S. 1909. The significance of the decreasing proportion of children. In *Race improvement in the United States*, ed. American Academy of Political and Social Science, 71–80. Philadelphia: American Academy of Political and Social Science.

Rothstein, William G. 1988. The botanical movements and orthodox medicine. In *Other healers: Unorthodox medicine in America*, ed. Norman Gevitz, 29–51. Baltimore: Johns Hopkins University Press.

Rubin, Bonnie. 1997. America's favorite healer. *Good Housekeeping*, November, 117.

Rumbarger, John J. 1989. *Profits, power, and prohibition: Alcohol reform and the industrialization of America 1800–1930.* Albany: State University of New York Press.

Rush, Benjamin. 1812. *Inquiry into the effects of ardent spirits on the human body and mind.* Middlebury, Vt.: T. C. Strong.

Rushing, William A. 1995. *The AIDS epidemic: Social dimensions of an infectious disease.* Boulder, Colo.: Westview Press.

Russell, A., R. B. Voas, W. DeJong, and M. Challoupka. 1995. MADD rates the states: A media advocacy event to advance the agenda against alcohol-impaired driving. *Public Health Reports* 110: 240–246.

Rutledge, Leigh W. 1992. *The gay decades from Stonewall to the present: The people and events that shaped gay lives.* New York: Plume.

Ruzek, Sheryl Burt. 1978. *The women's health movement: Feminist alternatives to medical control.* New York: Praeger Special Studies.

Ryan, Barbara. 1992. *Feminism and the women's movement: Dynamics of change in social movement ideology and activism.* New York: Routledge.

Ryan, Mary P. 1981. *Cradle of the middle class: The family in Oneida community, New York, 1780–1865.* Cambridge: Cambridge University Press.

———. 1979. The power of women's networks: A case study of female moral reform in antebellum America. *Feminist Studies* 5 (Spring): 67–85.

Saleeby, C. W. 1911. *The methods of race-regeneration.* New York: Moffat, Yard.

Salmon, Thomas W. 1910. Two preventable causes of insanity. *Popular Science Monthly* 76: 557–564.

Sanger, Margaret. 1931. *My fight for birth control.* New York: Farrar and Rinehart.

Sargent, Dudley Allen. 1909. The significance of a sound physique. In *Race improvement in the United States*, ed. American Academy of Political and Social Science, 9–15. Philadelphia: American Academy of Political and Social Science.

———. 1901. Gymnastics. *Harper's Weekly*, 2 January, 81.

———. 1897. Exercise and Longevity. 1897. *North American Review* 164: 5.

Scheidler, Joseph. 1985. *Closed: 99 ways to stop abortion.* Westcheter, Ill.: Crossway Books.

Schieffelin, William J. 1909. Safeguarding the sale of narcotics. In *Proceedings of the National Conference of Charities and Correction*, 208–212. Boston: George H. Ellis.

Schlafly, Phyllis. 1964. *A choice not an echo.* Alton, Ill.: Pere Marquette Press.

Schlesinger, Arthur M., Jr. 1950. *The age of Jackson.* Boston: Little, Brown.

Schlosser, Eric. 1994. Reefer madness. *Atlantic Monthly,* August, 1–26 (http://www.theatlantic.com/election/connection, last visited August 11, 1998).

Schneir, Miriam, ed. 1994. *Feminism in our time: The essential writings, World War II to the present.* New York: Vintage Books.

Schoepflin, Rennie B. 1988. Christian Science healing in America. In *Other healers: Unorthodox medicine in America,* ed. Norman Gevitz, 192–214. Baltimore: Johns Hopkins University Press.

Schroeder, Richard C. 1980. *The politics of drugs: An American dilemma.* 2d ed. Washington, D.C.: Congressional Quarterly.

Schulz, Ester D., and Sally R. Williams. 1969. *Family life and sex education: Curriculum and instruction.* New York: Harcourt, Brace and World.

Schwartz, Richard. 1970. *John Harvey Kellogg, M.D.* Nashville: Southern.

Scirvo, Karen Lee. 1998. Drinking on campus. *CQ Researcher,* 29 March, 242–263.

Segers, Mary C., and Timothy A. Byrnes, ed. 1995. *Abortion politics in American states.* Armonk, N.Y.: M. E. Sharpe.

Sellers, Charles Grier. 1958. *Jacksonian democracy.* Washington, D.C.: Service Center for Teachers of History.

Shattuck, Lemmual. 1850. *Report of the sanitary commission of Massachusetts: 1850.* Boston: Dutton and Wentworth.

Shaw, David. 1996. *The pleasure police: How bluenose busybodies and lily-livered alarmists are taking all the fun out of life.* New York: Doubleday.

Shew, Joel. 1855. *Tobacco diseases; with a remedy for the habit.* New York: Fowlers and Wells.

Shilts, Randy. 1987. *And the band played on: Politics, people, and the AIDS epidemic.* New York: St. Martin's Press.

Shipps, Jan. 1985. *Mormonism: The story of a new religious tradition.* Urbana: University of Illinois Press.

Showalter, Elaine. 1971. *Women's liberation and literature.* New York: Harcourt Brace Jovanovich.

Showdown in Atlanta. 1988. *Christianity Today,* 16 September, 44–46.

Shryock, Richard H. 1960. *Medicine and society in America, 1660–1860.* New York: New York University Press.

———. 1957. *National Tuberculosis Association 1904–1954: A study of the voluntary health movement in the United States.* New York: National Tuberculosis Association.

———. 1947. *The development of modern medicine: An interpretation of the social and scientific factors involved.* 2d ed. New York: Alfred A. Knopf.

Silent scream. 1985. *Newsweek,* 25 February, 37.

Simon, Rita J., and Gloria Danziger. 1991. *Women's movements in America: Their successes, disappointments, and aspirations.* Westport, Conn.: Praeger.

Sinclair, Andrew. 1962. *Prohibition: The era of excess.* Boston: Little, Brown.

Singer, Peter, and Deane Wells. 1985. *Making babies: The new science and ethics of conception.* New York: Charles Scribner's Sons.

Sloan, Don M., and Paula Hartz. 1992. *Abortion: A doctor's perspective, a woman's dilemma.* New York: D. I. Fine.

Smallpox and vaccination. 1902. *Current Literature*, April, 484–485.

Smith, David H. 1995. *Entrusted: The moral responsibilities of trusteeship*. Bloomington: Indiana University Press.

Smith, Geddes. 1941. *Plague on us*. New York: Commonwealth Fund.

Smith, Joseph. 1974. *Doctrine and covenants*. Salt Lake City: Church of Jesus Christ of Latter Day Saints.

Smith, N. Lee. 1979. Herbal remedies: God's medicine? *Dialogue: A Journal of Mormon Thought* 12 (3): 37–57.

Smith-Rosenberg, Carroll. 1980. Sex as symbol in Victorian America. *Prospects* 5: 51–70.

Snow, John. 1849. *On the mode of communication of cholera*. London: John Churchill.

Snowball, D. 1991. *Continuity and change in the rhetoric of the moral majority*. Westport, Conn.: Praeger.

Sokolow, Jayme A. 1983. *Eros and modernization: Sylvester Graham, health reform, and the origins of victorian sexuality in America*. Rutherford, N.J.: Fairleigh-Dickinson University Press.

Some cigaret figures. 1914. *Literary Digest*, 8 August, 238.

Spangler, David. 1971. *Revelation: The birth of a new age*. Forres, Moray, Scotland: Findhorn Foundation.

A standard of purity for drugs. 1910. *Outlook*, 1 October, 275–276.

Stanton, Elizabeth Cady, Susan B. Anthony, and Matilda Joslyn Gate, eds. 1969. *History of woman suffrage*. Rochester, N.Y.: Charles Mann.

Starr, Paul. 1982. *The social transformation of American medicine*. New York: Basic Books.

Sterling, Clarren. 1990. Drinking in pregnancy: A recommendation for complete abstinence. In *Controversies in the addictions field*, ed. Ruth C. Engs, 151–157. Dubuque, Iowa: Kendall/Hunt.

Stewart, Ella S. 1914. Woman suffrage and the liquor traffic. *Annals of the American Academy of Political and Social Science* 56 (November): 143–152.

Stewart, James Brewer. 1976. *Holy warriors: The abolitionists and American slavery*. New York: Hill and Wang.

Strauss, William, and Neil Howe. 1998. *The fourth turning: An American prophecy*. New York: Broadway Books.

Sullum, Jacob. 1998. *For your own good: The anti-smoking crusade and the tyranny of public health*. New York: Free Press.

———. 1996. What the Dr. ordered. *Reason*, January, 20.

———. 1995. A matter of taste. *National Review* 47: 55–57.

———. 1990. Invasion of the bottle snatchers. *Reason*, February, 26–32.

Sullum, Jacob, and Thomas Szasz. 1998. Drug trial. *Reason*, March, 22.

Sweet, Leonard I., ed. 1984. *The Evangelical tradition in America*. Macon, Ga.: Mercer University Press.

Synan, Vinson. 1997. *The holiness–Pentecostal tradition: Charismatic movements in the twentieth century*. Grand Rapids, Mich.: William B. Eerdmans.

———. 1971. *The holiness–Pentecostal movement in the United States*. Grand Rapids, Mich.: William B. Eerdmans.

———, ed. 1975. *Aspects of Pentecostal-charismatic origins*. Plainfield, N.J.: Logos International.

Tager, I. B. 1986. Passive smoking and respiratory health in children: Sophistry or cause for concern? *American Review of Respiratory Disease* 133: 959–961.

Tate, Cassandra C. 1995. The American anti-cigarette movement, 1880–1930. Ph.D. diss., University of Washington.

Taubenberger, J. K., A. H. Reid, A. E. Frafft, K. E. Bijwaard, and T. G. Fanning. 1997. Initial genetic characterization of the 1918 "Spanish" influenza virus. *Science* 275: 1793–1796.

Taylor, Humphrey. 1991. Has the fitness movement peaked? *American Demographics* 13 (10): 10.

Teenage pregnancy and birth rates—United States, 1990, 1993. *MMWR* 42: 733–737.

Teenagers and abortion. 1967. *Newsweek*, 12 October, 81–83.

Teller, Michael E. 1988. *The tuberculosis movement: A public health campaign in the progressive era.* New York: Greenwood Press.

Temin, Peter. 1980. *Taking your medicine: Drug regulation in the United States.* Cambridge: Harvard University Press.

Temperance almanac. 1833. New Haven, Conn.: Durrie and Peck.

Temperance almanac: Adapted to all parts of the United States and Canada. 1835, 1836, 1838. Albany, N.Y.: Steam Press of Packard and Van Benthuysen.

Temperance almanac of the Massachusetts Temperance Union. 1834, 1841, 1842, 1844, 1845. Boston: Massachusetts Temperance Union.

Temperance family almanac. 1835. Boston: Russell, Odiorne and Metcalf.

Thacher, James. 1826. *American modern practice: Or, a simple method of prevention and cure of diseases, according to the latest improvements and discoveries, comprising a practical system adapted to the use of medical practitioners of the United States.* Boston: Cottons and Barnard.

Third annual report. 1839. *American Physiological Society.* Boston: Marsh, Capen and Lyon.

This drug-endangered nation. 1914. *The Literary Digest*, 24 March, 687–688.

This is not a scarecrow. 1998. *Time*, 26 October, 72.

Thomas, Lewis. 1977. On the science and technology of medicine. In *Doing better and feeling worse*, ed. John H. Knowles, 35–46. New York: W. W. Norton.

Thomas, Robert David. 1994. *"With bleeding footsteps": Mary Baker Eddy's path to religious leadership.* New York: Knopf.

Thomson, Samuel. 1832. *New guide to health; or, botanic family physician. Containing a complete system of practice, etc.* Boston: J. Howe.

———. 1831. *New guide to health or botanic family physician. Containing a complete system of practice on a plan entirely new; with a description of the vegetables made use of, and directions for preparing and administering them, to cure disease, etc.* 3d ed. Boston: J. Howe.

———. 1825. *A narrative of the life and medical discoveries of Samuel Thomson. Containing an account of his system of practice, and the manner of curing disease with vegetable medicine, etc.* 2d ed. Boston: E. C. House.

Thurner, Manuela. 1995. Better citizens without the ballot. In *One woman one vote: Rediscovering the woman suffrage movement*, ed. Marjorie Wheeler, 203–220. Troutdale, Ore.: New Sage Press.

Ticknor, Caleb Bingham. 1972. *The philosophy of living; or the way to enjoy life and its comforts.* 1836. Reprint. New York: Arno Press.

Timberlake, James H. 1963. *Prohibition and the progressive movement, 1900–1920.* Cambridge: Harvard University Press.

Tissot, Simon André. 1832. *Treatise on the diseases produced by Onanism.* New York: Collins and Hannay.

To be young and gay in Wyoming. 1998. *Time,* 26 October, 38.

Torabi, Mohammad R., William J. Bailey, and Massoumeh Majd-Jabbari. 1993. Cigarette smoking as a predictor of alcohol and other drug use by children and adolescents: Evidence of the "gateway drug effect." *Journal of School Health* 63 (7): 302.

Torrey, John C. 1909. The prevention of infectious diseases. *Harper's Monthly Magazine,* March, 536–544.

Towns, Charles B. 1912. The peril of the drug habit and the need of restrictive legislation. *Century* 84: 580–587.

Tracy, James. 1988. The rise and fall of the know-nothings in Quincy. *Historical Journal of Massachusetts* 16: 1–19.

Trall, Russell T. 1972. *Physiology of sex: A scientific and popular exposition.* 28th ed. 1881. Reprint. New York: Arno Press.

———. 1855. *Tobacco: It's history, nature and effects.* New York: Fowlers and Wells.

———. 1854. *New hydropathic cook-book.* New York: Fowlers and Wells.

Trask, George. 1853. *Thoughts and stories for American lads; or Uncle Toby's anti-tobacco advice to his nephew Billy Bruce.* 5th ed. Boston: Geo C. Rand.

Treno, J. A., R. N. Parker, and H. Holder. 1993. Understanding U.S. alcohol consumption with social and economic factors: A multivariate time series analysis, 1950–1986. *Journal of Studies on Alcohol* 54: 146–157.

Troyer, Ronald J., and Gerald E. Markle, eds. 1983. *Cigarettes: The battle over smoking.* New Brunswick, N.J.: Rutgers University Press.

Trumbull, C. G. 1913. *Anthony Comstock: Fighter.* 2d ed. New York: Fleming H. Revell.

Turner, R., and L. Killian. 1957. *Collective behavior.* Englewood Cliffs, N.J.: Prentice Hall.

Tyler, Alice Felt. 1944. *Freedoms ferment: Phases of American social history to 1860.* Minneapolis: University of Minnesota Press.

Tyrrell, Ian R. 1982. Women and temperance in antebellum America, 1830–1860. *Civil War History* 28 (2): 128–152.

———. 1979. *Sobering up: From temperance to prohibition in antebellum America, 1800–1860.* Westport, Conn.: Greenwood Press.

Ulrich's international periodicals directory. 1998. New York: Bowker.

Underwood, Grant. 1986. Early Mormon perceptions of contemporary America: 1830–1846. *Brigham Young University Studies* 26 (3): 49–61.

Unexplained immunodeficiency and opportunistic infections in infants. 1982. *MMWR* 31: 665–667.

U.S. Department of Agriculture. 1999. Conclusions, *Healthy Eating Index* (http://www.nal.usda.gov/fnic/HEI, last visited January 3, 1999).

———. 1990, 1996. *Dietary guidelines for Americans.* Washington D.C.: U.S. Department of Health and Human Services.

U.S. Department of Commerce (USDC). 1991, 1995, 1996, 1998. *Statistical abstracts of the United States national data book.* Washington, D.C.: U.S. Dept. of Commerce.

U.S. Department of Health and Human Services. 1996. *National household survey.* Washington, D.C.: U.S. Department of Health and Human Services.
————. 1991. *National household survey on drug abuse: Main findings, 1990.* Washington, D.C.: National Institute on Drug Abuse.
————. 1986. *The health consequences of involuntary smoking: A report of the surgeon general.* Washington, D.C.: U.S. Government Printing Office.
————. 1984. *Smoking and health: A report of the surgeon general.* Washington, D.C.: U.S. Department of Health and Human Services.
————. 1983. *National survey on drug abuse: Main findings, 1982.* Rockville, Md.: NIDA.
U.S. Department of Health, Education and Welfare (USDHEW). 1979. *Smoking and health: A report of the surgeon general.* Washington, D.C.: U.S. Government Printing Office.
U.S. Department of Justice. 1997. *Crime in the United States.* Washington, D.C.: U.S. Department of Justice.
U.S. Department of Traffic (USDOT). 1998. *Fatal accident reporting system.* Washington, D.C.: National Highway Traffic Safety Administration.
U.S. General Accounting Office (USGAO). 1987. *Drinking age laws: An evaluation synthesis of their impact on highway safety.* Washington, D.C.: USGAO.
U.S. Office of the Assistant Secretary for Health. 1984. *Chronic obstructive lung disease: A report of the surgeon general.* Rockville, Md.: U.S. Department of Health and Human Services.
U.S. President's Council on Physical Fitness and Sports. 1977. *The president's council on physical fitness and sports: Organization, objectives, programs, situation report.* Washington, D.C.: President's Council on Physical Fitness and Sports.
Utah's "no smoking" signs. 1923. *Literary Digest,* 24 March, 14–15.
Van den Brandt, P. A., R. A. Goldbohm, and P. Van't Veer. 1995. Alcohol and breast cancer results from the Netherlands cohort study. *American Journal of Epidemiology* 141: 907–915.
Van Dussen, Gregory D. 1990. An American response to Irish Catholic immigration: The Methodist Quarterly Review 1830–1870. *Methodist History* 29: 21–36.
VanDyck, José. 1995. *Manufacturing babies and public consent.* New York: Macmillan.
Ventura, Stephanie J., Joyce A. Martin, Sally C. Curtin, and T. J. Mathews. 1999. Births: Final data for 1997. *National vital statistics reports* 47: 1–5.
Verbrugge, Martha H. *Able-bodied womenhood: Personal health and social change in nineteenth century Boston.* New York: Oxford University Press.
Vertinsky, Patricia. 1979. Sexual equality and the legacy of Catharine Beecher. *Journal of Sport History* 6: 38–49.
Wacker, Grant. 1984. Searching for Norman Rockwell: Popular evangelicalism in contemporary America. In *Evangelical tradition in America,* ed. Leonard I. Sweet, 289–315. Macon, Ga.: Mercer University Press.
Wagenaar, A. 1989. Alcohol beverage control policies: Their role in preventing alcohol-impaired driving. In *Surgeon general's workshop on drunk driving,* 1–14. Rockville, Md.: U.S. Department of Health and Human Services.

Wagner, David. 1997. *The new temperance: The American obsession with sin and vice.* Boulder, Colo.: Westview Press.

Wagner, Susan. 1971. *Cigarette country, tobacco in America: History and politics.* New York: Praeger.

Walters, Karen A. 1981. McLean County and the influenza epidemic of 1918–1919. *Journal of the Illinois State Historical Society* 74: 130–144.

Walters, Ronald G. 1993. The erotic South: Civilization and sexuality in American abolitionism. *American Quarterly* 25: 177–201.

———. 1978. *American reformers 1815–1860.* New York: Hill and Wang.

Warfield, Frances. 1930. Lost cause: A portrait of Lucy Page Gaston. *Outlook,* 12 February, 244–247.

Warner, Harry J. 1909. *Social welfare and the liquor problem: A series of studies in the sources of the problem and how they relate to its solution.* Chicago: Intercollegiate Prohibition Association.

Wechsler, Henry, B. Moykens, A. Davenport, S. Castillo, and J. Hanson. 1995. The adverse impact of heavy episodic drinkiers on other college students. *Journal of Studies on Alcohol* 56: 628–634.

Weil, Andrew. 1990. *Natural health natural medicine: A comprehensive manual for wellness and self care.* Boston: Houghton Mifflin.

———. 1983. *Health and healing: Understanding conventional and alternative medicine.* Boston: Houghton Mifflin.

———. 1972. *Natural mind: A new way of looking at drugs and the higher consciousness.* Boston: Houghton Mifflin.

Weir, Hugh. 1909. The American opium peril. *Putman's Magazine* 7 (December): 329–336.

Wernick, Robert. 1996. The know-nothings knew how to win . . . for a while. *Smithsonian* 27: 150.

West's encyclopedia of American law. 1998. Minneapolis/St. Paul: West Publishing.

What killed equal rights? 1982. *Time,* 12 July, 32–33.

Wheeler, Marjorie, ed. 1995. *One woman one vote: Rediscovering the woman suffrage movement.* Troutdale, Ore.: New Sage Press.

White, Ellen G. 1958. *Selected messages from the writings of Ellen G. White.* Book 2. Washington, D.C.: Review and Herald.

———. 1938. *Counsels on diet and food: A compilation from the writings of Ellen G. White.* Washington, D.C.: Review and Herald.

———. 1864. *Spiritual gifts: Important facts of faith, laws of health, and testimonies.* Vol. 4. Battle Creek, Mich.: SDA Publishing Association.

White, William L. 1998. *Slaying the dragon: The history of addiction treatment and recovery in America.* Bloomington, Ind.: Lighthouse-Institute.

White, William. 1972. *North American reference encyclopedia of women's liberation.* Philadelphia: North American.

Whitman, Alden, ed. 1985. *American reformers.* New York: H. W. Wilson.

Whitney, Leon F. 1934. *The case for sterilization.* New York: Frederick A. Stokes.

Whorton, James C. 1988. Patient, heal thyself: Popular health reform movements as unorthodox medicine. In *Other healers: Unorthodox medicine in America,* ed. Norman Gevitz, 52–81. Baltimore: Johns Hopkins University Press.

————. 1982. *Crusaders for fitness: The history of American health reformers.* Princeton, N.J.: Princeton University Press.

————. 1981a. Muscular vegetarianism: The debate over diet and athletic performance in the progressive era. *Journal of Sport History* 8 (2): 58–75.

————. 1981b. "Physiologic optimism": Horace Fletcher and hygienic ideology in progressive America. *Bulletin of the History of Medicine* 55: 59.

————. 1975. "Christian physiology": William Alcott's prescription for the millennium. *Bulletin of the History of Medicine* 49: 466–481.

Who's come a long way baby? 1970. *Time*, 31 August, 16–20.

Why the climb in crime? 1996. *U.S. News & World Report*, 27 October, 10.

Wilber, Sibyl. 1913. *The life of Mary Baker Eddy.* Boston: Christian Science Publishing.

Wilcox, Clyde. 1992. *God's warriors: The Christian right in twentieth-century America.* Baltimore: Johns Hopkins University Press.

Wiley, Harvey W. 1916. Little white slaver. *Good Housekeeping*, January, 91–95.

————. 1912. Drugging the baby. *Good Housekeeping*, October, 551–552.

————. 1907. Why headache remedies are dangerous. *Ladies' Home Journal*, February, 29.

Willard, Frances. 1889. *Glimpses of fifty years: The autobiography of an American woman.* Chicago: Women's Temperance Publication Association.

Williams, David E. 1996. The drive for prohibition: A transition from social reform to legislative reform, 1880–1920. *Southern Communication Journal* 61 (Spring): 185–187.

Wilsnack, Richard W., and Sharon C. Wilsnack, eds. 1997. *Gender and alcohol: Individual and social perspectives.* New Brunswick, N.J.: Rutgers Center of Alcohol Studies.

Wilsnack, Sharon C., and Linda J. Beckman, eds. 1984. *Alcohol problems in women: Antecedents, consequences, and intervention.* New York: Guilford Press.

Wilson, James Q. 1980. Reagan and the Republican revival. *Commentary* 70 (4): 25–32.

Wiseman, James. 1997. In vino veritas. *Archaeology* 89 (September–October): 12–17.

Wrobel, Arthur, ed. 1987. *Pseudo-science and society in nineteenth-century America.* Lexington: University of Kentucky Press.

Wuthnow, Robert. 1997. *The crisis in the churches: Spiritual malaise, fiscal woe.* New York: Oxford University Press.

Yamaguchi, K., and Denise B. Kandel. 1984. Patterns of drug use from adolescence to young adulthood. 3: Predictors of progression. *American Journal of Public Health* 74: 673–681.

Yarber, William L. 1987. *AIDS education: Curriculum and health policy.* Bloomington, Ind.: Phi Kappa Delta Educational Foundation.

A year of the Harrison narcotic law. 1916. *The survey*, 8 April, 58–60.

YMCA. 1998. Private communication with John A. Clark, Statistician. Chicago, National YMCA Headquarters.

York, Michael. 1995. *The emerging network: A sociology of the New Age and neo-pagan movements.* Lanham, Md.: Rowman and Littelfield.

Young, James H. 1992a. *American health quackery.* Princeton, N.J.: Princeton University Press.

———. 1992b. Two Hoosiers and the two food laws of 1906. *Indiana Magazine of History* 88: 303–319.

———. 1989. *Pure food: Securing the federal food and drugs act of 1906.* Princeton, N.J.: Princeton University Press.

Zentner, Joseph. 1974. Opiate use in America during the eighteenth and nineteenth centuries: The origins of a modern scourge. *Studies in History and Society* 5 (2): 40–54.

Zimmer, Lynn, and John P. Morgan. 1992. Prohibition costs—Always too high? Paper presented at the annual meeting of the Kettil-Brun Society for Social and Epidemiological Research on Alcohol, 30 May–5 June, Toronto.

Index

Sanger, Margaret, 147–148, 149
Sanitation movements, 89–92, 165–166, 174–175
Sanitorium movement, 168
Sargent, Dudley, 110–111, 112
Scapegoating, 12–13, 44, 221
Scheidler, Joseph M., 237
Schlafly, Phyllis, 231
Secondhand smoke, 205
Seventh-Day Adventists, 26, 28–32
Sex: education, 145, 233–234; extramarital, 62; marital, 61–62, 78–79
Sexual abstinence, 233–235
Sexual behavior patterns, 230–231
Sexually transmitted diseases, 62, 145–146
Sexual purity movements. *See* Purity movements
Sexual reform, 75, 77, 141–142
Sexual reform movements, 61–65. *See also* Purity movements
Shattuck, Lemmuel, 91–92
Shew, Joel, 96–97
Sinclair, Upton, 153
Six Sermons on . . . Intemperance (Beecher), 25
Sleep reform movements, 59–60
Smith, Joseph, 26, 27
Smoke-free environments, 133, 207
Smoke-free societies, 207
Smoking cessation programs, 206
Smoking education, 204–206
Social change, 3–4, 101–102, 184–185, 229–230, 239
Social engineering, 264–265
Social Gospel movement, 105–106
Social reform movements, 1–2, 4, 179–180
Spangler, David, 190–191
State health departments, 173
State legislation: abortion, 236–237; alcohol, 41–42, 215; alternative medicine, 197; drugs, 159; pure food, 152; tobacco, 134–135, 204, 207; tuberculosis, 169
Stepping-stone theory, 12–13
Stimulants, 42, 44–45

Student drinking, 217
Sullivan, Jacob, 256–257
Sunday, Billy, 109

Teetotalism, 39–40
Terry, Randall, 237
Theory of Evolution, 135–136
Thomson, Samuel, 94
Ticknor, Caleb, 57, 73
Tissot, Simon André, 57
Tobacco. *See* Antitobacco movements
Tobacco advertisements, 208
Tobacco industry, 208–209
Tobacco use patterns, 42–43, 132–133, 135, 202–203, 208, 209–210
Traditional medicine: alternative medicine and, 92–93, 192–193, 194–195, 196–197; Christian physiologists and, 56–57; physical fitness movements, 250; women's health movement, 227–228
Trall, Russell, 43, 78, 96–97, 114
Transcendentalists, 56
Transcendental meditation, 190
Treatise on the Diseases Produced by Onanism (Tissot), 57
Treatment of alcohol abuse, 211
Treatment of drug addiction, 156
Trudeau, Edward Livingston, 168
Tuberculosis, 166–167
Tuberculosis movement, 166–172
Typhoid, 175, 176

Underage drinking, 215–216
United States Public Health Services (USPHS), 173
United Way, 234
Upper class, 121, 122
Urine testing, 220–221

Vaccination, 175–176
Venereal diseases, 62, 145–146
Volstead Act, 127, 128
Voluntary health agencies, 169–171

Washingtonians, 40–41
Water cure, 30, 50, 95–96, 98

ABOUT THE AUTHOR

Ruth Clifford Engs is Professor of Applied Health Science at Indiana University, Bloomington. Dr. Engs has published numerous articles and book chapters and is the editor of several works including *Controversies in the Addiction Field* (1990), *Women: Alcohol and Other Drugs* (1989), and author of *Alcohol and Other Drugs: Self-Responsibility* (1987).

ISBN 0-275-95994-5

90000>

EAN

9 780275 959944

HARDCOVER BAR CODE